Policy, Program Evaluation, and Research in Disability
Community Support for All

Julie Ann Racino

The Haworth Press
New York • London • Oxford

The Haworth Press, Inc., 10 Alice Street, Binghamton, NY 13904-1580

Cover design by Jennifer M. Gaska.

Library of Congress Cataloging-in-Publication Data

Racino, Julie Ann, 1953-
    Policy, program evaluation, and research in disability : community support for all / Julie Ann Racino.
        p.   cm.
    Includes bibliographical references and index.
    ISBN 0-7890-0597-2 (hc : alk. paper).—0-7890-0598-0 (pbk : alk. paper).
    1. Handicapped—Government policy—United States. 2. Rehabilitation—Research—United States. 3. Handicapped—United States—Social networks. 4. Handicapped—Home care—United States. 5. Community health services—United States. I. Title.
HV1553.R24   1999
362.4'048'0973—dc21   99-17248
                                                                                      CIP

To my parents,
Augustine V. and Josephine H. (Bien) Racino

CONTENTS

ABOUT THE AUTHOR

Julie Ann Racino, MAPA, is Principal and President of Community and Policy Studies in Rome, New York. She has served as Associate and Deputy Director of the National Research and Training Center and its related national, state, and local projects at the Center on Human Policy at Syracuse University. Ms. Racino was selected for *Who's Who of Women in the World* and has over twenty years of experience in the policy, management, research, and development of community services. She is lead editor and primary author of the book *Housing, Support and Community,* and she has written over 100 articles in the areas of social policy and disability, organizational studies, and community services. Ms. Racino is a graduate of Cornell University and the Maxwell School of International and Public Affairs at Syracuse University. She has taught at the undergraduate and graduate levels at the Syracuse University School of Education and in the psychology department at The State University of New York at Oswego, and has lectured throughout the United States and the United Kingdom on public policy, community integration, and disability.

CONTRIBUTORS

James A. Knoll, PhD, is Associate Professor at Morehead State University in Morehead, Kentucky. As a graduate of Syracuse University, he has served as principal investigator, project director, and research associate of national projects in disability, community membership and support, and family support at Syracuse University, Syracuse, New York; Wayne State University, Detroit, Michigan; and the Human Research Institute in Boston, Massachusetts. As an educator, he is a prolific writer, and his national publications include *Emerging Issues in Family Support* (1992) for the American Association of Mental Retardation.

K. Charles Lakin, PhD, is Director of the Rehabilitation Research and Training Center (RRTC) on Community Living at the University of Minnesota, Minneapolis, Minnesota and principal or co-principal investigator of research and training projects contributing to the mission and effectiveness of the RRTC. Dr. Lakin has over twenty-five years of experience in services to individuals with mental retardation as a teacher, researcher, trainer, consultant, and advocate. Dr. Lakin has authored or co-authored more than 160 books, monographs, journal articles, book chapters, and national reports. President Clinton appointed Dr. Lakin to the President's Committee on Mental Retardation.

Dr. Lakin's work with academic and private research organizations has included both co-principal investigator of major national evaluations with Mathematical Policy Research (congressionally mandated study of separate educational settings) and MED-STAT (national education of Medicaid Community Supported Living Arrangements). He has been a frequent consultant to federal and state agencies in matters of policy, research, and evaluation, including the Assistant Secretary for Planning and Evaluation (U.S. Department of Health and Human Services), National Center on Health Statistics, Office of Technology Assessment (U.S. Congress), Congressional Research Service, General Accounting Office, Administration on Developmental Disabilities, Health Care Financing Administration, and Centers for Disease Control and Prevention.

Simi Litvak, PhD, is Senior Researcher and Policy Analyst at the World Institute on Disability (WID). Formerly the Director of WID's Rehabilitation Research and Training Center on Personal Assistance Services (PAS) and the Rehabilitation Research and Training Center on Independent Living and Disability Policy (ILDP), Dr. Litvak has completed research in the area of independent living and is a nationally known expert in independent living, personal assistance services, and health care reform as it impacts people with disabilities. Over the past fourteen years, she has contributed to juried and nonjuried journals, consumer publications, edited books, and publications on the subject of personal assistance services (PAS). She has provided technical assistance to states on PAS program design, trained advocates at national and state conferences, presented to policymakers and professionals working with various disability populations, as well as to undergraduate and graduate students, offered technical assistance to government and industry, and provided leadership in ideological and PAS system change.

Dr. Litvak received both a doctorate in Rehabilitation Counselor Education and a master's in Rehabilitation Facilities Administration from the University of Wisconsin, Madison, Wisconsin. She is also an occupational therapist and has over thirty years of experience in the disability field as a teacher, researcher, policy analyst, policymaker, and rehabilitation professional. She served as a member of President Clinton's Health Care Reform Task Force's Long-Term Services Working Group and the National Institute on Disability Research and Rehabilitation's (NIDRR) 1997-1998 Long-Range Planning Committee.

Gary Smith has been Director of Special Projects for the National Association of State Directors of Developmental Disabilities Services, Inc. (NASDDDS) since 1987. Prior to joining the association, he served as Deputy Director of the Colorado Division of Developmental Disabilities and held other senior government management positions in both Illinois and Colorado. Gary's technical assistance work and special studies on the management and delivery of support have taken him to forty-eight states during the past ten years. Gary is the author of several publications on the home- and community-based waiver program, supported living, and most recently (with John Ashbaugh of the Human Services Research Institute [HSRI]), *Managed Care and People with Developmental Disabilities: A Guide Book*. Gary serves as co-director of the Center for Managed Long-Term Supports for People with Disabilities, a collaboration between NASDDDS and HSRI in providing technical assistance to states. Gary lives and works in Littleton, Colorado.

Foreword

There was a time not too terribly long ago when center-based services were viewed as the only way to provide health care and treatment to those with disabilities. This was especially so for those with the most severe disabilities, who were viewed as the least capable and as having the least potential for community living. In the not too distant past, large institutions that held hundreds, and even thousands, of persons with severe disabilities were established throughout the world. There were also programs called intermediate care facilities where hundreds of persons with mental and physical disabilities predominated. Special day programs for adults with disabilities and segregated schools were the norm. The primary philosophy, until only recently, was one of the individual being incompetent and needing to be "fixed." This philosophy included assumptions about persons with disabilities that were cruel, erroneous, and even barbaric.

For example, the widespread sterilization that took place in many institutions was clearly a cruel, and many would consider barbaric, practice that was implemented for the stated principle of stopping persons with disabilities from being able to reproduce and be parents. Unfortunately, in all aspects of society, there were many negative misconceptions about individuals with disabilities, their rights, and their capabilities to parent.

In similar fashion, the large-scale dumping of persons with intellectual disabilities from institutions into nursing homes with hundreds of individuals who are aged, infirm, or otherwise significantly disabled was clearly wrong. The continued placement of persons with disabilities into sheltered workshops or adult activity centers is another long-standing practice that minimizes their life development potential.

Such practices have been extremely common in past decades and only within recent years have they begun to be denounced in the professional literature, through legislation, and by the courts, but it is a long and grueling process to change the day-to-day practices that service providers deliver to individuals with disabilities, that families come to expect, and, perhaps, tragically, that persons with disabilities believe in for themselves.

If individuals are continually told that they have no ability, no potential, and that they must go to the "back of the bus," after a period of time they will begin to have no confidence in themselves and to lose their pride, dignity, and ambition. This has been seen for centuries throughout the world, with all races and ethnic persuasions. It has been no different for persons with disabilities, especially those with significant disabilities. That is why this book by Julie Ann Racino will be a wonderful addition to the literature. This book highlights the means available to help persons with disabilities reach their full potential in their communities. It discusses making a difference, focusing on support, interdependence, and equality of life. This book challenges service providers to aspire to another level of performance, to not settle only for the status quo. The wonderfully crafted chapters in this book offer something for everyone who chooses to believe the best about persons with disabilities.

For far too long, society, as well as those who profess to be experts in working with persons with disabilities, has viewed the disabled population as being incompetent and as having limited potential; this book uses support as the underlying theme and assumes people with disabilities are normal human beings; that they can reach whatever level of potential they wish, based upon the nature and level of support that they are given.

For example, if a person who is given an IQ of 42 by the school psychologist after a Stanford-Binet test goes to a sheltered workshop, he or she will be viewed as being severely mentally retarded. On the other hand, if that very same person goes to work at a state library and is provided any necessary compensatory strategies, co-worker assistance, and job coach help, such supports will enable this person to earn $6.75 an hour with full state benefits, thus making him or her, at least in this work environment, normal. So we see that a person's abilities and potential are defined by the environment in which he or she is placed and by the overarching supports and interdependent networks that are offered. This is true for most people who have not been labeled as disabled.

The true strength and beauty of this book is that it provides numerous examples and illustrations of how community supports can work for people with a wide range of disabilities. It is an important reference that can be used for in-service training and as course reading for any of a number of graduate courses in such areas as social work psychology, rehabilitation, and special education. It is a true pleasure for me to give this work my highest endorsement.

Paul Wehman
Professor of Physical Medicine and Rehabilitation
Director, Virginia Commonwealth University
Rehabilitation Research and Training Center
on Workplace Supports
Richmond, Virginia

Preface

Beginning in the mid-1980s, new community services research began in the United States, as major research and training funding shifted to become more community-based for people with diverse disabilities. These changes resulted in the development of emergent literatures that reflected a movement toward personal autonomy and community membership, with the guiding paradigm of support and empowerment.

While the country moved toward community support, people with disabilities continued to organize, as did families and advocates, to correct the injustices and unfairness of service systems and societal practices. People with diverse disabilities, including people who stood a good chance of being confined to institutions, sought to become part of a new way of being in the world, later reflected in the aspirations of the landmark Americans with Disabilities Act (1990).

As a case study and evaluative research text, this book follows national qualitative research studies on new developments in community living for children and their families and for adults and elders with disabilities throughout the United States over a period of eight years (e.g., Racino, 1991a; Taylor, Bogdan, and Racino, 1991; Racino, 1995a). However, this book also highlights diverse disability constituencies, including people with physical disabilities; psychiatric survivors; people with brain injuries, mental retardation, and developmental disabilities; and people with multiple disabilities who may have hearing, speech, and visual impairments.

Beginning with a unique state policy research study representative of better approaches to community integration in states from the 1970s through the early 1990s, the book moves from the decade focus on de-institutionalization into economic, political, and social participation and life in the community. Personal assistance services (PAS), which are a high priority politically, yet remain underfunded at the local levels, are presented through the eyes of consumer experts. The hope is for direction by service users, universal access to support services, and community approaches open to all.

Ushering in a new decade of self-reflection and action based on research, the book shares the endemic problems of school exclusion and a reliance on out-of-home placements, as well as the gaps between the promise of family life, accessible and affordable housing, and community support and the status of today's established federal, state, and local systems. The dichotomy between the perspectives of people with disabilities and their workers offers a new framework of hope for future and better evaluations and understandings.

From theoretical and methodological perspectives, the book introduces and illustrates critical concepts in applied research in disability, with the central focus on qualitative research and its significant role. As part of the building of grounded theory in family, housing, and community life, the book marks a unique contribution in the fields of public administration, public policy, rehabilitation, special education, sociology, psychology, public health, anthropology, and social work, with relevancy in law, medicine, and allied health.

Written primarily for researchers, educators, disability constituencies, and community leaders of all walks of life, this book represents a major step toward community and naturalistic studies. Reflecting a support and empowerment paradigm, with pluralistic societies, the research highlights this paradigm as an analytic framework for new research and evaluation in and outside of the disability field.

Qualitative research, as a field versus a set of methods, has research paradigms, theories, interpretative and analytic frames, methodologies, and styles of its own, distinct from qualitative methods. Qualitative research is inclusive of participant observation studies, ethnographies, policy research, services research, life studies, and organizational studies.

Yet, the author recognizes the massiveness and complexity of the disability world and its integral ties to existing systems of primarily multimethod, quantitative-led evaluation and research. Holding promise for the future, the book is based solidly in the field of qualitative research on social, community, personal, organizational, and societal change and on the critical concerns that will face the disability field and its leadership in the decades to come.

Julie Ann Racino
President and Principal
Community and Policy Studies

Acknowledgments

Policy, Program Evaluation, and Research in Disability was written and edited at the home of my parents, Augustine and Josephine Racino, in Rome, New York, a city in the heart of central New York. My mother died on April 10, 1999, while the galley pages for this book were being edited. Thanks are extended to my parents for their hospitality during the preparation of this book.

In the 1970s and 1980s, I am indebted to Ellie Macklin, of Cornell University's Human Development and Family Studies, and Nat Raskin, Northwestern University Medical School, Clinical Psychology, for their training in field interviewing; to Norma Haan, visiting professor from California to Cornell University's School of Arts and Sciences for her seminar on moral judgment; to Paul Veilette, New York State Department of Budget, and the late Bob Iversen, of the Maxwell School of Public and International Affairs Mid-Career Program; Wolf Wolfensberger, Special Education, School of Education, Syracuse University; and Ken Reagles at Syracuse University's Rehabilitation Counseling Program, School of Education. Bob Bogdan and Steve Taylor are acknowledged for their national research and education in qualitative research methods at the School of Education, Syracuse University. For her leadership in disability research, thanks to Peg Nosek of the Independent Living Research Utilization, Baylor College of Medicine, in Houston, Texas, and thanks also to John Lord of the Centre for Research and Education in Human Services of Kitchener, Ontario, Canada, for sharing his approaches to community research. Thank you to Jack McCrea, the founding director of Transitional Living Services, a nonprofit, United Way agency in Syracuse, New York, and to many of the people previously or still associated with the agency, especially Richard Pratt, Margaret Hart, Aileen Jackowsky, Grace Flusche, the late Harry Maples, and William Remby (also of L'Arche).

Many people and organizations were involved in the research in this book, with particular thanks to Richard LePore, with whom I first worked in 1985, and Douglas Watson, Richard Crocker, and Donald Shumway, then of the New Hampshire Division of Developmental Disabilities and Mental Health. A tremendous debt of gratitude to the research informants, reviewers, and advisory board members on all projects, with particular thanks to Ray Blodgett, Jane Hunt, John MacIntosh, Chris Nicolletta, the Lakes Region self-advocacy group, Michael Cassanto, Don Trites, Sandy Pelletier, Ric Crowley, Jocelyn and Roberta Gallant, Gary Smith, Judith Heumann, K. Charlie Lakin, Richard Hemp, Patti McGill Smith, Alan Abeson, Nancy Ward, Michael Kennedy, Frank Laski, Perry Whittico, David Hagner, John O'Brien, Karan Burnette, David Merrill, Ginny Harmon, Freeda Smith, Mary Hayden, Sylvia Stanley, and Jan Nisbet.

For Part III, thank you to Simi Litvak and her former colleagues at the World Institute on Disability, the late Ed Roberts, Judy Heumann, and Steve Brown. Perry Whittico served as project associate on the personal assistance project with Community and Policy Studies and Lance Egley in the lead role for the World Institute on Disability. In Parts II and IV, the Center on Human Policy research team involved in these projects included Steve Taylor, Bonnie Shoultz, Susan O'Connor, Pat Rogan, Pam Walker, Zana Lutfiyya, Michael Kennedy, and Rannveig Traustadottir, with Robert Bogdan, Doug Biklen, Steve Murphy, and Connie Barna on related projects, together with all the center staff, associates, and former associates. These included Hank Bersani, Jan Nisbet, Alison Ford, Jim Knoll, Carol Berrigan, Michelle Surles, Janet Duncan, Stan Searl, Ellen Fisher, Susan Barclay, Maya Kaylanpur, Dianne Ferguson, Sue Lehr, Gordon Porter, Pat Killius, Marge Olney, and Deb Olson.

For the evaluations conducted in South Dakota (Chapter 13), thanks to Patti Miles, Tom Scheinost, Phyllis Graney, Jim Smith, David Merrill, and Gary Smith. For the evaluation in Milwaukee (Chapter 14), thanks to Marc Lucoff, Nancy Flax, and Diane Priegel of the Milwaukee Combined Community Services Board; Jim Esmeier of Christian Community Living Systems, Milwaukee County; and Dennis Harkins of the Wisconsin Developmental Disabilities Office. For the Idaho personal care evaluation (Chapter 14), thanks to John Watts of Idaho's Developmental Disabilities Council; Nick Arambarri of Region VI Office, Pocatello, Idaho; Reed Mulkey of the Idaho State School and Hospital; and Paul Swartzenberg and Lloyd Forbes of the Idaho Developmental Services and Medicaid Offices. For the evaluation of the family support organization (Chapter 12), thanks to Bernice Schultz of the Onondaga County Department of Mental Health, Barbara Weinstein of Seguin Community Services, and Jo Scro and Hillery Schniederman of Exceptional Family Resources.

Since the publication of *Housing, Support and Community* (Racino et al., 1993), many of the contributors to work in the disability reform field have died, including Cory Moore, Jerry Kiracofe, Ed Roberts, Ron Mace, Irving Zola, and Dick LePore; we are all better off for their contributions

in life. Thanks to the many people who continue to enrich people's lives
and who participated in these projects.

Research in this book was funded, in part, by several sources, including
two Research and Training Centers on Community Integration and the
Community Integration Project awarded to Syracuse University, Center on
Human Policy, through the National Institute on Disability Research and
Rehabilitation, U.S. Department of Education. Additional support was
obtained through a Research and Training Center on Residential Services
and Community Living at the University of Minnesota, the Research and
Training Center on Personal Assistance awarded to the World Institute on
Disability, and the New York State Department of Health through funding
from the Rehabilitation Services Administration. The project directors of
these centers and/or projects were Steve Taylor (Syracuse University),
Simi Litvak (World Institute on Disability), and K. Charles Lakin (University
of Minnesota), with William Reynolds representing the New York
State Department of Health. Family support demonstration funds were
provided to the family support agency by the New York State Office of
Mental Retardation and Developmental Disabilities. The interpretations
contained herein are those of the author, and no endorsement on the part of
the World Institute on Disability, Center on Human Policy, Syracuse University,
University of Minnesota, or the U.S. Department of Education
should be inferred.

Thanks to the staff of the Jervis Library and to the Franklin Press in
Rome, New York (especially Richard Fiore); the staff of The Haworth
Press, including Bill Palmer, Managing Editor, Melissa Devendorf, Administrative
Assistant, Marvin Feit, Haworth Health and Social Policy
Series Editor, Dawn Krisko, Production Editor, Karen Sweredoski, Copywriter,
and Jennifer M. Gaska, cover designer; Hannah King, then at
SUNY Health Sciences Center, and Rachael Zubal and her secretarial
colleagues at Syracuse University.

PART I:
INTRODUCTION

Chapter 1

Qualitative Evaluation and Research: Toward Community Support for All

Julie Ann Racino

INTRODUCTION

This book was the outgrowth of policy and practice research and evaluation in disability conducted from the mid-1980s through the mid-1990s in the United States. Centering around the time of the passage of the landmark Americans with Disabilities Act (1990), *Policy, Program Evaluation, and Research in Disability: Community Support for All* combines qualitative research case studies with methodological hints, analyses, and background readings on ongoing policy and programmatic concerns from the 1970s to the approaching decade, affecting the lives of people with and without disabilities.

Value-Driven Evaluation and Research

The case studies and evaluation research in this book can be classified as value driven (Linton, 1954, on universal human values), in being explicitly part of agreements to move toward the participation in community life of people with disabilities. Based in part on normalization principles begun in Sweden (Nirje, 1985) and Denmark (Bank-Mikkelsen, 1969), which have been highly influential since the 1970s in the United States and United Kingdom (Values in Action, 1990), the principles have been reformulated in the United States as social role valorization (Wolfensberger, 1985). The research in this book reflects shared values developed with collaborative groups in the 1980s, primarily in the United States (Center on Human Policy, 1987, 1989a).

As described in the shared values statement of the Rehabilitation Research and Training Centers on Family and Community Living (1990, p. 1), funded by the National Institute on Disability Research and Rehabilitation (NIDRR) of the U.S. Department of Education, these principles included the following:

- All people with disabilities will be able to live successfully in, and as part of, natural communities that provide them the supports they need.
- All people with disabilities will be recognized for the positive contributions they make to their families and their communities.
- All people with disabilities will benefit from enduring relationships with other people, including family members and community members without disabilities.
- All people with disabilities and their family members will be entitled to participate in decisions affecting the nature and quality of the services they receive.
- All people with disabilities will have access to services and supports that provide choice and promote full citizenship.
- Services and supports for people with disabilities will be individualized so as to be responsive to cultural and ethnic differences, economic resources, personal abilities, specific needs, and individual life circumstances.
- Public policy will stimulate opportunities for people with disabilities to enjoy productive and integrated lives.

Disability Politics and the Disability Agenda

Disability politics are complex (Hahn, 1985); they explicitly call upon people either to engage in self-examination of human values (Condeluci, 1996) from compassion to kindness or to identify one's own life in terms of disability (Shaw, 1994), as Parent, Disabled Person, Survivor, Advocate, or, more recently, Professional Parents. The former process is intimately tied to religious or spiritual practices and values, and the second, usually to political organizing. Excellent histories have been written of the disability movements, including from the perspectives of the disability community (Groce, 1992), in the historical tradition (Longmore, 1987), and within the framework of community integration and deinstitutionalization (Taylor and Searl, 1987).

Disability As an Industry

In the United States, disability is tied to a massive industry that supports governmental (local, state, federal) and for-profit- and nonprofit-sector workforces. Most governmental positions other than political appointments are governed by civil service, with standards determined on a state-by-state basis for most sectors. In the nonprofit sector, service-providing agencies may be independent living centers or parent-run organizations that may receive additional local funding from the United Way and other community-funding drives. The evaluation research industry (Haveman, 1987) involves university and private sectors that often interchange employees and consultants.

Independent Living and Self-Help Movements

With the birth of independent living in the United States in advocacy by students at the University of California at Berkeley, independent living became an international movement by people with disabilities to direct their own destinies (Zola, 1987). Words associated with the international movement have been empowerment, self-determination, and consumer control by people of all abilities. Similarly, Disabled People's International is a cross-disability movement (Zola, 1989); self-help movements, similar but distinct, are the survivor and ex-patient movements in mental health and head injury and self-advocacy in the field of mental retardation, its related conditions, and developmental disabilities.

Family Advocacy and Family Movements

In the United States, family movements began, in part, with efforts by parents to start some of the first services for their children with disabilities. Whereas political efforts are coalition-based, most family advocacy associations are organized by disability category (similar to funding streams), with separate groups of parents and "consumers" (e.g., the ARC, previously the Association for Retarded Citizens; Federation for Families in Childrens' Mental Health; National Head Injury Association). The late 1980s saw the formation of a new parents' organization based in Washington, DC, with a cross-disability focus, the Parent Network on Disability (P. Smith, 1994).

International Associations and Leadership

As with the rest of the world, disability politics are global (e.g., International League of Societies for the Mentally Handicapped [Dybwad, 1990]), with international leadership from the United Nations (1993a) through its statements in *Human Rights and Disabled Persons* to standards related to support services and equalization (United Nations, 1993b). In the United

States, the National Council on Disability (NCD) (1996) was designated as the contact point in the federal government for foreign policy in disability issues, with parent, educator, and provider associations (e.g., International Association of Persons with Severe Handicaps) advocating on behalf of particular groups. The economics of disability and the well-being of children and of elders remain as important gauges of the status of the condition of world health.

Public Policy and Disability

On an international level, disability has been distinguished from handicaps and impairments and, more recently, in classification schemes, by activities and participation and limitations in these areas of life. The intent of the new classification scheme was to move toward more neutral language and away from concepts of disablement (World Health Organization, 1997). Such an approach would more closely resemble the context described by Nora Groce (1985) in her study of hereditary deafness, which showed that the communities on Martha's Vineyard had incorporated deafness into everyday living.

In the United States, public policy concerning people with disabilities (Burkhauser, Haveman, and Wolfe, 1993) has primarily been considered part of health policy. Second, public access to housing, transportation, economic participation, education, recreation, employment, and all aspects of community life has become law, in part, through grassroots efforts. Federal laws, including the Americans with Disabilities Act (1990) (e.g., U.S. Department of Justice, Civil Rights Division and Equal Employment Opportunity Commission, 1997), have had a critical impact on states and localities [USDOJ, CRD and EEOC, 1997] ranging from accessible bus transportation to increased employment access. Sometimes, these changes are tied to federal programs, especially Social Security and Medicaid (see Congressional Review, 1990), which are driven, in part, by public policies toward elders (Burkhauser, 1991).

Citizenship for all people has been interpreted as the positive attributes and ideals of the society. These have included moral rights to employment, recreation, voting and political office, entrepreneurship and business ownership, homeownership, marriage and family, and a network of friends and acquaintances. However, full participation is not yet an integral part of the public policy schools, and disability studies programs remain sparse (D. Ferguson, P. Ferguson, and S. Taylor, 1992; Linton, 1998; Zola, 1992).

Segregation and inclusion continue as contradictory approaches to public policy in the United States, whether related to ethnicity, age, culture, social class, or disability. Central concerns of the disability community in public policy include income supports and disincentives to employment; the aging and diversity of America; movement of funding from institutions to community services; the culture of disability; services controlled by disabled people and their families; affirmative policies toward employment of people with disabilities; and participation as a citizen, with choice and without discrimination and stigma.

EVALUATION RESEARCH PRINCIPLES AND DIRECTIONS

Major principles and directions for evaluation research in this past decade were consumer or service-user involvement, collaborative research with diverse constituencies and key stakeholders, integration as a guiding value, the principle of diversity and multiculturalism, and the movement toward community research and quality of life.

Consumer or Service-User Involvement

During the United Nations Decade of Disabled Persons (1983 through 1992), a renewed interest in participatory action research (PAR), research with a social consciousness, evolved. Participatory action research, with its roots in qualitative research, sought the involvement of consumers or service users in all aspects of research design, data collection, analyses, evaluation and review, and dissemination of findings (Lord, Schnarr, and Hutchinson, 1987; Bruyere, 1993). This renewal was supported by the National Institute on Disability Research and Rehabilitation, U.S. Department of Education, with presentations and discussions with researchers, directors, and training directors through the leadership of William Graves.

Yet, the definition of consumer proved problematic (e.g., Pollitt, 1988; Thomas, 1993); to some major university research projects, it meant the rehabilitation and service agencies that provided services, and to others, it meant the parents of people with disabilities rather than the individuals themselves. The insight that all people are potential service users, or customers (Drucker, 1995), and, therefore, a critical component of evaluations was never systematically developed in the field. This was true even as new conceptualizations were formulated and research began comparing people with and without disabilities. Leading concepts were "consumer directed" (Doty, Kasper, and Litvak, 1996; Racino, 1995a) versus "consumer involvement" of service users, including people with significant disabilities; "family centered" (Nelkin, 1987), and "family directed" (Racino, J., O'Connor, Walker, and Taylor, 1991).

Collaborative Research with Constituencies

As part of the movement away from hierarchical organizations and structures (Martin, Harrison, and Dinitto, 1983), collaborative agreements between researchers and field administrators were viewed as ways of assuring research adoption and utilization (Weiss, 1972; Patton, 1997). Consensus methods (Fink et al., 1984), ranging from Delphi techniques and forms of structured group processes, brought together the perspectives of families and people with disabilities, including principles for collaborative research (Turnbull, Turnbull, and Senior Staff, 1989). These methods (e.g., focus groups) resulted in the identification of new areas of disability research (e.g., secondary and tertiary prevention as perceived by service users) (White, Gutierrez, and Seekins, 1996).

Public constituencies, with their diversity, are the province of evaluation research (Pulice, McCormick, and Dewees, 1995), resulting in the continuing ties with "stakeholder" approaches (Weiss, 1995; Patton, 1997). Yet, the politics of theory building and interpretation, presentation, and their relationship to utilization were overshadowed by research political concerns, including who would be funded, who would conduct the research, and what research agendas would be supported, with a perceived cost to services of any funded disability research.

Integration As a Guiding Value

Though the term integration in the disability field has been misused as a term and in practice, the intent was the participation of people of diversity in regular environments, the antithesis of exclusionary practices and models (Taylor, Racino, and Shoultz, 1988; Towell and Beardshaw, 1991). As conceptualized with people with disabilities, this means opportunities for, and participation in, schools, jobs, leisure, friendships, relationships, homes, and diverse interests and lifestyles. Community integration is an evolving definition of an understanding of full participation and acceptance in societies, which are, by their nature, culturally based, and represents a hope for better quality of life for all peoples.

Theorists have differentiated types and levels of integration in special education as physical, functional, social, community, and organizational integration (Ferguson, Ferguson, and Bogdan, 1987), and sociologically as a change of status (viewed through the concepts of luminality and rites of passage) (Calvez, 1993). In disability circles, integration became equated with doing something *to* people with disabilities instead of active pursuits *by* children, youth, adults, and elders with disabilities.

As Judy Heumann (1993), now a President Clinton appointee to the U.S. Department of Education and an independent living leader, explained,

"Forced integration doesn't work," and integration "must be on terms where we feel comfortable and equal" (p. 25). From integration, the field began to shift toward inclusion, with full membership of all (Stainback, Stainback, and Jackson, 1992) in classrooms in which not all children were yet welcomed. However, inclusion reflected a stronger emphasis on participation and diversity versus principles of social justice and power sharing, the latter requiring a change in the nature of our schools and institutions serving our youth (Jackson et al., 1993).

Diversity and Multiculturalism

Mario Cuomo (1994), the former Governor of New York who supported the "family of New York," described diversity as the right to be different and as one of the most powerful and unifying values. As one of the central concepts in a pluralistic or democratic society, diversity was reflected in a broadened, multicultural approach, based on the changing school populations, workforces, and the business, research, and policymaking communities.

Multiculturalism, including disability, was a proposed framework for approaches that encompassed ethnicity, culture, language, social class, social status, and gender (Traustadottir, Lutfiyya, and Shoultz, 1994). These frameworks differ from popular ethnographic and journalistic accounts of peoples in this country (Thom, 1976) and around the world (Carrier, 1992). They are distinct, yet related to approaches that are culturally sensitive, competent, and inclusive services and applied to people with disabilities and their families (e.g., Mackas, Marshall, and Wehman, 1997).

Quality of Life and Community Research

In the 1980s and 1990s, research began to move its focus from the comparison of types of settings, particularly institutional to community based, toward quality life in the community (Hughes et al., 1995). Quality of life could be defined by each person and sociologically constructed by individuals (Taylor and Bogdan, 1990). More commonly, quality of life is based upon principles of citizenship and community life (e.g., physical integration, personal growth and development, safety, health and comfort, social relationships, valued community participation, and personal autonomy; Lakin, 1988).

Research studies in the 1980s and 1990s continued to compare organizational or program types (e.g., life in foster care versus group homes), examining variables by organizational type (e.g., decision making and choice in group homes) and the costs and benefits of particular program models (e.g., early intervention programs, small homes in the community, and supported employment). However, research study designs remained in philosophical conflict on integration and segregation service models.

Health services research, including in the field of mental health, continued to proliferate, with two primary types of evaluation: evaluation of the mental health sector within the comprehensive systems of care and the evaluation of individual mental health facilities or types of care (Häfner and an der Heiden, 1991). Mental health policy research, though sometimes implying otherwise, typically does not include systems of care in developmental disabilities, mental retardation and related conditions, and brain injuries (see Friedman, Kutash, and Duchnowski, 1996). Similar reporting problems occur concerning financing and systems in physical disability and with functional impairments and disability; people with the most significant disabilities may be excluded in some analyses, for example, those which exclude people in institutions (e.g., residential schools).

As states faced new decisions regarding the futures of their public institutions (see Smith and Lakin, Part II, "Introduction," on institution-free states) and community infrastructure (see Knoll, Part IV, "Introduction," on empowerment), research on perceived problematic areas for community living remained in the forefront. These areas included people with behavioral challenges, school exclusion and integration, sexual offenders, violence and abuse, and children with medical and technological needs, epilepsy, or low-incidence disorders.

By the early 1990s, research was shifting into the community sector, as opposed to the disability sector (Taylor and Bogdan, 1994). This movement involved studies of community organizations, neighborhoods, employment and leisure, and aspects of community for people with and without disabilities. Sociologically, however, key concepts from grounded theory were presented as total institutions, stigmata, subcultures, and accepting relationships (Taylor and Bogdan, 1994), with an "insider's views" on a range of phenomena in community sites and families.

Although an important victory, the passage of the Americans with Disabilities Act (1990) continued as a minority group model (Biklen and Knoll, 1987b) in conflict on some tenets with the worldview of participation of all peoples in U.S. society. Another movement was toward support services separated from facilities (e.g., Bradley, Knoll, and Agosta, 1992; Racino et al., 1993; Taylor et al., 1987) and toward choice and self-determination, the latter reflective of citizens' rights in democracies (Cuomo, 1994).

The 1980s saw the emergence of the support and empowerment paradigm (American Association on Mental Retardation, 1992; Racino, 1992a; Smull and Bellamy, 1991) (see Table 1.1), together with a reframing of public policy toward supported employment, living, education, recreation, and families (Hibbard et al., 1989). Standards to guide support principles, suggested by outcome-based evaluators (Schalock, 1995), have included the following:

- Supports occur in regular, integrated environments *(which are a right of all people, including those citizens with disabilities);*
- Support activities are performed primarily by individuals working, living, or recreating within those environments *(with paid services and natural support);*
- Support activities are individualized and person referenced *(versus the supports movement toward person or family centered);*
- Outcomes from the use of support *services* are evaluated against quality indicators and valued, person referenced outcomes;
- The use of supports can fluctuate and may range from lifelong duration to fluctuating needs during different stages of life;
- Support *services* should not be withdrawn precipitously *(versus should be available as needed and desired, including for people with the most severe disabilities).* (p. 20, italics added)

In the 1990s, U.S. health care reform was dominated by "managed care," with greater control by the health care and insurance industries (General Accounting Office, 1993). A countereffort occurred to ensure that disability would not be defined in solely medical terms (Krefting and Groce, 1992). Unlike the decline in innovative programs reported in other fields (Freeman and Solomon, 1979), in disability, innovations and their study (e.g., best practices) continue to be viewed as valuable in terms of education, planned social change (Lord, 1984), and research (Taylor, Bogdan, and Racino, 1991; Racino, 1991c; Walker and O'Connor, 1997).

POLICY ANALYSIS AND EVALUATION RESEARCH

Policy analysis and evaluation research, which can occur independently, are fundamental in disability to the establishment, development, quality, and funding of programs. As explained by Haveman (1987), program evaluations were required of virtually every piece of social legislation, thus influencing the development of these practices in the human services field and the U.S. research industry. These research developments involve programs at public policy schools in the United States and in the for-profit- and nonprofit-sector research companies, including government-formed and -supported companies.

TABLE 1.1. A Comparison of the Rehabilitation, Independent Living, and Support/Empowerment Paradigms

Focus[c]	Rehabilitation paradigm[a,c]	Independent living paradigm[a,c]	Support/empowerment paradigm[b]
Definition of problem	Physical impairment, lack of vocational skills, psychological maladjustment, lack of motivation and cooperation	Dependence on professionals, relatives, and others; inadequate support services; architectural barriers; economic barriers	Attitudinal, political, economic, and administrative barriers to societal participation; inadequate supports within society
Locus of problem	In individual	In environment; in rehabilitation process	In society/environment; in rehabilitation process
Social role(s)	Patient—client	Consumer	Co-worker, community member, student, neighbor, so forth
Solution to problem	Professional intervention by physician, physical therapist, occupational therapist, vocational counselor, and others	Peer counseling; advocacy; self-help; consumer control; removal of barriers and disincentives	Redesign of schools, homes, workplaces, health-care systems, transportation, and social environments to include everyone
Who is in control	Professional	Consumer	People in alliance with one another
Desired outcomes	Maximum activities of daily living (ADL), gainful employment, psychological adjustment, improved motivation, completed treatment	Self-direction, least-restrictive environment, social and economic productivity	Pluralistic society inclusive of all people; quality lives as defined by people themselves; self-direction embedded in collaborative decision making and problem solving.

a Adapted from DeJong, G. (1978). *The Movement for Independent Living: Origins, Ideology, and Implications for Disability Research.* Boston: Tufts-New England Medical Center, Medical Rehabilitation Institute; and from DeJong, G. (1983). "Defining and Implementing the Independent Living Concept." In N. Crewe and I. Zola (Eds.), *Independent Living for Physically Disabled People.* San Francisco: Jossey-Bass.

b From Racino, J. A. (1992a). "Living in the Community: Independence, Support, and Transition." In F. R. Rusch, L. DeStefano, J. Chadsey-Rusch, L. A. Phelps, and E. Szymanski (Eds.), *Transition from School to Adult Life: Models, Linkages, and Policy.* Sycamore, IL: Sycamore Press.

c Lachat, M. E. (1988). *The Independent Living Service Model: Historical Roots, Core Elements, and Current Practices.* South Hampton, NH: Center for Resource Management in Collaboration with the National Council on Disability.

Evaluations and the Disciplines

Disciplinary-based evaluations, with a goal of multi- or interdisciplinary approaches, are common in disability. Primary disciplines are allied health, social work, education (and special education), rehabilitation, family studies, counseling, physical rehabilitation and medicine, human development, psychology, nursing and therapies, public administration, physical education and leisure studies, early intervention, and urban studies, among others. Each of these disciplines has its own training in evaluation and research, though usually with combined texts in the social or behavioral sciences (with behavioral sciences dominant in many fields).

Efforts to develop principles to guide evaluators have resulted in the identification of five areas for professional examination: systematic inquiry, competence, integrity/honesty, respect for people, and responsibilities for general and public welfare, with diversity of interests and values (American Evaluation Association, 1995). Evaluation frameworks and models are typically proposed based on categorical services: children's mental health, family programs in neonatal intensive care, statewide models in mental health for people of all ages, family support and developmental disabilities, and supported employment programs for people with traumatic brain injuries.

Sociological Perspectives and Research

Policy, Program Evaluation, and Research in Disability: Community Support for All highlights qualitative research, which has its roots in sociology and anthropology (Bogdan and Knoll, 1988; Bruyn, 1966). Qualitative research, as a field of its own, is generally acknowledged as having a crucial role in reinterpreting and reframing policy and in uncovering the positions and voices of those typically underrepresented in public policy. In relationship to the international community, a reframing of public policy to represent societies of "social acceptance" versus those of "world order" may be central to future societies.

Planning, Evaluation, and Change

Evaluation and research in disability have often been part of an ongoing strategic planning process (Neilson Associates Ply. Ltd., 1987; Towell, Racino, and Rucker, 1990), based upon values of community presence, participation, choice, respect and dignity, and competence (O'Brien, 1987). As described by Blum in health planning (1974), the levels of involvement in planning are local, metro, regional, state, federal, and international.

Evaluation research studies described and illustrated in this book are formative in nature, part of planned social change, and contributions to the development of grounded theory. Yet, this evaluation research remains targeted toward specialized populations and specialized systems in the disability world, but with goals of community integration, universal access, and community inclusion. These vary from internal action research approaches within organizations to evaluations at the community level.

Educational Evaluation Research

Educational evaluation research (American Evaluation Association, 1995) has encompassed within its boundaries community development and living, which are outside the traditional educational system, with its governing rules, standards, and professional criteria. Community research domains in education have involved funding for community programs with families and their children and with adults living, working, and recreating in neighborhoods and communities. Yet, "educative research" remains defined as education research in and for the field of education (Gitlin, Siegel, and Boru, 1989), not in, of, and for the community.

Basic Types of Evaluation

Schemata for research and evaluation range from the classic quantitative frameworks still prevalent today (Campbell and Stanley, 1963; e.g., preexperimental, quasi-experimental, experimental, and correlational and ex post facto designs) to qualitative schema. The latter may differentiate perspectives, paradigms, strategies for inquiry, and qualitative research designs (see Denzin and Lincoln, 1994; Wolcott, 1982, on types of ethnographies). More recently, values questions have been suggested as the primary organizers of evaluation types. Evaluators tend toward the use of multiple measures, indicators, and studies, especially in relationship to program, state, and/or constituency goals and objectives, which often involve questions of priorities, costs benefits, outcomes, and effectiveness. The following major distinctions often appear in research evaluation at these levels of community research:

Basic and Applied Research

Basic research, as in the hard sciences that are forms of art and insight, may not initially lead to applications in the field. Yet, for example, understanding how the mind works may eventually lead to innovations in various fields from computer technology to a cure for Alzheimer's disease to new communication techniques. Basic research is often tied to the more commonly used term knowledge generation. In contrast, applied research is designed for its applications, which may be technological, managerial, clinical, administrative, practical, and/or political, with demonstrable impacts. Applied research generally targets particular user groups, usually with multiple audiences (traditional research, training, and dissemination frameworks) and strong connections to marketability (business models).

Formative and Summative Evaluations

Formative evaluations have been known as process evaluations and have as their intent the development of the system, program, agency, or interventions being evaluated. Their focus is often on quality and on the relationships among the program's intentions, what occurs, and the outcomes. In contrast, summative evaluations have as their major purpose an evaluation of the status at the time of the evaluation and are sometimes used for decision making on whether to continue programs or funding.

Common measures, often used in summative evaluations, include cost-benefit analysis (e.g., Tines et al., 1990); cost-effectiveness and "value" (Gillis, Koch, and Joyi, 1989); impact evaluations (Rossi and Freeman, 1993); outcome, effectiveness and contextual analyses (Schalock, 1995), extent of achievement of goals and objectives (Weiss, 1972); unintended outcomes (Weiss, 1972); and consumer or user satisfaction (Kaufmann, Ward-Colasante, and Farmer, 1993; Reagles, Wright, and Thomas, 1972). Both formative and summative types of evaluations can be public in nature, or solely for internal use.

Outcome and Process Evaluations

In the 1980s, the field of disability moved toward outcome approaches as part of the major revision in standards (that apply to certified and licensed programs throughout the United States). Personal life quality and self-determination emerged as crucial outcomes, with increased expectations for better quality living, employment, education, leisure, and friendships in people's lives (Towell and Beardshaw, 1991). Outcome measures that tracked the movement of people between sites (e.g., homes versus hospitals and nursing homes) remained as priorities for reducing the institutional bias of the U.S. system. Yet, other groups promoted choice in (e.g., roommates, meals) and of any setting (e.g., cooperatives or group homes) versus approaches to community support. Methodologies moved toward approaches that incorporated consumer viewpoints in the evaluation research on a standard basis (Everett and Boydell, 1994), with attention toward community and ecological outcomes.

Performance Measurement and Evaluability Assessment

Performance measurement systems (see Wholey, 1983, for program performance indicators) were implemented by state and regional offices as one method of contracting for more integrated services and outcomes. These outcomes included community employment versus sheltered work or day habilitation at a segregated site (see, e.g., Wehman, Sale, and Parent, 1992; Kay, 1993, for indicators and outcome measures in employment). Evaluability assessment (Strossberg and Wholey, 1983), though not known by this term in the disability field, reflected the recognition that evaluation was worth the time, money, and effort on a major scale only when certain conditions were met, including a receptivity toward change on the part of the involved agency or entity. For example, some situations require management intervention and actions, but not necessarily full-scale evaluations. Creation of environments of receptivity, support, and information sharing was the mark of the preceding decade, which continued, however, to see change through adverse litigation in the field of disability.

Community Assessments and Focus Groups

Echoing the program evaluation techniques of the 1970s used by the National Institute of Mental Health, the late 1980s and 1990s saw a movement back toward community assessments (Robertson, 1988), with the identification of local community needs and barriers as they affected the lives of people with disabilities (e.g., World Institute on Disability, 1991a). Focus groups became a qualitative method of highlighting user perspectives (Diehl, Moffitt, and Wade, 1991; Schleien et al., 1995) and of reformulating basic research questions. Renewed emphasis was placed on the strengths of the method for uncovering how and why processes and changes come about (Morgan, 1988).

Exploratory Research and Pilot Designs

Qualitative research has been described as exploratory in nature, with the apparent assumption that it precedes the "real research." Although exploratory research is itself a major research endeavor (Hagner and Helm,

1994) to which some people may devote their lives, it is distinct from descriptive research and from pilots of methodologies and study designs. Its strength in research and development endeavors is its capacity to uncover hidden assumptions, relationships, and consequences that are not readily apparent or discernable. *Handbook of Qualitative Research* (Denzin and Lincoln, 1994) offers an overview of qualitative research and its underlying assumptions, with other tests also recently expanded and updated (Taylor and Bogdan, 1998; Bogdan and Biklen, 1998).

Qualitative Analyses of Quantitative Designs

Though articles have highlighted the qualitative analyses of quantitative designs (Bogdan and Ksander, 1980), research studies of this nature were not predominant during the period following 1985 in the disability field. These studies could include analyses of survey research as quantitative and qualitative strategies, comparative analyses, and the implications for future research. In particular, person-centered approaches to public policy and "individualized funding" (Snow and Racino, 1991) hold promise that has not yet unfolded in the quantitative or qualitative research fields.

Quasi-Experimental and Experimental Designs

The traditional research and evaluation texts (Campbell and Stanley, 1963) describe quasi-experimental and experimental designs, which are the basis for many research studies in the disability field. Most field studies tend to be quasi-experimental, sometimes with random assignment to conditions (e.g., traditional or innovative family support services) and with ethical issues often addressed by levels of services. However, experimental research studies may be embedded within field studies (e.g., outcomes of different types of therapy). These studies may be reported and analyzed by study type (pretest, posttest, nonequivalent control group designs, stratified sampling). Qualitative research, inclusive of naturalistic studies, has had its language assumed by quantitative researchers for community studies (Häfner and an der Heiden, 1991).

Longitudinal Studies

Longitudinal designs have been crucial to the community research agenda (e.g., Lowe, DePaiva, and Humphreys, 1986; White, Lakin, and Bruininks, 1989), due to the nature of the movement from institutional to community living and to the effects on lives over time. Longitudinal studies may be continuous in nature over a few years (three to five) or more, or they may involve periodic study over a regular interval of years. Quantitative designs tend to include diversity in structured interviews, together with on-site visits and observations, usually using instruments considered valid and reliable for field use.

Qualitative studies that are longitudinal in nature are called ethnographies, life histories, historical sociology, ethnographic studies, historical analyses, and related genres (multicase studies, e.g., Wolcott, 1982; Bogdan and Biklen, 1982). Interview methods in qualitative studies are generally open-ended and semistructured and are used together with participant observation, a primary methodology in the qualitative research field (Becker and Geer, 1957).

Survey Research

Survey research, which may involve questionnaires and telephone interviews, has been a primary methodology in national studies, especially for sampling done on a state-by-state basis. These surveys include ongoing data collection in states on a yearly basis over the decades (e.g., on the status of institutional and residential services in a field; Braddock et al., 1990) and status reports to strengthen younger services, such as family support (Knoll et al., 1992a). Such studies are distinct from federal data collection on federal laws (e.g., education of children with disabilities), disability and health surveys, such as the National Health Information Survey, and the census of the U.S. population (Thompson-Hoffman and Storck, 1991).

Policy Analysis and Evaluation

Policy analysis is intimately related to evaluation research, with policy products that may be used to aid in decision making (Florio, Behrmann, and Goltz, 1979). Policy itself can be defined in diverse ways and encompasses the decisions made by governments that have accumulated over time (see Guba, 1984, for eight definitions). Policy analysts may be producers of evaluation research (Smith, 1995), but more often are the users of such research, which may be qualitative and quantitative in nature. Timeliness to meet political demands has been a frequent criticism of policy research (Bruininks, 1990), as has been lack of responsiveness to the concerns of people with disabilities (Batavia, 1992). Policy research may be program focused; yet with strong roots in the theme "policy is personal." Person-focused evaluations (see Bradley and Bersani, 1990) and person-centered approaches to evaluation and policy analysis have not yet taken root in the methodological world of policy, holding promise for the future decades. Policy can be driven by "rough measures," for example, the overall effectiveness of a nation's health system as measured by health indicators (Häfner and an der Heiden, 1991), with evaluations found to have only a moderate influence on policy decision making (Florio, Behrmann, and Goltz, 1979).

Qualitative Research

Qualitative research is a field of its own, with its roots in sociology and anthropology and its own traditions, theories, methods, and emerging paradigms (e.g., see G. W. Smith, 1990, for a new epistemological/ontological paradigmatic combination). In their advanced handbook introducing the qualitative research field, Norman Denzin and Yvonne Lincoln (1994) describe the history of the research; the research process; the interpretative paradigms; feminism, ethnicity, and models of qualitative research; strategies of inquiry; methods of collecting and analyzing empirical materials; the art of interpretation, evaluation, and presentation; and the future ("fifth moment"), subsequently, the "sixth moment" (Denzin, 1997). These discussions vary from texts that are more strongly rooted in practice than in theory (Taylor and Bogdan, 1984, 1988; Bogdan and Biklen, 1982, 1988).

Qualitative research methods are naturalistic methods (Redfield, 1953), paralleling in some ways the naturalistic sciences, which are respectful of all creatures. Natural science shares with these methods the rigor of scientific endeavors such as field studies in natural habitats, and the time-consuming nature of an almost endless exploration of life in the universe. Naturalistic approaches (Guba and Lincoln, 1989), especially in the tradition of participant observation (Bruyn, 1966; Becker and Geer, 1957; Vidich, 1955), form the heart of sociological studies, fitting somewhat uneasily with the judgments of evaluation research.

Qualitative research has a strong history in the field of disability, from applied approaches to ethnographic studies and participant observation of diverse phenomena, including the use of ethnographic methods in the study of families and community sites (Taylor and Bogdan, 1981; Taylor, Bogdan, and Racino, 1991; O'Connor, 1995). The research methods are either aligned with political action (G. W. Smith, 1990) or in contrast to a cultural interpretive stance. Qualitative research remains a leader in highlighting both the perspectives of those underrepresented in public policy and the fundamental nature of social change (Lord, Schnarr, and Hutchinson, 1987).

This book is designed, in part, to highlight qualitative research methodologies and their contributions to community research (see Edgerton, 1988; Kemper, Applebaum, and Harrigan, 1987; Taylor and Bogdan, 1994). In particular, this book describes and illustrates the methods of participant observation, interviewing, snowballing techniques, and the use of negative cases; analytic methods, such as constant comparative analyses; the development of grounded theory and theoretical sampling; the strategy of the case study and its role in research; the design of multisite research; innovations in program evaluations; research ethics; and the politics of community research and public policy.

THE FORMAT OF THE BOOK

The book is divided into three major parts, with Parts II and III containing two separate qualitative research studies, with different, yet related, analyses, philosophical frameworks, and policy implications. The first major study's design is based upon the support and empowerment paradigm, and the design of the second is based upon the independent living paradigm, with analyses approached through a support and empowerment framework (see Table 1.1). Part IV integrates policy research studies, some conducted as part of statewide technical assistance agreements, with secondary agreements at local sites; other case studies are selected from national applied qualitative research studies.

Part II: Community Integration describes state policies and practices to support community and systems change. Organized as thematic case studies, this leading qualitative research study provides a historical overview of change in the state of New Hampshire, with a proposed framework for planning for change in the next decade. This study is introduced by Gary Smith, an evaluator of state programs and community services in developmental disabilities throughout the United States, and K. Charles Lakin, a national leader known for his research on deinstitutionalization at the University of Minnesota, Institute on Community Integration. These two advisory board members frame the New Hampshire study in the context of institutional closure and community developments in the United States.

Part III: Moving Toward Universal Access to Support is based upon consumer expert interviews with people with disabilities about the development of personal assistance services (PAS), endorsed by the United Nations (1993). Organized as combined highlights of the subfields of psychiatric disabilities, brain injuries, mental retardation, physical disabilities, and youth with disabilities, the research is designed to present public policy through personal perspectives.

Co-authored (with Julie Ann Racino) by Simi Litvak of the World Institute on Disability and one of the authors of *Attending to America* (Litvak, Zukas, and Heumann, 1987), Chapters 8 to 11 represent a selection of perspectives of "underserved" or "underrepresented populations" in relation to personal assistance services (PAS). Echoing the late Irv Zola's call for the universalizing of disability policy (1989), the interviews offer insight into future directions toward universal access and community approaches to PAS.

Part IV: Housing, Families, and Community Support presents a selection of excerpts from agency, regional, and state evaluation research, together with brief descriptions, reviews, analyses, and methodological descriptions. Introduced by James A. Knoll, an educator and national evaluator of family support programs from the university and private sectors, Chapters 12 through 15 highlight qualitative research case studies and evaluation research, based on work by Julie Ann Racino in such states as South Dakota, Wisconsin, Kentucky, Idaho, New York, Vermont, Massachusetts, Georgia, Minnesota, and Ohio. These studies reflect research and evaluation from both the research innovations and the technical assistance sides (often separate branches of policy units) as part of an ongoing change and developmental process.

The book leaves the reader at the point where the disability field moves toward community studies; neighborhood comparisons; studies of leisure and community employment sites, associations, and clubs; and the not yet reached community-to-community comparisons in some crucial areas of community life (Hollister and Hill, 1995). *Policy, Program Evaluation, and Research in Disability: Community Support for All* primarily examines the disability context and interpretative frames prior to their application by disability researchers to the "nondisability" world as part of the movement toward accepting societies. The concluding Chapter 16 describes the present status of the disability field, discusses trends in disability policy and planning, and presents hope for better futures for all of us.

PART II:
COMMUNITY INTEGRATION—
POLICIES TO SUPPORT COMMUNITY
AND SYSTEMS CHANGE

Introduction:
The New Hampshire Story—
Lessons That Are Still Important

Gary Smith
K. Charles Lakin

In 1991, New Hampshire closed Laconia State School and Training Center, thereby accomplishing what no other state had to date: it "just said no" to putting its citizens with developmental disabilities in a large public institution. In doing so, New Hampshire made a real and revolutionary contribution to public policy as it applied to people with developmental disabilities. The state demonstrated that type, severity, or any other feature of an individual's disability did not justify keeping that person from family, friends, and fellow citizens.

THE CLOSING OF LACONIA

The closing of Laconia State School sparked all manner of disbelief and denial from those who viewed large public institutions as core, and necessary features in a continuum of developmental disabilities services. Some were sure that the only way New Hampshire could close Laconia was to send people away to other institutions inside or outside the state's borders. They certainly did not believe it was possible to support people with severe disabilities or challenging behavior in the community. Others speculated (literally) that New Hampshire citizens with developmental disabilities must not be very disabled, for if they were, they would surely need an institution. Some were certain that the school closing would succeed only if New Hampshire allocated massive resources to pay for all the services Laconia residents required, services that could be provided far more economically in a large institution. This latter view was expressed by those who had no acquaintance with New Hampshire's storied reputation as one of the nation's most fiscally conservative states.

The closing of Laconia disconcerted those who believed that severe disability and institutionalization are largely inseparable, just as it was

25

reassuring for those who believed that institutions reflect the limitations of our society more than those of the people living in them. The former group, over the years, sometimes discounted New Hampshire's accomplishments by portraying it as an oddity. The latter group has sometimes viewed the closing of Laconia as an accomplishment more simple than those involved would describe it. This record of the closing of Laconia State School provides a useful summary of both the simplicities and complexities of a pioneering state's commitment to create a place in its communities for people with severe disabilities.

Since New Hampshire became the first institution-free zone, other states have followed suit. In New England, Rhode Island, Vermont, and Maine have closed their large public facilities (the irony being that these New England states were among the first to establish public institutions). Institution-free zones now exist outside New England—the District of Columbia, West Virginia, New Mexico, and Alaska. More states will follow in the future. New Hampshire was the first, but it is no longer alone.

Only thirty years ago, nearly 230,000 people with developmental disabilities were housed in large public institutions for persons with developmental and psychiatric disabilities. Our nation's response to developmental disability was to remove people from our communities. Yet, Laconia's closing was, to a considerable extent, an important, inevitable outcome. By the time Laconia closed in 1991, public institution populations nationwide were barely one-third of their 1967 totals. Between 1991 and 1998, state institution populations decreased from nearly 80,000 people to fewer than 52,000. In New Hampshire, by 1989, the number of state institution residents had fallen to just over 100 people, and average per-resident costs at Laconia had risen to over $90,000, an amount comparable to the national average in 1998, $98,500. Such forces are leading to state institution closures throughout the United States.

It is not difficult to close a public institution. One closes about every four to five weeks in the United States. Indeed, the closing of an institution is now merely noteworthy, not particularly newsworthy or revolutionary (except, of course, for all who are involved in the actual event).

It is extraordinarily much more difficult to become institution free. Even though large public institutions serve no unique or especially valuable purpose in meeting the needs of people with developmental disabilities, they still play a role of sorts in serving as the "placement of last resort" (aka, the "safety net"). Becoming institution free means that a state must confront problems that people have out in the community all the time. Being institution free means not having the institution to fall back on when problems arise.

Dick LePore was New Hampshire's Director of Developmental Services throughout much of the period when people were being placed out of Laconia and it finally closed. Dick passed away in 1998. Dick was a very wise and enormously caring person. He was resolutely dedicated to a straightforward proposition: people with disabilities, as much as any citizen, belong in the community, period. When asked what was the most important event in New Hampshire, Dick was quick to point out that it was not the closing of Laconia. To Dick, the vastly more important step was the decision in the mid-1980s to allow no more individuals to be admitted to the facility. That decision meant that New Hampshire had to figure out how to address people's problems within the community—the institution would no longer be available as a safety net. To Dick and others in New Hampshire, having a community service system meant having a system that would address the needs of everyone in the community all the time. Removing individuals from their community was no solution.

As extraordinarily difficult as it is for a state to become institution free, it is still not half as difficult as sustaining the vision that the most important task is supporting the community membership of people with developmental disabilities. Community membership is about people with disabilities being valued by, and connected to, their fellow citizens. It is about services not being an end in themselves but rather a means to weave the lives of people with disabilities into the fabric of the community.

There are many examples of people being moved from large institutions to smaller institutions. Relocation does not always mean that people's day-to-day lives are much improved. The Laconia closing could have been accomplished many different ways. People could have been shuttled out of their Laconia living units to more scattered group home living units in the community. Had this happened, the end result would have been to simply change who dictated how people spent their days. There is a world of difference between people with developmental disabilities merely being "in" the community and actually being members "of" the community.

The real accomplishment in New Hampshire was (and remains) the widespread allegiance to community membership as the overarching and abiding aim. Placing people in the community and closing Laconia was not good enough for New Hampshirites. It was an important step, but not the goal. What really counted was ensuring that services and supports fostered community membership, helped people take command of their lives, and assisted them in making connections with their fellow citizens. This meant no succumbing to expediency. Most important, it meant embracing a deeper vision of how the fundamental task of supporting people should be carried out in a public system.

The chapters that follow tell the truly important story of the New Hampshire experience. That story is mainly about a system transforming itself to embrace community membership for all its citizens with developmental disabilities. It is not so much a story of people leaving an institution as it is the story of the system that greeted them when they returned to their communities.

The New Hampshire vision of community membership led the state to create its network of area agencies that would draw upon the community to support people with developmental disabilities. It was once observed that "all services—like all politics—are local." New Hampshire's area agencies are proof that service systems can be bigger than they seem at first glance when communities and citizens are enlisted in support of people with developmental disabilities.

Another important part of the New Hampshire story is the enormous amount of collaboration that occurred at all levels in moving the state's vision forward. It is no simple matter to foster community membership for people with developmental disabilities. Old views about how people should be treated need to be unlearned. It is often too easy for impatience to gain the upper hand—to substitute expedient answers for the hard work involved in helping people make lasting, and vastly more valuable, connections to their communities. The following chapters recount this struggle from many different perspectives—not in a theoretical fashion but through the words of individuals who were directly involved, who had to rethink their relationships with people they support.

Another powerful aspect of the New Hampshire story is what went on inside the walls of Laconia itself. Too often, when an institution is being closed, the atmosphere inside the facility is dismal. It is very hard for staff to remain motivated. It is easy to forget that facility staff care deeply about the people they support and dread their separation from them. Chapter 4 describes enlisting people who care about those they support to view this return to the community as an outcome to celebrate.

Still another important part of the New Hampshire story lies in the managerial decisions that state officials made. In the early 1980s, the most common and safest way to pay for community placements from public institutions was to create ICF/MR (intermediate care facilities for people with mental retardation) group homes. New Hampshire officials followed a different course—they decided to move institutional dollars into the community through the then very young Medicaid Home and Community-Based Services (HCBS) waiver program. They did this because the HCBS waiver program was vastly more congruent with their vision of supporting people in the community than the ICF/MR program. At the time, this was a high-risk proposition because the HCBS waiver program seemed to have a highly uncertain future. New Hampshire made the right decision. Indeed, the New Hampshire experience taught officials in other states that the HCBS waiver program enabled tailoring services and supports to the needs and wants of people with disabilities. Smaller institutions did not need to be substituted for larger facilities. Today, twice as many people participate in HCBS waiver programs nationwide than are served in ICF/MR homes. These facilities—similar to public institutions—are beginning to fade away. As New Hampshire officials recognized in 1984, it is not wrong to expect the system—including the services offered and purchased—to operate in a fashion that is driven by what people want and find most useful rather than consigning them to prefabricated service models.

It would be wrong to pigeonhole as mere history what transpired in New Hampshire from 1980 to the closing of Laconia and beyond. In today's information age, we tend to remain always caught up in the moment, discounting the past as yesterday's news. The New Hampshire story would fit that category if, in fact, we could say that community membership is our field's commonly and widely accepted frame of reference. No doubt, our service systems are getting better at supporting people to enjoy everyday lives as valued members of our communities. We are better at listening to people. We are better at respecting and acting upon their dreams and aspirations. However, there is still a long way to go. It is too easy to slide back into thinking that the main task is finding someone a bed, assigning people to congregate residences based on their need for supervision, or being concerned that getting people real jobs in their communities would endanger the viability of sheltered workshops.

The value of the work that Julie Racino and her colleagues performed in applying qualitative analysis to the New Hampshire experience has been to capture not only the history but also the lessons that emerged. The following chapters are not yesterday's news. The lessons learned, so well distilled from qualitative analysis, are just as fresh and robust today as when these events first occurred. Vision has no meaning unless, and until, it is infused throughout a system of services and supports. Vision does not become real via proclamations, mission statements, or conference keynote addresses. It becomes real when state and local policymakers and officials, families, individuals, service providers, and advocates follow the dictates of the vision each day in every situation. The chapters that follow describe how challenging this is. Most important, they provide valuable lessons about how a vision of a community membership-based system can become reality.

What has happened in New Hampshire since these studies were completed? New Hampshirites will be quick to tell you that there have been rocky times, that New Hampshire is not necessarily Eden for people with developmental disabilities. Contentious debates have raged about the future of the area agency network, partly due to questions about its affordability. Proposals have been made to streamline the system. It is unclear how these debates will be settled. But, the debate in New Hampshire is not about returning to 1980; community membership is still the overarching vision. New Hampshirites are still very much engaged in figuring out better ways to achieve their vision. New Hampshire has pioneered home-ownership for people with developmental disabilities. It has broken new ground by sponsoring self-determination initiatives. Overall, the update from New Hampshire is that when a system embraces and adheres to community membership as its central vision, the work is never done; the vision constantly renews itself.

Chapter 2

New Decades, New Decisions: Community Integration and Deinstitutionalization

Julie Ann Racino

INTRODUCTION

We have learned that most often what people with developmental disabilities need has little to do with their disability and a lot to do with the environment in which they live, work, and play. They say they want opportunities to experience and choose those things in life that are not disability related. Yet all too often, due to their disability, their presence and participation in areas such as housing, employment, transportation, and social relationships has been restricted.

All people need safe and secure homes. All people need gainful employment. Everyone—from infants to older Americans—needs permanent and caring relationships. By addressing the needs of people who have developmental disabilities, by shifting away from cumbersome formal and specialized services, we reduce the risk of separating people and services from the larger community of all individuals who need support. Resources need to support individuals, not programs. Supports need to become more generic. Generic resources serve all people and are not limited to categorical application that is decided by the presence or absence of disabling conditions.

New Decades, New Decisions, 1991

This chapter is a modified version of Racino, J. (1993a). *An Edited Collection on Community Integration and Deinstitutionalization in New Hampshire.* Syracuse, NY: Community and Policy Studies. See Appendix B for research methodology for Chapters 2 through 7.

In the past decade, the mental retardation field has moved from research, training, and service framed by the debate of institutional versus community life to ways of supporting people with disabilities to be fully involved in regular homes, jobs, leisure, and community (e.g., Bradley and Knoll, 1993; Taylor, Racino, and Walker, 1992; Towell, 1988; Wehman, 1993). However, on the level of state policy research, in-depth studies of state systems remain scant (Research and Training Center [RTC] on Community Integration, 1990). Although a few case systems studies exist (e.g., McWhorter, 1986), most state policy studies focus on specific service programs or funding mechanisms within or across states (e.g., Kennedy and Litvak, 1991) or comparative studies of facilities or other research framed by the least restrictive environment (LRE) model (e.g., Hill et al., 1989).

Deinstitutionalization has been a notable exception, with more in-depth studies exploring the richness of the individual's experiences (e.g., Edgerton, 1988). A number of these studies also conceptually describe the meaning of community integration in practice, though often interpreting the data within the context of existing frameworks such as Nirje's (1980) levels of integration.

Many policy studies are methodologically based on telephone interviews and survey forms (e.g., Braddock and Mitchell, 1992) or on relatively limited on-site observations, or they are designed for specific formative or summative evaluation purposes (e.g., Taylor et al., 1992; Racino et al., 1989). Such studies also are often intended to serve the "world of action that governs the organization, process, funding and regulation of services" (Bruininks, 1990, p. 14) and may offer links among research, service, and social movements and local, state, and national leadership (Menolascino and Stark, 1990).

Yet, relatively little in-depth applied knowledge exists from a qualitative research perspective about state practices in areas such as community integration and deinstitutionalization, with major implications for public policy.

RESEARCH METHODOLOGY

The first purpose of this policy research study was to identify and describe practices and strategies that states use to promote community integration and deinstitutionalization (Research and Training Center on Community Integration, 1990). The second purpose was to better understand the nature of systems change and its relationship to individual life quality.

The policy research study reflects a more in-depth and systematic version of state evaluation research studies (Racino et al., 1989; Taylor, Racino, and Rothenberg, 1988; Taylor et al., 1992; Taylor et al., 1987a), developed as part of a national technical assistance effort on community integration with thirty-five states in the United States.

The policy research methodology has an interdisciplinary focus that draws on the disciplines of political science, sociology, psychology, rehabilitation, and other applied disciplines (Majchrzak, 1984). This methodology builds upon a long history of qualitative research studies, particularly in the field of mental retardation and is directed toward solving applied problems in the field (Weiss, 1978). The study relies on on-site semistructured interviews and observations, with a multicase thematic study design (Yin, 1989).

NEW HAMPSHIRE: A BRIEF OVERVIEW

The state of New Hampshire was considered to be one of the most conservative states in the United States. Located on the northeastern seaboard, it had no state income tax or sales tax and a strong belief in local control with minimal governmental intervention. Concord North is agricultural and divided by the mountains, and Concord South was more densely populated and "high tech" and located near the Boston corridor.

The statistics on New Hampshire support its consistent effort over an extended period to shift focus from institutional to community living for people with developmental disabilities. Over the period of 1977 to 1988, New Hampshire moved from twenty-fifth place in community services spending among states to eighth, while institutional spending remained constant (University of Illinois, Chicago, 1991). By fiscal year 1990, the area agency community system spent $59 million and served 3,218 clients at an average cost of $18,400 (New Hampshire [NH] Office of the Legislative Budget Assistant, 1991).

The concept of moving away from service systems and back to communities was a politically conservative notion. So, although New Hampshire moved in a direction considered progressive in the disability field, the movement toward communities was consistent with the "grain of a place like New Hampshire." They indeed managed to accomplish a great deal with relatively little money.

BRIEF HISTORY OF THE NEW HAMPSHIRE
SERVICE SYSTEM

Twelve or thirteen years before the study, "there was no community service system to speak of in New Hampshire." In 1979, the "system" consisted primarily of a "collection of sheltered workshops and [other] things started by parent groups; that's all there was, not a whole lot," and "a couple of group homes." The earliest community services were started largely by parents who visited Laconia, the state institution, and were "devastated by what they thought was the warehousing of people." They banded together with other parents, found volunteers, renovated or leased buildings, and developed the first school programs. Some of these parents then formed local chapters of the Association for Retarded Citizens (ARC), later joining the state association.

The basic state law governing the developmental disabilities service system, RSA-171A, was written in 1975 and had not been substantially changed since, except for modifications in the definition of developmental disabilities. The legislation called for the establishment of an area agency (regional) system and also provided for individual assessments and evaluations, "all that kind of standard terminology that nobody could figure out in 1975, but we all were committed to." In the mid-1970s, federal special education law PL 94-142, with the advocacy of groups such as New Hampshire's Coalition for Handicapped Citizens, was passed and implemented in state policy translations. Even though the law focused on children from birth through age twenty-one, these principles translated to adults, helping to create a vision of what was possible. Later, in the 1990s, adult services would begin to give back to special education by offering the next vision of the future.

Led by the New Hampshire ARC, in 1978, a class action lawsuit *(Garrity v. Gallen;* see Chapter 3) was filed by the residents of Laconia. A public trial was followed by a court order in 1981. The lawsuit came about because "two parents faced each other and realized that things were bad and something had to be done." The parents enlisted the support of New Hampshire Legal Assistance, and the Department of Justice later joined the effort. The basic state plan, Action for Independence, was accepted by the court. The key people involved within the state office/planning council in writing the plan remained as part of the implementation process over the next decade. In the late 1970s, in addition to parent advocacy, organizations such as the state's Protection and Advocacy Office were formed. The Independent Guardianship Program, considered to be developed through a "model statute," was written and implemented.

The next decade was marked by "an increasing sophistication and refinement of the service system (see Figure 2.1), particularly in the way finances are handled, [and] how services get paid for." New Hampshire successfully accessed the Medicaid Home and Community-Based Services waiver program (PL 97-35) for community services starting in 1983.

FIGURE 2.1. State of New Hampshire Developmental Services System

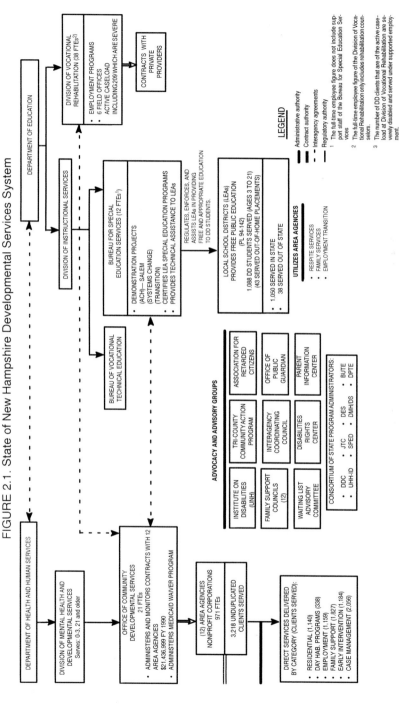

Source: New Hampshire Office of the Legislative Budget Assistant (1991, April). State of New Hampshire Developmental Service System Performance Audit. Concord, NH: Author, p. 11. Reprinted with permission.

In 1989, the concept of regional family support councils was established in New Hampshire Laws, Chapter 255 (RSA 126-G), following a report by a legislative task force on family support and grassroots organizing. These councils, one in each of the twelve regions, were a concrete representation of a beginning shift in the state to a new constituency base of families versus state institutional and community employees.

People with mental retardation, with assistance from organizations such as the state ARC and the New Hampshire Developmental Disabilities Council, formed People First of New Hampshire. In 1990, a statewide self-advocacy conference was held, and a contingent from New Hampshire traveled to the national conference in Tennessee. The Lakes Region self-advocacy group, which grew out of a previous state effort, was one of the earliest local groups, having been formed in the mid-1980s.

Laconia State School closed its doors on January 31, 1991, making New Hampshire the first state in the United States without a public institution for people with developmental disabilities. The closure itself was accomplished by people in a variety of sectors working together, including the Division of Mental Health and Developmental Services, the area agencies, the advocacy community, and staff from the institution itself. By the time it occurred, for all practical purposes, the area agency directors had the attitude that "nobody would go back to Laconia . . . and everybody would struggle with how to put things together so that didn't happen."

COMMUNITY INTEGRATION FINDINGS

The first set of findings describes state characteristics and major community integration practices and concerns. These are displayed in Tables 2.1, 2.2, and 2.3, respectively. Personal assistance services, of great concern to the independent-living movement (Litvak, Zukas, and Heumann, 1987), however, did not arise as a major service practice in this state. The second set of findings resulted in five thematic case studies on change within the state: the role of the courts in institutional closure, the management of the institutional closure, structural factors in community development (local agencies and Medicaid waivers), family support, and self-advocacy and guardianship. Four of these case studies are described in Chapters 3, 4, 5, and 6 of this book. A time line of major state developments (events) reported by the informants are in Figure 2.2.

The third set of findings, following the key leadership components of the system, is a brief analysis of comparative roles in the change process(es). The major roles were family leadership, external advocacy, progressive state and community leadership, roles of the media, and the role

TABLE 2.1. Critical New Hampshire Characteristics

Small Size

The state is small both geographically and in terms of population, with few people involved in the field. An informal talk network developed that made it easier to achieve agreement and to have both official and unofficial positions on issues, including controversial ones. People learned quickly who could be trusted; small efforts could have very large impacts, and the "best people" in the state could be brought together to personally address the most challenging situations.

Shared Values Base

Participants within the developmental disabilities system generally shared a common values base, and more emphasis was placed on the areas of agreement than on differences in degree, emphasis, kind, or position; the widespread belief existed that people were headed in the same direction.

State Leadership and Continuity

The continuity in key positions in sectors ranging from the advocacy community to the state administration had been extraordinary. Despite the small size, opportunities existed for people in all different sectors to play leadership roles, including at the state office, the university, the regions, family groups, advocacy organizations, and in the fledgling self-advocacy movement.

Reasonable Working Relationships

A highly significant factor was the degree of cross-collaboration that occurred over time. As an outsider familiar with many states shared, "The spirit of collegiality is extraordinary." Whether termed team, family, or collaborators, there was a real "solid group of people" who generally believed that one another "cares" and "wants to do better" even when things go wrong; this did not mean, of course, that "squabbles" or "battles" did not occur.

Commitment to Change

As the field changed, in New Hampshire, people tried to change too, not in the sense of following a fad, but of genuinely attempting to shift the system in that direction. They never became locked into one phase, remaining open to an interactive planning process of change.

Source: Racino, J. (1993a). *An Edited Collection on Community Integration and Deinstitutionalization in New Hampshire.* Syracuse, NY: Community and Policy Studies.

TABLE 2.2. Community Integration Practices

Family Support

In the early 1990s, family support represented the primary area of current energy and change. Probably more than anything else, the state division was trying to promote a family support attitude, that ownership of the system belongs to the families.

Supported Employment

New Hampshire's first individualization of programs in the 1980s, supported employment, was viewed as a demonstration of what people could do. Learning then transferred to other areas (e.g., community living), and responsibility was shifted to another state office.

Community Living and Homeownership

The University of New Hampshire has one of the Administration on Developmental Disabilities' A Home of Your Own Projects, which was in its very early development in 1991. Agency efforts existed to promote family and community connections and experiences with people with severe disabilities sharing apartments and homes.

Self-Advocacy

The ARC and Developmental Disabilities Council provided support for self-advocacy, including a 1990 statewide conference. New Hampshire People First was now formed.

Case Management

One area agency region was an early federal demonstration site for case management. Not all regions separated case management from the agency providing services.

Guardianship Program

The New Hampshire program has a number of characteristics that make it unique across the states. These include an independent versus a case management model of guardianship, use of a functional versus a medical definition of incapacity, and heavy reliance on limited instead of full guardianship.

Aging and Developmental Disability

In contrast to age integration, the division ascribed to the national movement of "cross-generational community participation of people of all ages." This meant that everyone lives and participates together, regardless of age, in community life, whether housing, recreation, or political life.

Source: Racino, J. (1993a). *An Edited Collection on Community Integration and Deinstitutionalization in New Hampshire.* Syracuse, NY: Community and Policy Studies.

TABLE 2.3. Community Integration Concerns

Eight major state issues and problems in community integration included long-standing issues (e.g., payment for education), those in which positive steps were being taken (e.g., children in out-of-home placements), and emerging ones (e.g., new population groups).

Educational System

Three areas of concern were funding education through local property taxes, especially in small towns; the need for better information on the educational rights of parents in this "entitlement" system, and more accessibility and relevance of adult education, including changes proposed in the Individuals with Disabilities Education Act (IDEA).

Supporting Children

The state had little experience with permanency planning, including foster care and adoption as components of a comprehensive system for supporting children to maintain permanent relationships with adults. New efforts in returning children home from expensive out-of-state placements were occurring.

The Waiting List

People were still not getting all of what they needed; some people were living at home without services, with elderly parents, or in the "back woods" depending on the kindness of other people in town. The waiting list issue was highlighted in the 1991 report of the New Hampshire Office of the Legislative Budget Assistant.

Community Transportation

Public transportation was not easily accessible, convenient, or even available for people, including those with disabilities who needed to rely on it to participate in community life.

Institutional Concerns

Although very little transinstitutionalization (i.e., movement to other institutions) had taken place, ideological compromises occurred (e.g., a new intermediate care facility). A private institution still was operating in the state; a few people were living in county or state homes for elders, hospitals, and age-inappropriate situations.

Restructuring Community Services

New Hampshire was examining ways to move from facility-based services toward supported employment and was also "breaking down the group homes." However, it was difficult to "keep going what you have, develop what is new, and then move to the new" without additional resources.

Housing

Reportedly, generic housing resources and subsidized financing were both underutilized. As of 1992, 60 of 125 properties funded by the division were owned by area agencies and mostly financed by banks at commercial lending rates.

Family Support and Part H

Family support, as reflected in federal Public Law 99-457, the Early Intervention Program for Toddlers and Infants with Handicaps, was described as tending to be service oriented, deficit based, professionally controlled, and based on a developmental framework. This contrasted with the intent of New Hampshire's early family support, which focused on support to participate in neighborhoods and communities.

New Population Groups

Particularly in the area of family support, people were reflecting on ways to address the needs of new population groups, including people with head injuries and significant emotional needs, especially during a time of scarce resources. As one state official said:

"What we really have to be about here is not a human service social system, but really changing how society, in general, responds to its people. . . . And that's got to be for everybody. It can't just be for 'DD' folks."

Source: Racino, J. (1993a). *An Edited Collection on Community Integration and Deinstitutionalization in New Hampshire.* Syracuse, NY: Community and Policy Studies.

of litigation and legislation/legislature in the change process. The final set presents diverse perspectives on change as one unified theoretical framework: change as an evolutionary process, critical turning points for change, the roles of new ideas, personal values, values-based training, personal relationships and systems, systems structure and change, and society and change.

KEY LEADERSHIP COMPONENTS IN NEW HAMPSHIRE

As background for a discussion of comparative roles in the change process, the following sections briefly highlight the key leadership components in the developmental disabilities system in the state of New Hampshire.

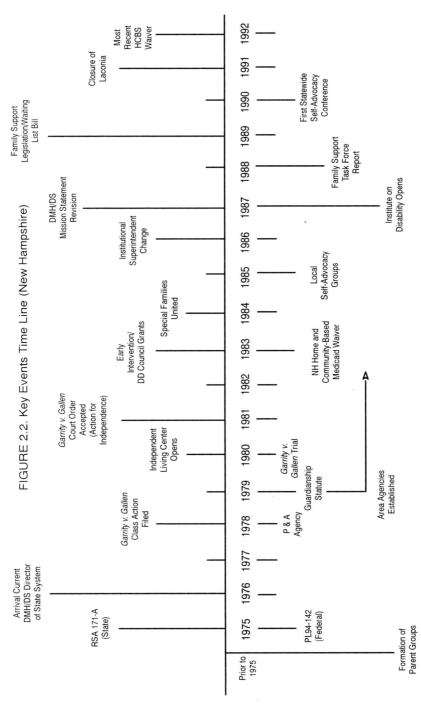

FIGURE 2.2. Key Events Time Line (New Hampshire)

Source: Racino, J. (1993a). *An Edited Collection on Community Integration and Deinstitutionalization in New Hampshire.* Syracuse, NY: Community and Policy Studies.

41

Division of Mental Health and Developmental Services

The Division of Mental Health and Developmental Services (DMH/DS) was statutorily responsible for a comprehensive service delivery system for people with developmental disabilities in the state. It developed and managed the system through contracts with twelve regional, private, nonprofit organizations and maintained communication with the legislature, governor, area agencies, communities, and families.

Family Leadership

In addition to the Association for Retarded Citizens, other family groups, such as Special Families United, have come into existence for periods of time. A family leadership series, sponsored by the Institute on Disability, University of New Hampshire, brought together diverse families. The family support task force led to the state's family support legislation and family support councils, for which families were playing new leadership roles. Table 2.4 highlights the principles underlying the family support legislation.

Area Agencies

The state's twelve area agencies may provide services directly or contract with vendors for services such as case management, residential, employment, habilitation, and family support. They were the primary recipients of state funds and responsible for an internal program of quality assurance. The New Hampshire system cannot be understood without knowledge of how these area agencies work.

Institute on Disability

The Institute on Disability, also the university-affiliated program (UAP) at the University of New Hampshire, was created by the leadership in the state in the late 1980s. The functions of the UAP included bringing additional resources into the state, leveraging change as an outside catalyst and conscience, serving as a training resource, and pushing systems, especially the educational system, in positive directions.

Advocacy Organizations

A functional system of external advocacy existed in New Hampshire, with long-term leadership positions in such agencies as the Protection and

TABLE 2.4. Family Support Legislation—1989 Laws of New Hampshire (Chapter 255)

Statement of Purpose:

The general court, in recognition of the findings of the New Hampshire legislative task force to study family support needs, accepts the following principles relative to supporting families who have children with disabilities:

(a) All children, regardless of disability, belong with families.
(b) Families must receive the support necessary to care for their children at home.
(c) Family support must focus on the entire family.
(d) Family support must be sensitive to the unique needs and strengths of individual families.
(e) Family support must build on existing social networks and natural sources of support.
(f) Families must have access to appropriate services to meet their needs.
(g) Family support is needed throughout the life span of the individual who is disabled.
(h) Family support must encourage the integration of people with disabilities into the community.

Approved May 26, 1989
Effective July 1, 1989

Source: State of New Hampshire (1989a). *Family Support Legislation—1989 Laws of New Hampshire,* Chapter 255.

Advocacy Organization and the Office of the Public Guardian. Other catalysts for change included the Developmental Disabilities Council, the Disability Rights Center, and the Alliance for Values-Based Training.

Institutional Leadership

The superintendent who started at the institution in 1985 was "brave" and spoke out against the institutional conditions. The second superintendent, arriving in the mid-1980s, was credited with transforming the values base in the institution, an action which played a pivotal role in Laconia's closure. The union and staff within worked toward closure, and the institutional parent group, a branch of the ARC, continued in the community as a watchful safeguard.

Legislature

The state legislature was distinct in being one of the "largest legislative bodies in the world," with "400 people in the House and 24 Senators." This meant that almost everyone personally knew a legislator and could even themselves end up becoming one someday.

COMPARATIVE ROLES IN THE CHANGE PROCESS

This section highlights strategies for change by role and function, based upon experiences within the state. These include grassroots organizing by families, external advocacy, progressive leadership, the media as a consciousness raiser, litigation as external pressure, legislation and policy as setting expectations, and the shifting power base for community services.

Family Leadership: Traditional Grassroots Organizing

The passage of the family support legislation and the actions surrounding it were "pretty traditional organizing," that worked. What was notable was that it was done well (people "stuck together"), at the "right" time (paired waiting list and family support legislation), with the "right" people (including new families and people inside the system), and with broad-based support for the desired outcomes. The strategies used (e.g., inviting legislators to meet your child; thematic balloons) were aimed at personalizing the issues and keeping people involved, while doing a "professional job."

External Advocates: "Keeping Things Honest and on Track"

External advocacy by parents was critical to the start of a massive systems change involving consciousness raising, the development of the community services system, and changes within the institution. It was insufficient, however, in itself, for the development of the community system or for the closure of the institution, which required "committed" allies from within. External advocacy roles were achieving a built-in tension that kept "things honest and on track," challenging complacency with what existed, and serving as safeguards to keep the "floodgates from opening on something that's terrible."

State and Community Administrators: Progressive Leadership

State and local leadership ("the most progressive state agency and . . . by and large, very progressive community directors") played a critical role in the change processes. The state leadership developed, influenced, and shaped policy and managed the system. Essential functions beyond a management view of their roles included keeping a consistent message out in the field, supporting choice and experimentation, spending time with people who were doing the work, supporting and working with community leaders, effectively solving problems, and helping move people along toward "real system change."

Media: "Consciousness Raiser"

The media in New Hampshire, particularly its coverage surrounding the *Garrity v. Gallen* court order and exposé, played the role of "consciousness raiser" and "muckraker." The original stories were "a masterpiece unveiling of what the story was, what the issues were and what could be," which set the stage for an editorial position for the newspapers and media that was very supportive of the change from institutional to community life. The major perceived role of media was to "be a force to help us pinpoint really negative things."

Litigation: External Pressure to "Do the Right Thing"

Litigation provided the external pressure necessary to obtain resources to make changes that the bureaucrats wanted to do, but were unable to; it was a consciousness-raising tool, highlighting serious problems that existed and potential solutions, it led to legislation and other policy, and it clarified and strengthened the values of those who participated in the litigation process, particularly as witnesses. The institutional litigation was considered absolutely essential to Laconia's closure and a "catalyst" to the evolution of the community system, remaining an active force for over a decade.

Legislation and Policy: Baselines and Expectations

The three most important legislative/policy pieces in New Hampshire that proved historically significant were state law RSA-171A, which established the developmental disabilities services system ("stood the test of time"), the state's special education law ("gave people hope and excitement," provided for due process, and was the clearest embodiment of civil rights that set an "expectation baseline" for community development and deinstitutionalization), and Action for Independence, the major planning document that embodied the planning concepts of the federal Developmental Disabilities Act. Policies that simply emanated from the state office without tangible discussion at all levels throughout the state of New Hampshire were viewed as often leading to dissension and becoming a barrier to change.

Legislature and Shifting Power Base: The Future Power Balances

One of the major changes identified as critical to the future was the initial shifting power base in relationship to the legislature and, consequently, to the state office. The traditional power base of an administrator was the size of the budget and the number of buildings and employees, which translated into influence with the legislature and budget. This meant that the state's "customers" were state employees or agencies, while the new power base was "the families," with families and family support changing from innovations to business. This shift represented a new balance of power that has yet to be fully achieved.

PERSPECTIVES ON CHANGE

Change As an Evolutionary Process

> Systems change, real systems change, takes a long time. It is not an overnight thing. If you are going to hire somebody and say, "We are going to turn this thing around in three years," it can't happen. It won't happen.

Community integration was not viewed as a product or goal to be achieved, but as an evolutionary change process ("I think that state and area agency people must understand that change is part of the process, that you are never done.") The complexity of making changes on the community and person levels in "real life" meant that a long process was necessary for "real" systems change.

Critical Turning Points in the Change Process

> We got a commitment to, and a trust of, a more integrative life in the service system. And again, there were certain individuals who really

made that happen, who really saw it, really felt how it could be. . . . We had come along far enough that we could take the flight of imagination and belief that was required in really seeing what a person's life could be. Things were approximating it enough so we could start moving toward it.

The change process had critical events or turning points, some, such as the *Garrity v. Gallen* court order, had high public visibility, and others reflected a visible shift in ways of thinking and believing on the part of a group of people. This latter shift involved not only changes in structures, systems, or places but a change in the nebulous qualities of human beings, such as trust and commitment. A few people (visionaries, leaders) saw, felt, and knew the possibilities and "made it happen." Enough concrete changes took place (e.g., jobs) so that a new picture of community life could be viewed and experienced as "real."

The Role of New Ideas in the Change Process

Real organizational and systems change . . . is setting up an environment where people change over time, change their attitudes, and change the way they do things.

The guided change process came about, in part, through the infusion of new ideas and concepts, their constant repetition in diverse ways, and the real-world attempts to implement these ideas in practice. The process brought in people from around the country to help people to get excited, raise their expectations, and become energized enough to try to make the changes. Some people gradually shifted as the vision became more of the norm or the general expectation. This occurred in an environmental context that created opportunities and supported the people who were really interested in being leaders (i.e., "the experimenters").

The Role of Personal Values in the Change Process

We are all human. . . . What do you do if you are an area agency director, in (your) late forties or fifties, been there for eight or nine years, it's pretty comfortable, salary's good, you get along pretty well, but now you need to restructure? And you begin to look at it, and if you are honest at all, you see there are things I have to do to undermine the empire, and can people do that? It is hard.

Part of how systemic changes came about was that people viewed themselves and others in new ways and came to believe in themselves and in new possibilities for the future. Personal beliefs represented the basis for all the daily decision making, which influenced a person's experiences as a service user. Yet, it was also difficult for people (e.g., leaders, directors) to take apart what they had previously created.

The Role of Values-Based Training

> It was the largest group that I have ever seen of people in one place. It was a critical mass of people who had heard this stuff. And quite a strong group of people . . . kind of emerged from the institution.

Values-based training was viewed as integral to the systems change process, including the institutional closure ("it was a critical mass of people who had heard the stuff"). In this research, values-based training helped people to "get off of the academic mark," to start acting and then to reflect critically on the meaning of their actions. The hope was that people could get past their fear of failure and desire for perfection. A subculture also existed which grew out of PASS (Program Analysis of Service Systems) (Wolfensberger and Glenn, 1975) and personal commitments and which performed effective and important work that the formal organizations did not always view as valid.

The Role of Personal Relationships and Systems

> And if you are going to change a system, you convince . . . one staff member this is a good idea. You do something on behalf of one person with disabilities. . . . We have to recognize the power of small change as very significant compared to large change strategy.

Personal relationships were viewed as either facilitating "good things" to occur for people with disabilities or standing in the way. One of the hidden factors in the final closure of Laconia was that the institutional superintendent and the state community services leader "played" in different arenas. Sometimes changes occurred through the avenue of personal relationships with people with disabilities (e.g., "there is no substitute for relationships with people with disabilities") partially because systems themselves were so complex and unwieldy.

Systems Structures and Change

> I think systems can set a direction, set the tone, and set up parameters to facilitate individual movement, but systems themselves don't do anything.

Five areas related to the nature of systems structures and change were the limitations of systems, thereby increasing the importance of individual actions; the increasingly outdated nature of traditional systems planning processes; the tendency to assume that state and federal policy and visible structural changes necessarily lead to better individual life quality; the tendency of professionals to become "enamored with concepts" without really knowing what was going on at the client level; and the need to move from a Band-Aid approach to systems change ("white knights") to new approaches based upon a better understanding of the experiences of people with disabilities and their families.

Society and Change

> The pessimist, in terms of society, would say that society always needs a certain kind of underbelly, whether we devalue mentally retarded people, poor people, or people who have blue eyes.

Within this framework, change in the lives of people with disabilities in communities was viewed as meaning that society must also evolve. This evolution would require very different ways of interacting with people in communities than the typical ways staff were used to, and a recognition that neighbors, co-workers, and industry may actually have more capacity to accommodate differences than people within human service systems believe. It would involve changes in U.S. social policy, which continues to have an underlying punishment perspective, and changing the social forces affecting people's lives, instead of focusing solely on programmatic structures.

A LOOK TOWARD THE FUTURE

Today, New Hampshire is facing new issues, since the major motivating force of movement from the institution to the community has now to a large extent been achieved. As discussed in this book's opening epigraph which explained the mission:

> We'll know when we've been successful when there is evidence that people with disabilities are participating in their community, working at meaningful jobs, involved in integrated employment situations, and enjoying the simple opportunities for life and recreation the rest of the world take for granted.

New Decade, New Decisions, 1991

While numerous areas exist for further study, the following represent several emerging themes to explore.

Informal Talk Networks and Working Relationships

Since systems change may be tied with the individual or person level of change, a more in-depth investigation of relationship patterns and how they "work" may be beneficial to the field. This study suggests that many changes are on the horizon; practitioners of this decade will be in the role of making challenging decisions that will call not only on their professional skills but on their personal and interpersonal strengths.

Grassroots Coalitions/Shifting Power Base

This appears to be a major mechanism for substantive societal change and an in-depth investigation of the patterns and effects in the disability field may be useful. How, and if, such realignments occur can affect the nature of the relationship between service users and agencies in the decades to come.

Patterns of Shifting Practices

The patterns and processes of shifting practices in the field are worthy of further study both from the perspective of causative factors and of the relationship of the shifts in emphases (e.g., from employment to family support to homeownership). In particular, there is a need to pursue how and why these changes come about, including their ties with financing, lead agency, technical assistance, and philosophical changes in the field.

The Role of New Ideas

It is unclear how new ideas come to the attention of people in the field, including policymakers, and how they also fade from view. Understanding these dynamics is critical to long-term, fundamental changes versus surface or transient changes. This area also holds important implications for the replication framework currently predominant in the disability field, suggesting instead an evolutionary approach to change.

Leadership

Although leadership has been an area of intensive study, many aspects of it are still not well understood. In particular, the nonhierarchical roles of individual people, the ways in which women and those from diverse multicultural backgrounds lead, and the fusion of personal and professional strengths need to be better explored and articulated.

How Systems Work

Probably the most important aspect of this study is to explain "how systems work," not only as presented by those in control of these systems, but also from diverse viewpoints. This can provide the information to help people better understand how to work together in the transition to the next generation of community life. It can also assist in identifying specific target areas for change, such as "ossification" of service systems, and critical areas for skills development, such as administrative skills in "dismantling" what exists.

Interrelationship of Categorical Groups

There are indicators in this first study about the importance of enlarging the research scope to include cross-population research, inclusive of people with head injuries, elders, and those involved with the mental health systems. Issues for competition for resources and implications for cross-systems reorganization are critical areas for further examination.

CONCLUSION

The upcoming decade may call for new ways of working together—parents, people with disabilities, community members, policymakers, researchers, business and community leaders—to achieve change, which may involve changes in communities, not simply in human services.

It was an exciting time to be an observer in New Hampshire, to capture the feelings of accomplishment, but even more important, to consider the questions about what the future might hold. Here, one sees glimpses of what might come to pass as people begin to reflect on new definitions of community life, new roles for agencies and family support councils, a new vision of what is possible, and the changing constituencies and alliances that will carry the spirit of the next generation.

Chapter 3

Garrity v. Gallen:
The Role of the Courts
in Institutional Closure

Julie Ann Racino

INTRODUCTION

When he was about ten and a half or eleven, we made the decision
for the Laconia State School. . . . So with our backs against the wall,
we took him up there. That was one day that neither of us ever
recovered from; it was without question the worst day of our lives. . . .
It was just a horrible experience, and it took quite a while to get over
it so we could even talk about it.

He took a lot of abuse up there, as did some of the others who
would not defend themselves. Sam was kicked in the testicles so
much that he was herniated from it, and that had to be repaired
surgically after a few years. And they would find him unconscious.

We were always searching for something better for him. But if we
thought we found a place, either it wasn't what we expected or we
couldn't afford it because this kind of care can become pretty expensive if you are footing the bill. . . . And we just didn't have those
resources so we had to stay with the state of New Hampshire and the
Laconia State School.

We came to feel a certain sense of security there, feeling it was a
state-operated institution. So as long as the state was functioning,

This chapter is a modified version of Racino, J. (1993a). *"Garrity v. Gallen:* The
Role of the Courts in Institutional Closure." In *An Edited Collection on Community
Integration and Deinstitutionalization in New Hampshire.* Syracuse, NY: Commu-
nity and Policy Studies.

why there'd be a place for our children; plus there was nothing else anyway. . . . Many parents, including ourselves, then resisted their children leaving the state facility because of the stability and security, even though there were many things that weren't right and were unpleasant.

Everyone has been out of Laconia now for a year. . . . [The region] promised us great things, but we have been promised great things many times, but nothing ever happened. So we took it all with a grain of salt. . . . They have done everything they said they would do. And if we can find anything to ask for, which isn't much, they are right on it.

It just worked out; it's [as if] just something we could even never dream of just happened. A few years ago we couldn't have even imagined Sam in this situation, but thank goodness it happened. . . . He is living like you and I live or anybody else, in a home. And he has recreation and activities and cleanliness and he is not being beat up on and kicked every day. It is a normal form of the way a person should live. And he is able to experience that now, when for a long time he couldn't . . . so he has had to learn a whole new lifestyle. . . . It takes a long time to relax and not be on guard for twenty-four hours a day.

Sam's father and institutional parent group leader, 1991

In January 1991, New Hampshire became the first state in the United States without a public institution for people with developmental disabilities. This chapter highlights some of the key features of the early litigation, including the national battle, led by leaders of the Association of Persons with Severe Handicaps, between two different philosophies about how people with disabilities would live over the next decade. Though the role of the courts has changed markedly through the years, this research is relevant as new conflicting philosophies emerge about *who will determine how people with disabilities will live their lives?*

BRIEF HISTORY

In 1977, the Pennhurst case was considered to be the first "frontal assault on an institution seeking community relief"* in the United States.

---

*All quotations in this chapter are from the reseach case study on *Garrity v. Gallen;* for methodology, see Appendix B.

Based on findings of federal and constitutional violations, Judge Broderick issued an order in March 1978 requiring community placements and services for the class of about 1,200 people at the Pennhurst state institution in Pennsylvania (see Figure 3.1).

Meanwhile, New Hampshire Legal Assistance was approached by the New Hampshire State Association for Retarded Citizens (ARC) to "file a lawsuit" regarding Laconia, the state's only public institution for people with developmental disabilities, because of the horrendous conditions and the growing feeling that there was a "dumping of people in inappropriate placements." New Hampshire Legal Assistance was reluctant to take on the case, having just completed extensive prison litigation.

In September 1977, New Hampshire Legal Assistance held its first major retreat, inviting their clients, staff, the director, and others representing their cross-disability constituencies to determine what the priorities would be for their legal assistance. The Executive Director of the ARC and the State ARC President were the two key outsiders there. Largely through their advocacy efforts, the decision that Laconia should be the priority was agreed to unanimously, including by AFDC (Aid for Dependent Children) clients, because the conditions were so very bad.

In April 1978, the Laconia complaint was filed, making it the first federal institutional lawsuit after Pennhurst. That filing was significant because the lawyers were able to use "the claims very specifically modeled after Pennhurst." The interaction between Pennhurst and Laconia included overlap in witnesses and experts, the role of the Justice Department, and specific references to court orders and opinions between the cases.

The period of litigation between 1978 and 1981 was very antagonistic, the whole discovery process being "very hard ball" with "depositions and interrogations and expert witnesses by the busload, truckloads of paper." The public trial lasted from April 1980 through June 1980, making it "the longest civil trial in New Hampshire history."

The decision from the federal district court judge came in August 1981. While he did not order community placements, he found that people had a right to habilitation. He also found that discrimination had occurred against people with the most severe handicaps. The findings on special education and on the ability of people with significant disabilities to learn and benefit from the right kind of setting were also significant.

The state was ordered to produce an implementation plan by November 1981. The implementation plan was the window of opportunity taken by state planners who "developed" four plans: A, B, C, and D, with plan C masterfully designed as the right choice. Plan C called for significant

FIGURE 3.1. New Hampshire Closes Its State Institution: Leadership in the United States

NH Mental Health System Leads U.S.

State to Be First to Close Institution for Retarded

By JOHN DiSTASO
Union Leader Staff

CONCORD—Even while bracing for a 1991 budget battle in economically difficult times, the state director of services for the mentally retarded is quietly leading a celebration of another New Hampshire "first-in-the-nation" event.

Within the next two weeks, New Hampshire will become the nation's first state to close its institution for the mentally retarded and operate its treatment program entirely through community-based residential and workshop programs.

The move comes 10 years after a huge legal battle over the Laconia State School and Training Center, in which the facility was portrayed as a glorified warehouse whose residents were often restrained physically and deprived emotionally while being mentally unchallenged and unstimulated.

In 1981, a federal judge ordered the system overhauled.

The Laconia State School housed about 1,000 in the early 1970s. When the federal class action lawsuit was tried in the spring and summer of 1980, the population was about 700. Today, there is no state school to speak of.

In its place is a statewide system of group homes, including one on the Laconia site housing about a dozen today and only six by year-end. Last week, plans were unveiled for the future of the 400-acre tract. They included a new minimium-medium security state prison, a state park and social service programs.

Donald Shumway, the director of the Division of Mental Health and Developmental Services, says it is a true success story written by the experts in his division, lawmakers and governors, advocates, parents, the clients themselves, and a state which has, in general, become much more accepting of the developmentally disabled than it was 10 years ago.

A leading expert in the field, Dr. David Braddock, director of the Institute for the Study of Developmental Disabilities at the University of Chicago, told state officials, advocates and students at a UNH

LACONIA STATE SCHOOL, Page 5

LACONIA STATE SCHOOL
(Continued from Page 1)

seminar last month that the progress the state has made in treating the retarded was "truly remarkable," an example for other states.

Shumway said treatment of the mentally retarded has been an issue that for the most part has stayed above the political fray. While advocates for the mentally retarded are often stereotyped as liberals, in New Hampshire, Shumway noted, conservative lawmakers and governors turned out to be advocates, too.

"Our policies were put in place by Republican governors and Republican Legislatures, and we have the best developmental disabilities system in the nation," he said. "I don't believe it's a partisan issue. It's an economic issue."

But with the state facing budget shortfalls, Shumway said he knows the Legislature "is going to be challenged" in the 1991 session, and necessary programs will compete for some of the same budget dollars.

But deinstitutionalization has been shown to have economic benefits while being the morally right thing to do, according to the director.

"I take a retarded person out of a $90,000-a-year program, which is what Laconia cost the taxpayer per person served, and place them into a community program which costs $40,000 a year. But because the person is now in the community, he often will be employed, perhaps at a part-time job, bring in $8,000 a year and pay taxes. That is incredibly productive outcome for the state, especially compared to the past."

Shumway said about 1,000 people are in state-run community residential services at a cost of $37 million during fiscal 1991. He said it would cost about $90 million to treat them at an institution. In all, 3,100 people are served by the state, more than 2,000 of them living in their own homes, on their own or with their families.

The endeavor has not been inexpensive, although Shumway says that adjusted for inflation and taking into account the growth in population, the per-patient cost has actually gone down as the population of the state school has decreased.

In fiscal 1977, the total budget for mental retardation was $9.2 million, more than two-thirds of which was designated for the institution. By 1981, the cost was $18.2 million, two-thirds of it still for Laconia, with nearly 700 people in the institution and fewer than 300 in community programs.

In 1983, with about 1,000 people in the system, half were at the state school and half in the community, with the total budget $32 million. All but about $5 million was state money.

By 1988, with a total budget of $62 million, there were about 900 people in community programs and about 100 at the state school. Of that budget, about $40 million was state money and $22 million was federal, most of it obtained through waivers granted for Medicaid funds designated for the institution.

Shumway said that obtaining those funds requires a special technique at which New Hampshire officials have become more adept than their counterparts in other states.

Shumway has requested $52 million and $55.3 million in state money for fiscal 1992 and 1993, respectively. For the first time, all of it is designated for community services. The Laconia line item is zero.

Ten years ago, only the most optimistic advocates envisioned a system without a Laconia State School. A deinstitutionalization plan drawn up by the state in the late 1970s under the threat of the lawsuit envisoned a permanent facility for about 50 of the most severely retarded and medically handicapped clients.

John MacIntosh, a Concord lawyer who as a staffer with New Hampshire Legal Assistance led the plaintiffs' legal team, said that as it turned out, "The most severely medically involved people are all out. It was an evolution. The state and the parents gained confidence in the quality of the placements, and as it went on, those with the most challenging behavioral prob-

lem and medical conditions seemed to do better out of the institution than in and in some cases better than less involved people."

In 1981, U.S. District Court Judge Shane Devine ordered the state to place each Laconia State School resident in the least restrictive environment possible based on each person's individual needs. He did not order the institution closed, recognizing that for some retarded people, perhaps the institution would be the least restrictive environment possible.

The advocates claimed victory, but so did state officials, who argued that the judge had done nothing more than order them to implement their own plan.

Source: DiStaso, J. (1990). "NH Mental Health System Leads U.S." *The Union Leader,* December 17, pp. 1, 5.

community placements and the building up of all important community infrastructure. Some of the people who wrote or contributed to the plan continued with implementation through the time of the institutional closure in 1991.

The judge's decision was "Solomon-like," with everyone winning. The state was ordered to plan, which is its role, and was given federal court support to develop the community services system. The plaintiffs won their lawsuit, and the state was to implement or deliver on what the plaintiffs had asked for. In many views, the judge came up with "just the right thing."

From the administration viewpoint, the court order had three foci: institutional improvement, developing community service options within available resources, and making special education responsive to youngsters with severe disabilities. By 1985, the community placements of approximately 225 were done and the basic institutional improvements were made.

After the decision, the state reported monthly to the court to accomplish the order. This method, versus the use of a court monitor, was viewed as key by state officials for the flexibility required to adjust to changing practices within the disability field.

By the mid-1980s, placements had slowed down as community agencies became more involved in local issues and legal handles (i.e., possible legal actions) for community placements had eroded. In 1986, the institutional superintendent changed, and a sustained effort from within the institution contributed, in part, to its closure in January 1991. The court order was still active in 1992.

The litigation is almost universally recognized within the New Hampshire disability field as an absolutely necessary condition for the institutional closure and the development of the community services system. Unlike most litigation, there were also very few negative impacts of the legal actions with tremendous benefits ranging from public education to financial support for the development of community services.

KEY FACTORS CONTRIBUTING TO POSITIVE OUTCOMES

This section of the case study describes a number of the significant factors surrounding this litigation that contributed to its positive outcomes.

Poor Institutional Conditions

One of the key factors was that the institutional conditions were "horrendous." As with other institutions in the country, Laconia had become very overcrowded; at the same time, the governor was making staff cut-backs. At Laconia, about half the buildings were certified as intermediate care facilities (ICF/MR) and half were not, although the certified ones were described as "only a bit better." The Powell building, which housed "presumably the most severely involved" was remembered as the worst. In the Powell building, each ward had a sleeping area of forty by fifty feet with maybe thirty beds lined next to each other, a day room of fifteen by twenty-five feet with benches around the perimeter, and mass bathrooms where people were hosed down. One lawyer described the conditions as follows:

> People were enclosed, sticking their heads into toilets, the smell of feces and food and vomit mixed together in an environment that was not ventilated sufficiently and staff overwhelmed and demoralized by the experience. . . . The eating situations . . . were a circus type of affair. People being fed; folks who had more skills stealing from those who were less skillful. People who were at the institution presumably for residential purposes assisting people with more se-vere disabilities because the staff weren't available in sufficient numbers to do that. It was a deplorable thing.

The building closed in June 1978, two months after the lawsuit was filed. However, people were moved into other older buildings that then became "equally inhumane because it created an even more overcrowded situation." Between 1975 and 1978, the institutional superintendent re-portedly had done a good job of reducing the use of seclusion and re-straints, so there were not as many shock treatments, papoose boards, or ten-point restraints visible. Over 40 percent of the residents at the time of filing, however, were on some form of psychotropic medications.

A Clean Slate: No Community Services

One way to view the New Hampshire community services system at the time of filing the complaint was as a "clean slate" with "very little, good or bad, that was occurring in the community." No community services existed in New Hampshire, except for several group homes for people with mild handicaps and scattered sheltered workshops or day habilitation sites. Community services were still young nationwide; Eastern Nebraska Community Office of Retardation (ENCOR), (see Taylor et al., 1986) a regional system in eastern Nebraska, and Macomb-Oakland, Michigan, were all "doing part, but not complete, systems of community services." New Hampshire's neighboring states of Maine and Vermont would have been considered considerably ahead of New Hampshire in terms of community development. No regional structures (i.e., area agencies; see figure 6.1) existed in New Hampshire, only Laconia, the state institution. The community services budget "hovered around the $250,000 figure." Although the developmental disabilities legislation, RSA-171A, was "on the books for two to three years, it had not been funded."

"Timing is Everything"

The Laconia agreement slipped through during the proverbial window of opportunity, just as the litigation victories were beginning to turn against community placements. The Pennhurst orders had been very favorable toward community placements, but they were being overturned by the Supreme Court. Because the legal context was uncertain, the state of New Hampshire was hesitant to take a "strident stand." Yet others said, "Unlike a half dozen other suits filed around the country at that time, Laconia was one of the few that carried through the trial, to an order, and through implementation."

Significant Legal Features: Nondiscrimination Against People with Severe Handicaps

The New Hampshire case was modeled on Pennhurst, which has as its most significant feature the direct claim of the right to community services derived from the Constitution, Section 504 of the Rehabilitation Act, and state law. The essential constitutional theory was that based on the Fourteenth Amendment, *as a matter of due process, one should not be confined to an institution or restrictive setting if there are less restrictive alternatives available.*

From the viewpoint of counsel for the plaintiffs, the basic case had aimed at three points: indicating what a terrible place Laconia was, showing the potential of a person with mental retardation, and demonstrating that no matter what the person's potential, he or she could live in a community setting. One of the plaintiffs' lawyers described the state of the art as follows:

> There were good examples that (Marc) Gold [1980] would refer to in terms of persons with the most extraordinary disabilities, assembling parts at NASA. And (there were) inclusive education programs, though we didn't call them that at the time, in Madison (Wisconsin) and other places, but none of it in any kind of coherent singular location.

The defense was threefold: First, it doesn't make any sense to court-order x, y, or z when there is so much disagreement in the field. Second, all these community programs are not really what they are cracked up to be. Third, the state had made improvements in the institution (though they didn't defend the institution itself) and was planning to move in that direction anyway (the plan called Action for Independence). The plaintiffs' lawyers agreed that the state had some potentially good arguments, he explained:

> The state could effectively say that what the plaintiffs have pointed to are isolated examples of where people with extraordinary commitment and values have made it succeed, but that is neither the pattern or what represents the mainstream of professional judgment.

The ultimate battle was fought over people with medical and behavioral needs. As one attorney explained, "The state knew it had an indefensible case, though they perceived our view to be arrogant. They said they would develop community services for some, but not all of the people. . . . The irony is that the people who are the easiest to move and the safest to move are the people with medical needs. If you've survived an institution, you are probably pretty hardy."

A major strategy used by counsel for the plaintiffs was to "have the state identify people whom they thought needed an institution and we found a *developmental twin* in the community. We found surprising, but isolated, pockets of wonderful school efforts in New Hampshire where there were both cultural and geographical reasons why they did not want kids sent down to the institution. Keene (one of the regions) also had developed some different alternatives for individuals."

In a very important finding, the federal district court judge concluded that *it was not all right to discriminate between those with or without severe handicaps*. He basically said that the state could not provide a different quality or set of services based upon severity of disability. The state was required to address the problems of those who were the most severely handicapped. New Hampshire was important in a legal sense nationally in convincing the courts that community placements were beneficial.

The Class of Plaintiffs

The six complainants represented a spectrum of disabilities at Laconia as well as with the state Association of Retarded Citizens. As one observer explained, "Compared to some other states, the plaintiffs were a group of families who were really very unhappy with Laconia." The class itself was "fairly loosely circumscribed in the court order." The vagueness was of benefit to those who support community living because the class could be interpreted to be defined as "all those who had been institutionalized and all those who would be in danger of being institutionalized." Operationally, the class was defined not only as the 620 to 640 people living at Laconia, but also those who were at risk of going in or who were on "unconditional discharge status" for a total combined class of about 750.

Public Nature of Trial: The Role of the Media

The fact that a visible, public trial took place instead of a consent decree had an enormous impact on the future development of community services in the state; it was a milestone process. As one lawyer expressed, "There's nothing like a trial to educate the judge and the public about what is going on." Articles appeared virtually daily in the newspaper during the lengthy trial in part because of the potential cost to taxpayers. Before the trial, the press concentrated on the institutional conditions and on the settlement. As the plaintiffs' lawyers explained:

> At the time, this attracted enormous media attention. If the plaintiffs win, it will cost $150 million in income tax. We were beaten up for two and a half years by the conservative press for being undemocratic and by the liberal press for the strident position on closure. Twelve weeks of trials changed people's attitudes. You could see it in the editorials. *The Union Leader* said, "We (the community) have done wrong. We need to do the right thing." The stories were so horrible.

In particular, an intuitive cub reporter from *The Union Leader,* the only statewide newspaper in New Hampshire, was in court almost every day and ultimately influenced the reporting that occurred. He was a "high quality professional" who "had incredible talent and did some superlative reporting." As a state official expressed:

> We lucked out, had some very great reporters. . . . [They] did some reporting that was superlative and challenged the editorial views of their own editors. [This then] . . . became a masterpiece of unveiling of what the story was, what the issues were, and what could be. And then set the stage for an editorial position for the newspapers and media that became very supportive of change.

Outside Experts

Because New Hampshire was a small state, the outside experts were
able to "really deluge the state." As one TASH expert noted, "We were
young enough to just constantly say that the state of the art was the only
way to go." Aided by the visibility of the public trial and the relatively
"clean slate" in the community, an important philosophical and practical
base was at stake for the future development of the service system. The
trial clearly showcased for a long time two distinctly different philosophies of how to view people with disabilities. As one professional described these developments:

> those (two philosophies) were probably best represented by TASH
> (the Association of Persons with Severe Handicaps) (which sup-
> ported community services) . . . and others. . . . who were of another
> era . . . who felt that without any experience to back this up, that
> there were those who were so neurologically involved, so complex .
> . . so behaviorally damaged that they could never leave the institu-
> tion or would die.

This was one of the first times that one of the TASH founders, a noted
figure in the field of special education (Lou Brown, e.g., Brown et al.,
1981), testified in an institutional legal case. Recalling one of his first
conversations with this national leader, a lawyer for the plaintiffs recounted, "He said, 'I won't help if you want to fix up the institution. If you
want to close it, I'll put you in touch with every expert you'll need.'"
This TASH leader also recalled his visits around the state, saying that
the strategy was not to characterize people as bad, but to try to find some
good examples. The lawyers took this witness to a high school with jun-
iors and seniors, "pretty severely handicapped kids," who were working
in the local drugstore, grocery, and hardware store with job coaching and
relying on the owner to help out:

> We wanted to have positive community displays to the judge. So we
> went around looking in New Hampshire for some good things and
> we found a couple. . . . It was such a small state and they put their
> money into institutionalization, essentially, denying services to
> people. . . . [Due to little or no community development] it was easy
> to build the right stuff to start from state of the art, and to guide it.

More, however, was at stake than the specific trial. The Association of
Persons with Severe Handicaps (TASH), which first developed as a con-

cept around 1971 to 1972, had an enemy to fight. As one of its leaders, who was strongly committed to community life for people with the most severe handicaps, saw the challenge, "We had the best young talent in the field and they didn't . . . they thought they were hot stuff, and we just beat them badly. To me, that's very, very important." The experts for the plaintiffs testified that everyone can live in the community.

No Court Monitor or Master: Maintaining the State Roles

State officials strongly believed that having a court order in place instead of a court monitor was a key factor contributing to long-term success. According to one state administrator, the state "worked real hard to not have a court monitor . . . the fact that we didn't have a court monitor allowed us to keep trying innovative programs, trying new things, changing direction." The order of compliance kept the state responsible for doing its job in planning and developing, while still being held accountable. One state official indicated it would have been considered insulting and offensive to have a court monitor, which is what the plaintiffs' lawyers had requested. Upon reflection, one lawyer shared it was "probably helpful not to have another level of state bureaucracy" and the struggles between the judicial and executive branches, such as occurred in Connecticut with the court monitor (see chapter on Connecticut in Bradley and Bersani, 1990). It was also unnecessary because there was not a recalcitrance on the part of the state or strong vested interest groups fighting to retain the institution. Because the federal court ordered the state to plan, this could be viewed as a "kind of mediation" which toned down the legalistic aspects, allowing the policies and implementation to go forward with strong financial and judicial support. One state official described the situation as follows:

> They gave us license to come forward with the right thing, or at least what we thought was the right thing, and then the court ordered it, put the weight of the federal court behind what the executive branch said it wanted to do, [and to] which the plaintiffs could agree. . . . That has been of enormous importance.

Commitment and Leadership

This effort was successful, in large part, because of the courage and tenacity of the parents who filed the suit, the commitment of the lawyers to the causes they were advocating for, the leadership of state planners and area agencies in implementation, and the wisdom of the judge.

Plaintiffs' Lawyers

The lawyers worked hard, fought aggressively and steadfastly, became educated and spent time educating others, and were available to the families. They provided guidance and advice, used the opportunity to reshape the service system, and collaborated effectively with the Justice Department.

The Justice Department

From the point of view of the plaintiffs, the Justice Department was enormously helpful, with experience, resources, and money for experts. Their involvement was a significant factor in making the lengthy trial possible.

The State Planners

They played a critical role in the pretrial, trial, and after-trial phases. They wrote the plan Action for Independence, which became the plan that was eventually implemented in the state. This gave the state Division of Mental Health and Developmental Services an authority and license that was key to managing and guiding the creation of the community service system. The state leadership had to maintain good relationships with all parties.

Area Agencies

The area agencies played several different roles that contributed to the successful outcomes, including providing information, acting as experts, demonstrating that good community services could be done, and developing their own political support. The state had no control over the private, nonprofit sector that provided information to the legal sector. One of the results of the lawsuit was that the providers gained confidence in serving people with severe handicaps, making substantial progress with people who were "developmentally disabled and mentally ill" at the New Hampshire Hospital. During implementation, the placements were generally successful ("They were good and the parents were happy.").

The Wisdom of the Judge

The federal district court judge, who was recently appointed to the bench and new to these kinds of cases, was educated by the plaintiffs' attorneys. As one attorney explained, "He had to get angry about abuses and the devastation to families, why the community was necessary." The judge was described by another of the attorneys as follows:

> [He was] a moderate to conservative Democrat. He knew this was a case that he wasn't going to get rid of for a long time. He also knew it was going to be scrutinized for a long time, morally, politically, and legally. He also didn't trust the state. . . . In my view, [he] felt that community was the way to go. But, [he was] judicially suspect of whether the constitutional law mandated that. Not surprisingly, he cajoled and threatened the other parties involved to settle the case, but we couldn't.

A great deal of respect was paid to the federal district judge for the way he managed the case (kept the momentum going) and for the wisdom he showed in his win-win decisions. He allowed the ten-week trial because he knew it was important ("He gave us that opportunity."). In many ways, the judge came up with an ideal solution, sorting through the longest civil trial in New Hampshire's history. As one state official surmised:

> The judge cut the baby in half perfectly. It was a Solomon-like decision. The judge ordered us to plan. So that the plaintiffs won; but we won. . . . So the state gets to implement the way it wants to implement provided that it delivers on what the plaintiff outcome is. It was a very cohesive concept of a court order.

Cooperation

Probably the most important aspect of change was that people were located both within and outside of the system who had a common goal. This resulted in lots of "strange kinds of cooperation" between people, even among those who were alleged adversaries, whereby benefits accrued to all. This cooperation was not eroded by the adversarial process, and adversaries continue to speak highly of one another's roles today. In their "heart of hearts," state disability officials believed that people with severe disabilities could live in the community, though, politically, the attorney general was safeguarding the legal position of the state. The focus of a number of key people, both inside and outside the system, was on finding a way to move forward so that change could occur to better the lives of people with disabilities. As one state administrator explained, "It is really a situation where people have to say we've got to change and we've got to work together and we've got to give each other information that will help this go forward."

Once the litigation phase had passed, the opportunity arose to rebuild healthy relationships, which was relatively easy in a situation in which people were "reasonable" and "wanted to do the right thing." The foundation was a shared belief among both the state planners and the plaintiffs that people with disabilities can live in the community. In essence, "that is the difference" between this situation and many other instances of institutional litigation. Once the court made clear that people were going to leave the institution, even the attorney general's office joined forces in fighting back most, if not all, efforts by communities to resist deinstitutionalization.

Minimal Organized Opposition

Unlike a number of other states, organized opposition in New Hampshire was minimal. To some extent, this stemmed from the fact that it was "unusual to advocate in New Hampshire" since it was not an "active consumer state." An attempt by the attorney general's office to create opposition parent groups such as at Willowbrook (New York), Pennhurst (Pennsylvania), and Connecticut's Southbury was reported. The lawyers wanted to subdivide the class and say that the plaintiffs did not represent all of the Laconia residents. There also was no reported opposition from the local state union, which was not part of a larger organization such as AFSCME (American Federation of State, County and Municipal Employees). One professional describes this lack of opposition:

> I remember in New York seeing a billboard near Troy that said, "When institutions close, everyone loses" put out by the union. Nothing like that ever happened here. There were also certain values in the union. They were friends. I knew them. They didn't want to be on the bad side. They didn't want to be perceived as supporting the state.

Other Key Factors

Other key factors contributing to the closure and community development were the redefinition of institutional admissions requirements to be more stringent; the lack of a public external closure plan to minimize opposition and retain flexibility; shifting of finances, including federal Medicaid, to the community; and an individual planning process. Underlying each of these was the development of an attitude that no one would go back to the institution and people would work together, whatever their place and role in the system, to see that everyone would remain in the community.

LITIGATION, INSTITUTIONAL CLOSURES, AND COMMUNITY DEVELOPMENT

Across diverse areas inside and outside of the state, people unanimously agreed that the litigation and court order were absolutely essential conditions for the closure of Laconia within the state of New Hampshire. In their experience, without the litigation, at best, it may have stayed open with a "residual population," or even have grown in size. Informants also were convinced that the community system would not look at all the same, since the lawsuit was viewed as a catalyst for the development of that system ("the genesis . . . of the modern system.").

The litigation was critical partially because of the conservative nature of the state, the need for educating the legislature and citizenry, the reluctance of the state to become involved in "big services, big community systems," and the need for people to "get ready," to clarify the governmental roles that would be consistent with the state's philosophy of live free or die, independent living, self-determination, and a strong community base.

The litigation "made it possible for people inside and outside the system to really bring about change." The education of, and obligations on, the legislature were extremely important and created a force that lasted over the decade of community services development. One leader shared:

> It brought a measure of authority to the whole process so that in a constant process of competing interests of different issues—and I don't just mean one human service against another, but highways against human services, or low taxes against human services, or whatever—it established a clear compelling willingness in this area, that in part was public understanding, in part was judicial authority, and that has stayed with us through more than a decade and that has been extremely valuable.

Overall, New Hampshire experienced few negative impacts of the legal actions. As an imperfect tool for social change, litigation, by its nature, does result somewhat in a two-class system with differential benefits. However, the effect of this lawsuit was greater than for most lawsuits, and as one lawyer recounted, "We were able to accomplish more than one can normally hope to accomplish in these sorts of things." Yet another person added, the fact that this should happen in New Hampshire "of all places, says to me that it can happen anywhere."

CONCLUSION

In the 1970s and 1980s, the community-institutional debate was the primary driving force behind the development of community services. In New Hampshire, as elsewhere in the world, the 1990s have been marked by differing philosophies about how people with disabilities will be viewed in the next decade. *Who will determine how people with disabilities will live their lives? Who will control the resources, be the active agents of change and "own" the service system?*

DOCUMENTS REVIEWED (*Garrity v. Gallen*)

1. Complaint, Civil Action 78-116.
2. Motion of United States for leave to file complaint in intervention (August 1978).
3. Composite final order (11/16/81).
4. Memorandum opinion (8/17/81).
5. Defendant's proposal for negotiations in settlement.
6. Plaintiff's submission, draft proposed consent decrees.
7. Alternatives for approaching *Garrity v. Gallen* court order, Plan C (November 5, 1981).
8. Memorandum on amendments (Addition to *Garrity* court order).
9. Amendment to United States complaint in intervention (July 26, 1979).
10. Summary, *Garrity v. Gallen.*
11. Correspondence NH Attorney General to Department of Justice (June 29, 1979); Cohen to NH Attorney General (July 27, 1979).
12. Defendant's report pursuant to paragraph two of the order of implementation (November 1, 1982).
13. Correspondence, Cohen to Miller (July 27, 1978); NH Attorney General to Cohen (October 24, 1978).
14. Overview of Attorney General's commitments made to Justice Department.
15. *Garrity v. Gallen* fact sheet for interested citizens.
16. Proposed agreement, *Garrity v. Gallen.*
17. Mental Disability Law Reporter (January-February 1979).
18. Final report to U.S. District Court by State Board of Education (July 15, 1985).
19. State of New Hampshire *Action for Independence. ARCFACTS.* Arlington, TX: Association for Retarded Citizens.

Chapter 4

The Closing of Laconia:
From the Inside Out

Julie Ann Racino

INTRODUCTION

When people understand these are the right things to do, even if it comes at a personal cost, they don't stand in the way.

Ray Bardley, Institutional Superintendent

On January 31, 1991, Laconia Developmental Services (LDS) closed its doors, making New Hampshire the first state in the United States without a public institution for people with developmental disabilities. This is part of the story of two people employed by the state of New Hampshire, Ray Bardley and John Simmons, who worked from within the institution to close it. This chapter details some of the personal struggles and professional dilemmas they faced.

Ray, who was institutional superintendent at the time of the closure of Laconia, returned to New Hampshire from his supported employment agency director role in a western state. He previously worked as a community services planner in New Hampshire and returned to this new role based on the suggestion of his previous secretary.

John Simmon's arrival at Laconia in August 1988 was considered to be a wonderful stroke of luck. After a tumultuous period with one of his

This chapter is a modified version of Racino, J. (1993a). "The Closing of Laconia: From the Inside Out." *An Edited Collection on Community Integration and Deinstitutionalization in New Hampshire.* Syracuse, NY: Community and Policy Studies. See Appendix B for research methodology. All names used in this chapter are pseudonyms unless otherwise indicated.

board members, John departed from his position as one of the state's twelve area agency executive directors. Because he was the "valued person in the system you hate to see leave or hurt," he was hired to work part-time at both the state division office and at Laconia in a flexible role.

This case study shares their perspectives on what they learned, including efforts toward respecting all people, inclusive of staff members and residents who lived in the institution during the closure process. As one of many diverse stories that form a composite picture of the inside view of the Laconia closure, it is particularly meant to be shared with those who are working within for change.

INTERNAL CONSIDERATIONS IN INSTITUTIONAL CLOSURE

Probably as many different ways exist to examine the internal experience of the closure of Laconia as there are people who were involved in the process or who viewed it from the outside. Through the eyes of an administrator working within the institution, four major areas were particularly critical in the internal process of closing Laconia: revisions in the personnel system, caring for and about staff members, restructuring and reorganizing the institution as it became smaller, and maintaining institutional quality during the closure process.

Revising the Personnel System

From an administrator's view, the closure of an institution is a tremendous personnel job with the lives of many people, both staff and residents, affected by the decisions that are made. Several critical strategies were used that affected how the personnel system operated during the closure process. These included taking direct control of the personnel system, investing in staff values-based training, and revising the performance outcome system.

Taking Control of the Personnel System

When one of the first building closures at Laconia occurred, the institutional management team met to discuss the staffing decisions that had been made. At Laconia, as in many institutions, the staff members from that building had been reshuffled to other buildings and locations within the institution, and no actual staff reductions had taken place. Ray shared the following:

I said, Well, I guess we can talk about reducing the staff because that building closed and there [were] so many people associated with it." My managers . . . weren't up to this. . . . Everyone played dumb. What happened to the staff? Of course, what happens in a lot of large organizations. People had been moved around and buried in different sorts of ways.

In response to this situation, Ray decided to take direct control of the personnel system so that no decisions for the rest of the closure process were made without his involvement. He established a Thursday morning personnel management meeting, which came to be known as the "cut and slash committee," during which the hard decisions regarding staff reductions took place under his direction. The participants included himself, the personnel team, and two business office personnel. These meetings were viewed as suspect by the program staff who did not feel represented, even though Ray said he was a program person. Although he viewed this forum as an effective management strategy, Ray described the emotions that were involved in the decision making that occurred:

> Those little cut-and-slash meetings. People used to think we sat up there and kind of in an aloof, unfeeling manner destroyed people's lives by laying them off or whatever. . . . Those were awful meetings. . . . There was crying in there.

Investing in Staff Values-Based Training

The original design of the personnel system at Laconia was viewed by one of the administrators as "a very punitive, capricious type of system." Such a system resulted in a lot of time being invested in appeals meetings with the labor board in Concord, the state capital, about the way employees were treated.

One strategy considered to be an essential part of the institutional closure process was to revamp the disciplinary structure, making it less punitive, with training and counseling as the responses to disciplinary issues. As part of this new focus on training, money was invested in values-based training in areas such as PASS (Program Analysis of Service Systems) (Wolfensberger and Glenn, 1975) or PASSING (Program Analysis of Service Systems' Implementation of Normalization Goals) (Wolfensberger and Thomas, 1983), which are founded on the principles of normalization. As Ray continued to explain, "This theme was woven into all aspects of training, including driver's ed[ucation], nursing, everything." At one time, over seventy staff, including all of the top management, the middle managers, and even some direct care staff, had attended this training. This educational effort was so successful that in 1991, the key leadership in New Hampshire's Alliance for Values-Based Training was former institutional employees who were working to get people out of the institution. As Ray explained, the staff "were doing what was expected of them, and when we changed those expectations and gave them some training and some values, a lot of people changed."

Revising the Staff Performance Outcome System

Although the personnel system was revamped to become more focused on staff development and training, by 1988, performance standards were raised, deficiencies in staff performance were made known to other staff members, and a series of steps to respond to disciplinary issues were put into place. The performance standards were not about quality per se, but about doing your job and meeting objectives within a certain time frame. If people were consistently appearing on the deficiency list, "a disciplinary process [would begin] which started with counseling, questioning, asking if they needed more training and support, and could get very serious. We ended up terminating a few people."

Caring for and About Staff

Probably more than anything else, the personnel changes and strategies were all based on principles of valuing and caring about and for the staff. Specific strategies included creating a future for professionals, appreciating the environmental context of the staff's work, fairness in employment, and finding people jobs and staff support.

Creating a Future for Professionals

One creative idea in gaining the support of key professionals and managers was the development of a cutting-edge adaptive equipment center on the grounds of the institution, which became a state support center. Creating a future for the professionals, Ray explained that they stayed working at the institution during the downsizing process:

> We had very little problem after the first year with professional staff because I created a future for OTs [occupational therapists], PTs [physical therapists], speech pathologists. . . . It is the adaptive equipment center, which is now a state support center. We had no problem.

Key managers who would be necessary throughout the process were told that every effort would be made to preserve their jobs. An effort was made to ask them what they wanted in the future and to make arrangements to see if that could happen for them. Ray is satisfied that "all of them really ended up doing exactly what they asked for, except for one, and she kept changing what she wanted so it was hard to orchestrate. . . . I orchestrated it for everyone."

Appreciating the Environmental Context

Unlike the negative images often portrayed of institutional staff, the administration believed in these employees. When given the opportunity to do "wonderful things" such as going to Dunkin' Donuts with one of the residents for coffee or going out to buy clothes, they just loved it. As Ray explained, "There are a lot of people here who are very good people, very committed, very dedicated to what they are doing, but have never been given the tools or the information to do anything other than what they are doing."

Ray explained that many of the longtime staff members who came to the institution could not believe the conditions at Laconia. However, they eventually adjusted because it was what everyone was doing. Ray understood that it was hard, if not impossible, for people to hold beliefs that are incompatible with their personal experiences. The staff members adjusted to what many originally felt was an abnormal environment and over time came to see those conditions and actions as routine. However, instead of portraying the institution itself as a bad place, Ray described the problem more in terms of dormitory living with thirty people not being a comfortable, permanent lifestyle for any group of people.

Fairness in Employment

As the downsizing process took place, one critical element was to ensure that management was fair to the employees on what was a fair day's work so that "employees were not pushed over the brink." This required a knowledge about the specific jobs that people did so that reasonable demands could be placed upon people. The underlying administrative belief, according to Ray, was "if a person has accepted employment and they understand the conditions of it, we have a right to expect a reasonable day's work. . . . You wanted to be fair."

When jobs changed as reorganization took place, people were invited to restructure their jobs. A lot of this job restructuring was done with the issue of maintaining quality in mind.

Finding People Jobs and Staff Support

The management tried to create a situation in which the staff felt that they were being paid attention to, treated fairly, and related to on an individual basis. There was a concerted management effort to try to recognize people's strengths and skills. Other strategies used included aggressively managing attrition, working with remaining staff on transfers to other state agency or community jobs, and attempting to respond to individual employee situations by relocating the person within the system and supporting those who needed support.

Each staff member was viewed as having his or her own life story, and management tried to know, to some extent, what was going on in staff members' lives. People noticed management's efforts to take care of them, and that contributed to improved morale. Time was spent simply talking with staff, letting them know what was going on as far in advance of official notices as possible so that plans for jobs could be made. Ray described this as one of the most sensible things that they did:

> We were nice. I think part of it was I talked with everybody . . . there wasn't a person who was afraid to say something. I was just a regular person and I talked to people; they talked to me.

Of the reduction of 650 positions to effect closure of the institution, 450 were managed through attrition, and ultimately, only twenty-two of the remaining people did not end up with jobs. Those people were direct care staff with less than two years of experience. Even when these staff members were laid off, the institutional management continued to work with them to find community jobs. Some people who had "bumping rights" transferred to other state jobs, others retired, and "there were some people who ended up making more money, and that didn't hurt either." A few of the institutional staff continued to work for state-operated residential programs. Few institutional staff went to work in the community services system because the pay and benefits differential made such a move unaffordable.

Restructuring and Reorganizing

Three important strategies for change during the closure process were reorganization of infrastructure, creation of a culture for closure, and maintenance of cooperative relationships with the union.

Reorganization of the Infrastructure

During the course of the downsizing and closure, at least eight major staff and program reorganizations occurred within a period of four and a half years. This involved conceptual and structural changes and reorganizations when key people left.

The psychology unit, for example, was reorganized several times, always with attention to maintaining high-quality, up-to-date professional services. Initially, the unit had been unitized and oriented toward "writing behavior plans versus assisting staff with client learning styles and troubleshooting [problems]." The unit was departmentalized, new leadership brought in, and staff retrained. When that supervisor left, the state management contracted out for psychological supervision and returned to a mixed, unitized department structure.

The restructuring itself was very hard and demanding, partly because the same managers who had created and refined the institutional ICF/MR system basically needed to undo their own work. Ray explained as follows:

> Restructuring is hard . . . one of the things I found here is that I [had] inherited a group of managers who spent their lives from 1975 to 1986 building up this ICF/MR system and getting the kinks out of it and restructuring this, and changing this, [and] polishing that, and really working to get it as good as they could after ten or eleven years only to have me come in and say we are going to rip it apart.

Creating a Culture for Closure

One of the important activities that people did was to try to create within the institution an atmosphere of moving forward, of being part of the future, and of doing something worthwhile. Staff planned and organized celebrations to commemorate the closure of institutional buildings. Another effort was to create a sense of openness so that the institutional service delivery system was open to everybody's purview. Service delivery work group meetings were set up so that everyone could come and put anything on the agenda. This gave direct care people a voice in what was going on and helped to maintain quality, for example, Ray's comments:

> And I chaired those meetings, and it was in those meetings that somebody who was a direct care staff person . . . who was working with a client who had occupational therapy needs, could say in front

of the department head of occupational therapy, "Your therapists aren't coming in on time. They haven't shown up for two weeks, and we don't know why." . . . I would then turn [to the department head] and say, "How about that?"

Maintaining the culture also meant striving to pay attention to each of the residents. As the institution headed toward closure, particularly during the last year, this became more and more difficult as the attention of staff began to focus on the community.

Working with the Union

The union issues were not as difficult as in many states, because the state did not have a major union such as AFSCME (American Federation of State, County and Municipal Employees). Potential problems were averted by keeping the leadership informed and by acting fairly, which avoided grievances and the feeling that people were being treated unfairly. Only one formal labor management consultation occurred, which, under the collective bargaining agreement, was set up as needed.

The institution began to send laundry to New Hampshire State Hospital when the laundry operations at the institution were closed down. The president of the local employee's union coordinated the dirty and clean laundry and its shipment between the institutions. This meant that she was around the grounds and at the various buildings talking to everybody on campus all the time. Management kept in touch with her by informally responding to her questions and exchanging information, as well as through formal channels.

Maintaining Institutional Quality During Closure

A critical internal focus of the closure strategy was to maintain the quality of institutional living for people who continued to reside there while the closure took place. In addition to values-based training, this was accomplished by improving the direct care staff ratios from 1:7 to 1:4, thus maintaining programmatic quality and meeting federal standards for continued funding.

Even though the ratios for both professional and direct care staff were better than three years earlier, staff members still felt worse. This may possibly be because the absolute decrease in numbers of people was noticeable and adversely affected staff morale. The reductions in support staff were the greatest, and although the ratios of staff increased, the demands in terms of programmatic quality also increased.

The staff tried to maintain a "clean bill of health from the feds [federal service teams] without compromising values." This was done by interweaving into the individual service plans (ISP) community-based objectives, functional skills, and partial participation (not common in an intermediate care facility, particularly of institutional size). The quality was maintained so that at the exit interview of the last federal look behind (i.e., monitoring visit), "the HCFA [Health Care Financing Administration, responsible for the federal Medicaid program] people said they had never seen a place so well run. They never even sent us a piece of paper."

KNITTING AND CONNECTING

John Simmons held a very different role within the institution, serving as a liaison, "knitter," or "switchboard operator" among three elements of the state's system: the state division in Concord, Laconia Developmental Services (LDS), and the community service system represented by the area agencies. He was sometimes on the phone for the entire working day, calling and talking with people, helping people from the community and institution get to know one another."

In bureaucratic terms, John's job was mainly a liaison or "personnel" job, and he influenced the placement process, though he did not have any specific responsibility, accountability, or authority for either the process or the supervision of staff activities. At the institution, he worked closely with the director for quality assurance who was responsible for the supervision of social workers and program coordinators. John was on the management team of the state division office, but not on the management team in the institution.

On another level, John's role was a very intuitive versus structural one, involving helping others to recognize and act on good opportunities and to negotiate agreements based on the uniqueness of the region, the person with a disability, his or her family, and others involved. The role he created for himself was described by Ray as "really quite a stroke of masterpiece." John interacted in a way that facilitated and supported the social workers and the program coordinators to communicate with community case managers and case manager supervisors about people rather than adhering to a defined placement process. He also had an ability to work among the area agencies, the state division, and the institution, knowing that everyone had an important role to play.

The Placement Process

The process of community placement in New Hampshire was formalized in regulation, "made sense early on," and basically worked, though it became less functional over time. What John accomplished, together with others within and outside the institution, was to facilitate improved relationships between the community and institutional staff and to focus on the individual person and his or her family so that, "even in the end, [we still] made some really good placements."

John used and built upon many of the standard structures already put in place at Laconia through Ray's management efforts. The standard team process at Laconia was more highly evolved than the team process in many regions, already incorporating future planning, attention to relationships, functional skills, and community participation. There were high expectations for staff and the necessary management support and values base that made the realization of these values possible.

STRATEGIES FOR CHANGE

The primary strategies for creating these changes included shifting the attention of the area agencies to the people remaining in the institution, building trust and sharing expertise between the community and institutional systems, finding the window of opportunity, reinvigorating the internal process by building on the knowledge and skills of institutional staff, and planning with individual people. The first four strategies are highlighted in this section.

Shifting Attention Back to the Institution

Following the court order, the area agencies and state personnel made a very strong effort to bring people out of Laconia, but placements reached a plateau by the mid-1980s. As the community system solidified, people in the area agencies (i.e., the regional structures) focused less on the people in the institution and more on their own backyards. The community staff were working hard on the stability of their system, on problem solving of people in jeopardy in the community, and on keeping people out of the institution. As ordinary turnover took place among case managers and community staff, "people at the institution got lost. They just weren't a priority," partially because of the distance from their home communities.

However, it was frustrating, especially to institutional administrators, when money was being pulled out of the institution to build up the community but placements were not occurring on schedule. This placed the institutional superintendent in the position of losing credibility and at risk of having reduced quality within the institution (resulting in decreased life quality for people living there). He explained that although people in the community and institution basically wanted the same thing, a lot of conflict occurred around these kinds of placement issues.

The state division (responsible also for community services financing) had increasing pressures in the community. Because of the slowing placement rate, a lack of belief existed at all levels that the institution would really close. Thus, part of what needed to occur was to "raise people's consciousness again" that there were still a lot of people in the institution, that the job was not done. According to state regulations, people in the institution were still the number one priority, so efforts had to be made to get people back in touch, to get the area agencies to lead, and to help people with disabilities live again in the community.

Bridging the Institution-Community Gap

One fundamental problem revolved around the gap in worldviews between the institutional and community staff. As John noted, staff members, each with his or her different experiences of an individual, needed to work together across community and institutional lines to design the right supports.

Overcoming the Evil-Good Dichotomy

One of the most important steps was overcoming the community's image of the institution staff, including recognizing the strengths of the people who worked there. The Laconia staff "were tremendous" because they knew the people who were to move into the community, could bridge the gap with the families, and could offer some very practical training to providers. John explained why this exchange between community and institutional staff seldom happened before:

> [A belief seemed to evolve] that the institution was evil and the community was good, and the role of developmental services system around the court order was to save people from the institution. Therefore, it was a bad place and all the people who were there were probably bad too, or even if they were not bad, they were probably so institutionalized they aren't going to change. None of that was true. It was not true largely because Ray had done a lot of work in getting people [to develop good] skills [and values].

Connecting Community and Institutional Staff

John described his role as helping the institutional and community staff to recognize one another's expertise and, especially, their "lack of expertise." One of the ways John attempted to connect people was by writing and calling the community case managers to let them know which people were still in the institution. After telling them about the people who remained, he then invited community staff to visit and asked the institutional staff to serve as hosts. John purposefully avoided being viewed as the person who could answer questions about residents at Laconia so other people would correctly be seen as the experts.

The rule or framework they used was to try to identify the person in the institution who knew or cared for the person the most. This same approach was used in identifying which staff in the institution would visit the region. "It didn't matter if it was the janitor, [kitchen staff], or the program director, or whomever. Who seems to care the most about this person?" That person was then empowered to "go explore that community setting or go to the meeting or whatever and come back and tell us what [her or she thought] about it." That person's role was to try to figure out if that would be a good place for someone to live and he or she was able to be very vocal about "whether or not it was a good idea . . . always with the question, what would it take, what was needed to support this person?"

Finding the Window of Opportunity

John saw a kind of window of opportunity to ask the question, "What would it take, individual by individual, for this person to succeed in the community?" He felt people didn't understand that question so he explained that if these issues were not addressed, the person would be perceived as having failed. He then devised a questionnaire of twenty-three "supports/needs" questions about the kind of supports they would need, not what skills. This questionnaire included areas that must be paid attention to:

> Do they take medications? Do they have seizures? Do they take seizure medications or psychotropics? Is there an active nursing care [plan] or some attention to detail like communication, sign language? Do they use a wheelchair? . . .

Most of the questions concerned what was likely to go wrong if people ignored these issues and what assistance the individual would need to keep him or her from being at risk. "The attempt was to shift the philosophy away from the incapacities and deficits of people to building capacities of community systems, the capacity of staff, or whatever." The question was not whether an individual was "ready," but what would it take for that person to do well?

From the beginning of his work, John tried to personalize the process. The institutional staff asked people in the community to visit in groups of no more than two or three people—"no entourages." As John said, "You cannot come to a meal unless you are going to have a meal. There is not going to be anyone sitting around observing." A concerted effort was made for people from the community agencies to meet individuals who were moving from the institution. Before anyone moved, they always visited a couple of times and stayed overnight at the home where they would be living back in the region.

Reinvigorating the Placement Process

Internally, the placement process was reinvigorated as people began to see one another and themselves differently. "It really did happen." Over the next two years, John helped develop "a reasonable collaborative process. It wasn't without its arguments. It was just a nicer process between peers working to solve this problem."

John's priorities for placement were the youngest, then the oldest, then people with the most severe disabilities. It did not work out that way ultimately; yet, it was a safeguard to avoid picking people who were seen as easy. The people who were the most difficult to match or to figure out ultimately had some of the most "individualized placements." Advantageous to all concerned, this meant placements like regular homes with in-home staff support for people with "real behavioral challenges" or "lots of physical needs." The focus was always on the individual person.

Money was moved as necessary from one region to another; a regional contract or divisional money was not appropriated and available for x number of people to go to the community. The idea of region of origin was abandoned for people who had been in the institution for thirty-five years or more and who had no ties to their region of origin. As John explained:

> What made more sense was finding a place and a program that was (sic) very compatible. It wasn't whether they belonged to Manchester or belonged someplace else.

The placement process itself just snowballed. In "the first year, placements were 115 percent of contract. In the second year, 137 percent of contract. And for the previous several years they were less than 40 percent or 50 percent of contract. We exceeded our best expectations." It turned out that everything was so far ahead of schedule that no one actually believed it, or even fully realized it, until one day somebody said, "this [closure] is really going to happen."

At some point, it became competitive, too, a sense of personal "disgrace" if the regional director did not make some contribution to this effort. However, placement toward the end was the most difficult, not because of the needs of the people, but because the community system itself was becoming saturated. The effort had been high, people were tired, and more avenues needed to be explored.

John said he was not particularly significant in the process. He said, "I just asked . . . why don't you come up? Is there anything we can help with? . . . Would you like us to give his mom a call?" By asking if there was anything he could do to help (the answer was virtually always no), it did mean that people then felt obligated to do it. He found it was important to keep a very high profile, maintaining high activity levels so that people knew that someone was concerned about this situation and would follow up on their conversations to find out whether things had been accomplished.

Other critical areas that contributed to the internal efforts in the closure of Laconia included how the money worked, the advantages of not having a formal closure plan, working with parents, developing individualized placements, and a capacity to make compromises, solve problems, and overcome the search for perfection (Racino, 1993a).

CONCLUSION

Since the research for this case study was collected, Ray and John have both assumed new roles within New Hampshire's State Division of Mental Health and Developmental Services. John shared, "I was very glad to be a part of something . . . like that. And, in some ways, it was a culmination of my career of twenty-five years." Ray also reflected back on his personal experience:

> There were a . . . [lot of] tears here and a lot of pain. There was a lot of consternation at the individual level; we were changing their jobs . . . . They had their individual troubles, but they could relate to the bigger part. . . . It wasn't easy.

Although it is likely that not everybody is totally satisfied, the "state office" received very few complaints about the way the closure and placements were handled. Today, though it was not easy, New Hampshire has become one of the nation's leaders in moving people to good places within local communities, in part because of the work of people from within the institution.

Chapter 5

A Qualitative Study of Self-Advocacy and Guardianship: Speaking for Oneself

Julie Ann Racino

I really feel strongly about self-advocacy because no one can speak as effectively for an individual human being than that individual human being.

A New Hampshire Advocate

INTRODUCTION

Self-advocacy is part of a growing movement across the United States and is discussed here as a counterpoint to the beginning shift in New Hampshire from a service system dominated by providers and state employees to one in which families are recognized and supported.[1] This case study raises the question "How will this shift to family-centered systems include what people with disabilities want and need?"

This qualitative research case study includes a brief overview of the status and development of self-advocacy in New Hampshire, describes the

---

This chapter is a modified version of Racino, J. (1993a). " A Qualitative Study of Self-Advocacy and Guardianship: Views from New Hampshire." Syracuse, NY: Community and Policy Studies. In *An Edited Collection on Community Integration and Deinstitutionalization in New Hampshire.* See Appendix B for research methodology. All names used in this chapter are pseudonyms, except for T. J. Monroe and Ruth Sinkowitz-Mercer.

1. For more information on family support development in New Hampshire, see Shoultz, B. (1992b). *Like an Angel They Came to Help Us: The Origins and Workings of New Hampshire's Family Support Network.* Syracuse, NY: Syracuse University, Center on Human Policy, Research and Training Center on Community Integration.

state's guardianship program, and highlights areas of concern for people with disabilities. In particular, the research reflects upon the meaning of self-advocacy, its development in New Hampshire, local self-advocacy groups, the role of advisors and supporters, future issues, and desired outcomes of self-advocacy.

THE MEANINGS OF SELF-ADVOCACY

Self-advocacy has a variety of meanings to people with and without disabilities based on both their personal experiences and their beliefs about what advocacy means. Self-advocacy in New Hampshire has three primary components: (1) enabling people with developmental disabilities to speak for themselves, (2) joining together with others to achieve systems changes through advocacy strategies, and (3) sharing social and personal support (known as peer support in the independent living movement) offered by local self-advocacy groups.

Speaking for Oneself

In one sense, self-advocacy is about speaking for oneself. This may be as simple as calling the vocational rehabilitation counselor for the first time. For another person, it may mean indicating by nonverbal expression that she would like a glass of water. Some people might not call these actions self-advocacy. However, these are steps in building a person's own confidence that he or she knows best what he or she wants and can translate these desires into actions.

Self-advocacy is about decision making and self-worth and is one of the ingredients to becoming more self determined. Being part of a self-advocacy group means that a person may be able to get what he or she wants, whether that is an apartment, a job, or simply being heard. The hope is that people with developmental disabilities will learn more about what they want, express it, and have at least some of their desires met.

Joining Together

Self-advocacy also means joining together with others to achieve systems change that affects the well-being and lives of others. As the treasurer of one self-advocacy group described, this means using legislative advocacy strategies, such as writing letters to Congress, "to get the government behind you":

> Self-advocacy . . . is a way to get your problems solved . . . if you get the government behind you 100 percent. I think writing letters to Congress is going to improve a lot . . . because we're going to get what we need. . . . We've done our part. So now it is up to them to do theirs.

In this view, self-advocacy means that people with disabilities can "fight" for the services that they want. It is based on a framework that the government should provide these services, particularly in instances where such services have been previously denied by virtue of institutionalization.

People can become involved with self-advocacy for many reasons, including the wish to "make a difference" ("you could help other people make better lives for themselves"). As one man who has been involved in the movement described:

> Yes, I think we've made a difference. I think we've gotten people moving . . . excited. . . . I think we've made the point for some people who need to have . . . a little bit more help than others.

From the viewpoint of professionals, one of the reasons self-advocacy is important is because legislators listen more to people who are directly affected by, and who care about, an issue. Self-advocacy allows professionals to play a background role by providing information, education, and resources, while the people most concerned are in the forefront. As one advocate illustrated:

> If I go to testify to the state legislature [about] . . . motorized wheelchairs . . . who cares? Why don't we get some people who use motorized wheelchairs to go? Why don't we alert them and say, "Do you know the state is considering not paying for that anymore? . . . I just thought I'd pass that information on to you."

Social and Personal Support

Being part of a self-advocacy group also means having a place to meet other people, to make new friends, to unite with old friends, and to be independent. For parents, it may also be an opportunity for their son or daughter to be out of the house participating in a different activity.

In self-advocacy, a "group behind you to guide you along" in making choices and decisions offers support. This is similar to the concept of peer support in independent living which helps to "kind of gear someone up or put a little fire in them" to make decisions and face issues in their lives. These social and personal support aspects of self-advocacy groups are illustrated further in the section on local groups.

DESIRED OUTCOMES OF SELF-ADVOCACY

The desired outcomes of self-advocacy vary; however, they include the following: marriage and family, a "dream" career, a comfortable place to live, freedom to come and go, housing, adult education, positive results of individual service plans, clothes and equipment, and transportation (see also Racino with Whittico, 1998; Racino, 1993a). This section highlights housing, education and transportation.

Housing: Congregated and Living Together

Staff at the Granite State independent living center (ILC) noted that housing for many people with disabilities was a big issue. Accessible, subsidized apartments were congregated together in units, which was not the way people with disabilities would choose to live. As an independent living advocate described her state:

> Housing is a pretty big issue in this state. Pretty much what they've done is they've grouped; they've sort of ghettoized. . . . You live in a twenty-four-unit [building]. Everyone has a disability . . . or just like an elderly-disabled mix. . . . They wouldn't choose to live there on their own.

This may contrast with housing through the developmental disabilities services system in this state, whereby people commonly live with just a few other people, by themselves, or with a roommate, as described by one advocate:

> You'll find very few people in this state with developmental disabilities who live with more than two or three other people who have developmental disabilities. That's a real step forward in a setting where you can get somebody to pay real solid attention to you, alone, yourself, for periods of time.

Education: The Individuals with Disabilities Education Act

One self-advocate expressed concern about how the Individuals with Disabilities Education Act (IDEA)—passed by Congress and signed into law by Gerald R. Ford in 1975—was designed and what would be the implications for her own life. She believes the law should be expanded to include adults with disabilities over the age of twenty-one, as well as children, especially for people who had been institutionalized ("it's a very unfair law"):

> I am not happy with the way Congress in Washington had designed . . . [part of the] legislation called the Individuals with Disabilities

> [Education] Act, and I'll tell you the reason why. . . . It's very unfair to
> people like me . . . who were denied a good foundation, a basic
> elementary and high school education, against our will by the state
> while we were at Laconia State School for so many years.

She explained that existing adult education programs did not meet her
needs because they concentrated more on socialization ("like little children") than on basic skills such as spelling or reading that she would need
to obtain a good job or drive a car.

Transportation

Transportation was repeatedly underscored as one of the major issues
faced by people with all types of disabilities. The public transportation
system in New Hampshire was described as practically nonexistent, particularly between towns or in the more rural areas. One woman who
advocates for this issue described the problem this way:

> The entire state of New Hampshire really ought to have mass trans-
> portation, period, especially for those who do not drive around. . . . It
> is a hell of a problem, period.

This self-advocate described strategies to advocate for change, such as
her participation in a federal hearing on transportation held in Maine. She
said nothing happened as a result of her efforts, partially because the
federal and state government tend to ignore problems ("This is true. They
have a tendency to ignore problems"). An op-ed article she wrote for *The
Monitor* is shown in Figure 5.1.

Transportation problems extend to getting to self-advocacy meetings
and to activities, including vacations. While the Lakes Region area agency
office, in particular, has been generous with the use of their vans, getting
access to this valuable commodity is not as easy as people would like. As
one self-advocate from the region described:

> We need to have those vans and if we need to have them, we've got
> to have them. . . . We can't force people to do that for us, but we need
> those vans. Because otherwise, we wouldn't be able to get to meet-
> ings, . . . we wouldn't be able to do our . . . dances, we wouldn't be
> able to get to places that we need to go.

The lack of one's own transportation can negate community recreation and
work as viable options ("Maybe there aren't a lot of recreational opportunities everywhere, but if you can't get there, it's almost a moot point
anyway"). One of the women at the state's independent living center
described the situation as follows:

FIGURE 5.1. One Self-Advocate's View of Transportation in New Hampshire

People with disabilities need buses on nights and weekends

By ROBERTA GALLANT
For The Monitor

Monitor Forum

Board of contributors

I am the secretary of the Concord Area Self-Advocacy Group. The purpose of this group is to advocate for ourselves and others with disabilities. All of our members have disabilities.

One issue we have in common is a need for public transporta-

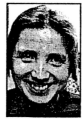

Gallant

tion. Concord is fortunate to have a bus system, but CAT needs to be more available than it is now.

The Concord Area Transit recently conducted a survey of its riders. Among other facts, the survey found out that 24 percent of the people who use the regular bus system own cars; nearly half use the system to get to work or to go shopping. Many others (42 percent) use the system to go to doctors' offices.

The Concord Area Self-Advocacy Group conducted its own survey on the problem of transportation. Here is what we learned:

• Two-thirds of us use the regular bus system. Only one of us uses the para-transit.

• One out of three members has a driver's license or access to a vehicle.

• One out of three members is working. Nearly half of us are looking for jobs.

• We all do our own shopping, and half of us use a laundromat to wash our clothes.

• A third of us have to get to places that aren't on the Concord Area Transit bus line.

• Two-thirds of us wish the bus could run at night, to 10 or 11 p.m.

• Three-quarters of us wish the bus

could run on weekends.

What does this mean?

For those of us who use the bus and are looking for work, our job choices are limited. We can't take night or weekend work, and we can't take a job in a place to which the bus doesn't go.

For those of us who are church-goers, we have to get rides to Sunday services. This can be difficult in bad weather or if we're in a new neighborhood or church.

For us, shopping is a problem on weekends or after work hours during the week. Washing and drying our clothes at the laundromat in time to get the last bus home is very difficult.

We need a transportation system that will give people with disabilities as much access to the community as drivers enjoy. We need a regular system that can be used by people in wheelchairs.

We need route maps, schedules and bus signs that are understandable, even if we have visual impairments or are non-readers. We need the bus drivers to assist us if we ask for help.

The bus system is good, but it could be much better than it is now for people with disabilities. It's not that we want special service from the transportation system. It's just that we want the same results that people without disabilities get.

(Roberta Gallant, a member of the Monitor's board of contributors, lives in Concord.)

Source: Gallant, R. (1993). "People with Disabilities Need Buses on Nights and Weekends." *The Concord Monitor,* April 13, p. B6.

Because there is none in the state, it pretty much means your own transportation, and that is either a van or a modified car. For some people, it even means a driver, and there is no funding in the state for that right now.

THE DEVELOPMENT OF SELF-ADVOCACY IN NEW HAMPSHIRE

In October 1984, the New Hampshire Developmental Disabilities Council, in cooperation with the Center on Human Policy at Syracuse University, sponsored a conference on self-advocacy, which was held on the seacoast. The conference inspired a young woman, who together with another woman case manager, recruited people for a self-advocacy group in the Laconia region. The group started about March 1985, mainly as a social group, and she became their advisor.

The Lakes Region self-advocacy group, described as the strongest in the state, has been meeting since then and has had a number of other advisors, including a man who was the pastor at Laconia State School and who then worked at New Hampshire State Hospital. One coadvisor previously was with Speaking for Ourselves from Pennsylvania, a nationally known self-advocacy group.

The New Hampshire Developmental Disabilities Council (DDC) was the springboard for a number of local groups that met statewide every month in the mid- to late 1980s. The project then faded on the state level until January 1990 when the council and the state ARC (previously the New Hampshire Association for Retarded Citizens) decided, at the request of an energetic young woman in Concord, to assist people to meet again.

A statewide conference was held in Manchester in June 1990, with over 100 self-advocates in attendance. As one advocate described the event, "It was amazing . . . messy, disorganized, and so powerful I couldn't believe it." All the presentations were given by self-advocates, including sessions on how to be an advisor, on how to start a self-advocacy group, and on understanding the Americans with Disabilities Act (ADA).

T. J. Monroe, a national leader in self-advocacy, was a guest speaker. He was described as very charismatic and able to energize the audience. Microphone time was set up afterward so people could discuss their own issues too. T. J. listened and gave a personal response, which was a very dynamic aspect of his presentation. Another keynote speaker was Ruth Sinkowitz-Mercer, from Massachusetts. One advocate described reactions to the presentation as follows:

> She talked about being . . . at Belchertown in Massachusetts and being written off. . . . People started standing up spontaneously in the

audience and saying this happened to me at Laconia State School. . . .
The bureaucrats like us, were just, jaws were dropping. It was just
very, very powerful listening to people share their experience and
needing to be validated, to have somebody listen and say, "Yes, I
understand where you are coming from."

After the first conference, a group of six self-advocates from three local
groups and three or four bureaucratic-type people met on a Saturday for a
"marathon" meeting. The group decided to have another conference,
assemble a "help team" to assist people in forming groups, and determine
if people needed leadership skills training, such as how to run meetings.
Though the help team had not yet materialized, the second conference was
being planned (and has since been held) and a newsletter was published.

The group also decided to ask about applying for a grant from the
Administration on Developmental Disabilities (ADD) in Washington, DC.
They made a videotape of a letter and sent it to the woman in charge
"because some people don't have writing skills and they decided everybody should have a chance to be included." As one eyewitness reported:

> So they started to put their own ideas together and added them in,
> and they came up with a draft letter. . . . Donna was reading sections
> of it, and she can read sort of well, but every once in awhile, she
> would come to a word she didn't know, and then there would be this
> kind of consultation. . . . And people would say s, i, t—I know what
> that word is. . . . It was wonderful.

The Commissioner of ADD responded and told them "it was fine" to go
ahead with the grant application. As one person said, "Wouldn't this be
amazing if this group of self-advocates puts a grant together and goes up
against this group of PhDs and comes away with it?"

Every fourth Saturday, local representatives continued to meet in Con-
cord. The group was now officially incorporated as People First of New
Hampshire, with a board of directors, voting and nonvoting members, and
a part-time executive coordinator. She was the previous advisor in the
Lakes Region, and her position was funded by the Association for Retarded
Citizens (ARC) through a grant from the Developmental Disabilities Council.

LOCAL SELF-ADVOCACY GROUPS

Local self-advocacy groups in New Hampshire have at least three basic
functions. The first is to provide opportunities for people to discuss issues
and problems, particularly in relationship to services. The second is to

provide opportunities for people to connect with others socially and personally. The third is to present opportunities for people to develop leadership and organizing skills.

Both the state and local groups consist of people with handicaps. In People First of New Hampshire, all the local groups come together and share ideas with one another. The groups are "mainly the same" in that all of the local groups like Laconia, Concord, Keene, and all the surrounding towns "are attached to the statewide group." However, groups vary from one another and can experience different trends through the years, as explained by one advisor:

> Sometimes we really focus on what our goals are, and sometimes we really talk about what is on people's minds in meetings. . . . And we've been most productive when we've listened to a person in a group meeting talk about some of the problems [he or she] might be having with staff, and the group tries to come up with resolutions for that person's problems, and the next month we ask what has transpired.

Social Activities

Social activities, such as dances, were an important part of the Laconia self-advocacy group's activities. Dances seem to have several different benefits: the enjoyment of the activity, the challenge of achieving a successful outcome through group effort, and fund-raising. The dances also form a part of the historical story of the group. The group's treasurer described their decision making about the last dance:

> We hired a group called the Boys to play for us. . . . They're terrific. . . . We went ahead and talked about these dances at our meetings. We talked about how we were going to do it, you know, who is going to buy what . . . who handles the money . . . who's going to help set up, who's going to decorate, that sort of thing . . . What we did; we all put our strength together.

Self-advocates go to dances for the same kinds of reasons that other people do, judging the dances by the same standards, such as how many people attended, if the music was good, and whom they met while there.

Activities of Local Groups

As described by the members, the Laconia group was also thinking about hosting a booth at the Plymouth craft fair in addition to the one they sponsored at the commemoration of the closing of Laconia. The group developed a telephone tree so that members could keep in touch with one another. Two group members also testified to the legislature about eliminating the waiting list, while others prepared together for presentations at the self-advocacy and case management conferences. The Laconia group publishes newsletters and meets with other groups that are forming to share some of its information with them.

Roles Within Groups

In the Laconia group, the officers, elected by the group's members, played a central role. The group has two chairpersons, both women, a secretary, a treasurer, and a gavel keeper. One chairperson described being in charge as a new experience for her:

> **B:** Well, I like being a cochairperson. I like being in charge. I didn't think I would, but I do like it, and they do listen.
>
> **JR:** What does it mean to be in charge?
>
> **B:** Oh, it means like being a boss, like in a job, someone in charge of other people, and just being in control.

Being a leader was equated in part with formal roles for this woman, though other characteristics were also associated with it. She might now be able to define herself as a leader, which was different from when she first started with the group.

As several members of the group explained the different roles, the treasurer "keeps the money and the bankbook and keeps you up to date on how much money is taken out for food . . . and how much money is put in." The secretary "does the flyers" for the dances and "new manuals." The group also has a "gavel keeper," which "is an important role for her," and yet another woman who organizes the refreshments.

Roles of Advisors and Supporters

For people familiar with self-advocacy, roles of advisors in these groups are often complex and challenging. Describing one of the talented advisors of the past seven years in New Hampshire, one advocate shared the following:

> She's thought hard and struggled with the role of the advisor, how to help people make decisions without making them yourself. I watched her in action. She'd be sitting on the edge of her chair, but waits until someone asks for help. She works at shutting up and not taking control.

This advisor, also the mother of two young children, was described by one of the women with disabilities as "a pretty nice person to talk to." In describing her own role, the advisor referred back to the self-advocacy conference she attended in 1984:

> I liked the way the advisors sat in the background and gave subtle clues whenever necessary. . . . I always tell them [people in the self-advocacy group] to shut me up when I talk too much, but whenever our local group is in a crunch, that's when I will step in and try to help guide them into a direction that seems meaningful to them, or when I am asked.

People in the self-advocacy group have their own ideas about what advisors do, and part of their role is viewed as overseeing or "keeping an eye on things," giving suggestions and working with people:

> An advisor is someone who . . . keeps an eye on things, making sure that . . . we don't spend too much. . . . I have an advisor working with me. He comes along with me when I go to the bank. He makes sure that we don't take out too much money.

An advisor keeps the group together and makes sure that people do not make mistakes or get off track. As one young man explained, the advisors are essential, help the group to avoid major problems, and keep people on important issues that can make a difference.

FUTURE ISSUES IN SELF-ADVOCACY

Self-advocacy was in its early stages in New Hampshire, more so than in some parts of the country. While immediate issues abound, such as formation of groups, issues of control, roles of advisors, and so forth, the interviews also raised some emerging areas, which are highlighted in the following research.

Can Everyone Speak for Themselves?

One of the questions informants were asked was what self-advocacy meant in the lives of people with very severe disabilities, who may not speak or move much or who may have very little ability to process information. One advocate described how she always tried to assume that people "have opinions, ideas," explaining that she "would rather be safe than sorry." She takes the position that "they have desires and needs and wishes and preferences," though sometimes people need to develop an ability to listen with more than their ears. She sees self-advocacy as approaching people in ways that support self-determination for everyone.

Family-Driven Service System and Self-Advocacy

People with disabilities involved with self-advocacy were not yet an active force in New Hampshire. Yet, the state was pushing toward a family-driven system, and the question of where adults with disabilities fit was not yet a crucial part of open discussion. As one reflective professional explained:

> This is practically heretical to say in this state at this point, but I happen to know that there are a substantial number of people who are probably living at home who don't want to live there. . . . I do not want resources to go to family support at the expense of even greater support needed for adults who are out on their own.

Parents may be reluctant for their children to move out of their home. As one independent living center staff member shared, "I think sometimes parents will take a risk or a chance for themselves, but they wouldn't necessarily sort of allow, which is a terrible word, but they wouldn't maybe create a situation where that young adult would perhaps want to take the same risk for [himself or herself]." The Lakes Region advisor was trying to find a way to reach teachers who could contact the parents to promote their son's or daughter's involvement in self-advocacy.

Self-Advocacy and Control of Money

Financial resources continued to flow into the systems, with only a small proportion of the money reaching the people for whom it was intended. In discussing the reasons why money was not given directly to consumers but to agencies instead, one administrator explained our lack of trust and need for control:

> People fear the lack of control. They'll do bad things, go buy booze, or something. The controls that we put through governmental social policies are more or less statements that we don't trust these people will make good judgments, and in fact, they may not. . . . And we'll have forty-five people to manage that 5,000 dollars.

The more immediate financial issue was the one faced by People First, which had funding on a six-month basis at the time of the last research visit. Describing a problem of all advocacy groups, the director said, "I want to make sure that the direction of People First isn't my direction,

[that] it is what the people want. . . . I've got to make sure that wherever I get my money, they don't have hidden agendas for People First too. That will be crucial."

The Disability of Mental Retardation

People with mental retardation, head injury, or any type of actual or perceived mental or cognitive disability are often stigmatized, including among other people with disabilities. There is a tendency for people to compare themselves to one another, and this happens even in rehabilitation hospitals, where people will construct a hierarchy based on disability.

People with mental retardation or mental illness face social and physical barriers every day, as illustrated by the following comments of a physically disabled woman:

> I don't actually feel disabled until I come upon a barrier. . . . My apartment's all accessible so I don't think about the fact that I'm in a wheelchair . . . until I get to a place [where] . . . there's stairs and I can't get in. But I would imagine that . . . if it is mental retardation or mental illness, and that the barrier is that . . . I run into this person in the lobby of my building every day [who is] always condescending to me. . . . That's a barrier you're faced with every day.

On the opposite side of the coin, people with mental retardation may view people in wheelchairs as the ones who need more help. As one man explained, "We're trying to make these people in wheelchairs feel like . . . they've done something, making them proud of themselves. And someday, live on their own."

NEW HAMPSHIRE'S GUARDIANSHIP PROGRAM

Since self-advocacy is tied closely to choices and decision making, the way in which guardianship operates remains intimately connected with a person's freedom. From the viewpoint of the program director who has been involved with the state program since the late 1970s and who has served as President of the National Guardianship Association, the New Hampshire program had a number of features that made it fairly unique among the states. These include (as presented in Table 5.1) the independent versus case management model of guardianship, use of a functional versus a medical definition of incapacity, and heavy reliance on limited instead of full guardianship, as well as other features to promote time-limited use of this alternative.

TABLE 5.1. Central Features of Guardianship in New Hampshire (1991)

Creation of the Independent Guardianship Program

The guardianship program was created by a lawsuit in which the state supreme court concluded that for people in an institution, specifically the state psychiatric hospital, or Laconia, who were incapacitated, the state must pay for and ensure provision of an independent guardian (when no family member is willing or able to be appointed). A separate independent corporation was established to provide both guardianship services and "less restrictive services" such as money management, representative payee, conservatorship, durable health care powers of attorney, and other surrogate functions.

Functional Definition of Incapacity

The law in New Hampshire specifically disregarded medical definitions and was interested solely in what a person could or could not do. This means instead of a finding of incapacity based on IQ or the presence of a certain disease or condition, the law was built around functional assessment. The law also required that a guardian be given authority only over the areas in which the person was actually incapacitated.

Limited versus Full Guardianships

In New Hampshire, about 90 percent of the guardianships were limited at the time of the study, whereas the director's experience in other states was that only 0 to 10 percent were limited. In New Hampshire, for people with developmental disabilities, whoever had the primary responsibility for providing services to the person (e.g., area agencies) also had the responsibility of determining whether a guardianship petition should be filed. The two key factors for filing for guardianship were that a severe incapacity existed and that incapacity had to lead to the likelihood of harm.

Independent versus Case Management Model of Guardianship

In New Hampshire, according to the state law, no one who worked with a person on an individual professional level could be a guardian. When public guardians were used, for example, when family members were unavailable or inappropriate due to abuse, guardians were prevented by law from providing services. The guardian was considered free to be a decision maker instead of a case manager to the extent that feasible conflicts of interest were minimized. Three common concerns were (1) the use of the person's money to control his or her actions; (2) different rules of service providers and foster families not located in the same communities; (3) guardians who treat people like children and continually ask people to prove themselves and act according to the guardians' standards instead of their own.

Source: Racino, J. (1993a). "A Qualitative Study of Self-Advocacy and Guardianship: Views from New Hampshire." In *An Edited Collection on Community Integration and Deinstitutionalization in New Hampshire.* Syracuse, NY: Community and Policy Studies.

Changes in "Guardianship World"

At the time of the 1970s' *Garrity v. Gallen* legal actions, a large number of guardianship petitions were filed, partially because some people had been subjected to a lot of abuse in the institution and may even have been abandoned by their families, who relinquished all responsibility for their sons or daughters. Compared to other groups, people with developmental disabilities are now a smaller proportion of the caseload of the Office of the Public Guardian, and it continues to decrease as years go by.

Most of the changes in the "guardianship world" were coming from the population of vocal elders who used grassroots legislative advocacy to force legislators to look at these issues. Especially as people started to live longer and tended to die of chronic as opposed to acute illnesses, guardianship issues potentially can affect everyone. Recent changes that occurred, such as in money management programs, though targeted at elders, could also positively affect people with developmental disabilities or mental health labels.

CONCLUSION

Whether viewed through the lens of self-advocacy, through the decisions and concerns of people with disabilities, or through the efforts to limit guardianship intrusion in people's lives, this case study suggests that, in New Hampshire, the future roles of people with disabilities in their own lives are still largely unknown, probably more so than in any other area (see Table 5.2). The following illustrates the course that was being traveled in New Hampshire, with the bend still not turned in the road:

> The change occurs because you are traveling along a road, as a metaphor, and every step you take changes the horizon because you are looking at it from a different place. That's how it occurs. You cover a stretch of road; you look up and say, "I didn't know the river was down there. . . . Maybe I better get ready to fjord it." And then you travel a little further and maybe you cross the river and say, "Oh my gosh, there are mountains up there. It's going to be cold up there, and I'll need to find a way through the mountains." That's how it happens.

TABLE 5.2. Relationships and Advocacy: An Excerpt from the Story of Josie and Jessica

I like her. I don't know why people like the people they like. She embodies and is affected in her life by things that people like me don't see coming when we are in the middle of social change. They hit people like Jessica right in the middle. . . . We spent ten years planning for Laconia, but for Jessica, it happened in the space of a morning.

Josie, state advocate, 1991

In describing her relationship with Jessica, whom she met at the Laconia State School (See Chapters 3 and 4), this advocate reflects on her own roles, on how Jessica changed her life, and what the future might hold. Josie, who was working as a case advocate [who would visit Laconia], met Jessica when she came up to her and said, "Are you the lady who gets people out of here?" And as Josie explained, "We've been friends ever since."

Jessica and her older sister spent about twenty-three and a half years at Laconia, having arrived there as young children. As Josie explained, "She re-members very vividly her mother giving her her favorite toys and packing them up, taking them there, and having them all taken away from her. . . . She re-members being exploited for her labor."

Moving to the community also was not easy for Jessica, to the point where Josie experienced terrible guilt and anguish, questioning whether what she did was the right thing. Jessica was so unhappy her first five years, facing changing rules ("like [she] grew up in Tibet and [you] dropped her in Times Square"). There was a lot to deal with all at once, "and we just kind of dumped it in her lap and said deal with it."

Over time, Josie's and Jessica's relationship evolved, as disagreements occurred without the loss of the friendship. This climaxed in a situation in which Josie tried "six ways from Sunday" to dissuade Jessica in her personal decision. And finally, Josie decided to try to find a way to support [Jessica's decision, while disagreeing with it]. Josie explained it was a matter of develop-ing faith and trust [in Jessica], and for Jessica [to believe] that Josie would not leave because of her decision.

Source: Excerpt from Racino, J. (1993f). *Monograph on Deinstitutionalizaton and Community Integration in New Hampshire.* Syracuse, NY: Community and Policy Studies, draft, pp. 42-43.

Note: Changes in brackets based upon review by Josie, 1998.

Chapter 6

People Working Together:
Local Control, Health Care Financing,
Federal Regulations, and State Policy

Julie Ann Racino

The issue, to me, that stood out is people working together. Here in New Hampshire, and as I have seen elsewhere, there is a strong potential for fragmenting philosophies and directions and a strong antagonism that can come from that. . . . We had the potential, but it didn't happen.

Robert Schultz, New Hampshire State Director

INTRODUCTION

Working together throughout the course of this decade's development of the community services system, New Hampshire has had a remarkable consistency in state administration, regional services, and other parent and advocacy leadership in the area of developmental disabilities. This "enormous consistency" has allowed people to "learn from each other" and to "build trust" in a way that "became a very self regenerating process."

This chapter highlights two key milestones in the development of the New Hampshire community service system: the concept of the area agen-

This chapter is a modified version of Racino, J. (1993a). "Critical Structural Features in Community Services Development." In *An Edited Collection on Community Integration and Deinstitutionalization in New Hampshire.* Syracuse, NY: Community and Policy Studies. See Appendix B for research methodology. All names used in the book chapter are pseudonyms unless otherwise indicated.

cies and the use of the Medicaid Home and Community-Based Services
(HCBS) waiver program, a major federal financing source for community
services. Combined together, these features have aided the development of
the community system from the 1970s, facilitating community integration
and deinstitutionalization. The final section of this chapter compares two
frameworks for thinking about regulations.

As with all retrospective accounts, history is remembered somewhat
differently by each person who participates in its making, partially dependent on factors such as her or his role, personality, and the nature and level
of involvement. Presented from the perspectives of Robert Schultz, a state
director, George Leskin, a middle manager, and Tom Bradon, the Medicaid waiver manager, this case study is particularly meant to be shared
with those working within or with state government in creating positive
change in the lives of people with disabilities.

AREA AGENCIES:
THE REGIONAL STRUCTURES
AND LOCAL COMMUNITIES

The area agencies, as a milestone event, as a policy construct, have
been fundamental. I wouldn't change it much at all.

Robert Schultz, New Hampshire Commissioner (1991)

What I was really interested in, really wanted a commitment to, was
the concept of area agencies, the concept of a private, nonprofit
system of providing services external to the state system because I
really wanted to see if that could work.

George Leskin, New Hampshire State Administrator (1991)

The twelve area agencies in New Hampshire (see Figure 6.1) are nonprofit corporations designated to provide services for individuals with
developmental disabilities in each region of the state. An area agency is
the organization that receives funds from the state division for providing
services (either directly or through vendors/contract agencies) in areas
such as case management, residential, employment, habilitation, and family support, and for conducting an internal quality assurance program. Each
area agency is governed by a board of directors and is subject to redesigna-
tion by the Division of Mental Health and Developmental Services (DMH/
DS) every four years. State program specialists are the liaisons between

FIGURE 6.1. Area Agencies in the State of New Hampshire

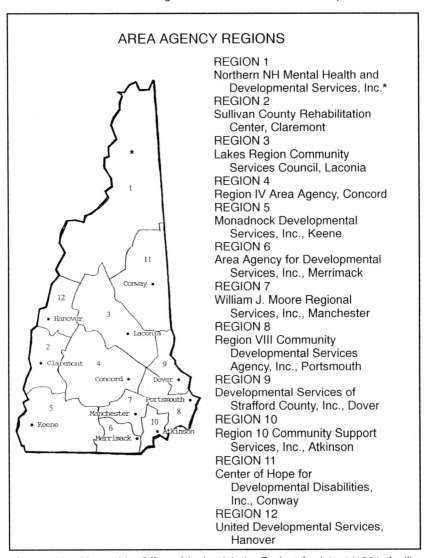

AREA AGENCY REGIONS

REGION 1
Northern NH Mental Health and
    Developmental Services, Inc.*
REGION 2
Sullivan County Rehabilitation
    Center, Claremont
REGION 3
Lakes Region Community
    Services Council, Laconia
REGION 4
Region IV Area Agency, Concord
REGION 5
Monadnock Developmental
    Services, Inc., Keene
REGION 6
Area Agency for Developmental
    Services, Inc., Merrimack
REGION 7
William J. Moore Regional
    Services, Inc., Manchester
REGION 8
Region VIII Community
    Developmental Services
    Agency, Inc., Portsmouth
REGION 9
Developmental Services of
    Strafford County, Inc., Dover
REGION 10
Region 10 Community Support
    Services, Inc., Atkinson
REGION 11
Center of Hope for
    Developmental Disabilities,
    Inc., Conway
REGION 12
United Developmental Services,
    Hanover

Source: New Hampshire Office of the Legislative Budget Assistant (1991, April). New Hampshire Developmental Disabilities Services Performance Audit. Concord, NH: Author, p. 96.

* Region 1's main office is located in Conway, part of Region 11.

the area agencies and the state office, and regular statewide meetings were held in Concord.

Brief History

The area agencies were first authorized in law as single points of entry (into service systems) in 1979 and became operational by 1983. However, none formally came into existence until 1981 when the state division was mandated, through the *Garrity v. Gallen* court order, to establish these agencies in accordance with the law (New Hampshire Office of the Legislative Budget Assistant, 1991). Summaries from case studies of two area agencies are presented in Tables 6.1 and 6.2.

The area agencies may have been the brainchild of one of the early division directors who believed in the private, nonprofit sector. The concept seemed to have two central aspects: a single, fixed point of referral and the need for a new entity to minimize altercations among the different competing groups. The area agency concept required an area board with family membership with groups of citizens forming boards that would develop regional services.

Because of the nature of community development during the early years, the area agencies developed in a fragmented way, piece by piece, as funding and other resources became available. The Developmental Disabilities Act and the federal dollars that came with it were "really big money" at the time "equal to or greater than the community services budget." Robert explained how the community services system came "on line":

> They had to turn to their communities and put on-line a community service system. . . . [It was] like going out in the cold with one boot, one sock, a hat, three gloves, and a coat because that was what we could fund this year and you really need[ed] more. . . . So they had to . . . deliver on a very spotty development concept and make it work. . . . They did a great job of it.

The regional boundaries were determined partly by natural geographic ones and partly by political compromise based on the existing relationships between directors.

Action for Independence was the key state planning document that guided community development and included the definitions of area agencies, program models, planning principles and process, and budgets. Consultants assisted in restructuring the community service system through a systematic and conscientious planning process that included public forums and intensive interviewing. About 1983, the area agencies and division

TABLE 6.1. Monadnock Developmental Services: Region 5, New Hampshire

---

This region was visited because it was described as having the best examples of supported employment in the state of New Hampshire, serving, for example, in 1986, as one of the area agencies selected for the development of community employment. The case study report of the region,* which served about 350 people with a $6.5 million budget in the southwestern part of the state, highlighted the following factors associated with the change process toward integrated employment:

- *Workshop closure.* As of summer 1992, the region had disbanded their two sheltered workshops.
- *RFP (request for proposal) process.* All community service providers needed to submit proposals and interview to obtain contracts, resulting in three providers defunded and five remaining providers in the region.
- *Performance review and quality assurance.* Developed jointly with the area agency, these reports are reviewed by outside consultants three or four times a year.
- *Money tied to people.* Interpreted as a fee-for-service system whereby day and residential service agencies will only be paid for units of services provided.
- *Person-centered planning and individualized job placement.* Each of the three agencies visited described a commitment to "individualized job placements" and center planning around "getting to know the person and learning about their dreams."
- *Natural supports.* All agencies said they had an orientation toward natural supports, which was described as the term used to mean "support provided by job site personnel and/or other non–human service people."
- *School-to-work transition.* Described as relatively new for school and adult agencies to work together to facilitate movement of students from school to postschool work and living.
- *Providing only work-related supports versus other support.* Emphasis was to keep the focus on employment, including marketing, though two agencies were required to serve people six hours a day.

---

* For the case study report on this region, see Rogan, P. (1992). *Integrated Employment for All.* Syracuse, NY: Syracuse University, Center on Human Policy, Research and Training Center on Community Integration.

came together at the University of New Hampshire and developed a mission statement for the system. Every area agency board adopted the mission statement, though sometimes incorporating changes within its framework. As one state administrator explained, "It really helped us be really consistent and to measure ourselves and our programs against what our vision of the future was going to be like for people with developmental disabilities."

TABLE 6.2. Deinstitutionalization to Support: Region 6, New Hampshire

This region was nominated for study because it was considered to be one of the strongest in the state, especially in relationship to case management, family support services, and quality assurance.* Region 6 encompasses the cities of Nashua and Merrimac and, in 1991, served 400 people with a budget of $9 million. According to the case study report, the following are examples of key regional practices:

Case management
- Use of action plans instead of standard use of the ISP (individual service plan) meeting for people who dislike this process.
- Use of beeper for case management availability and efforts to develop backup supports with vendor organizations.
- Use of an advocacy orientation for a person with disabilities by case managers in instances of disagreement or conflict with vendors and/or the person's parents.
- Redefinition of the job as a benefits technician.
- Assisting people who have developmental disabilities and mental health labels residing in mental health institutions.

Family support services
- Approximately 200 families receiving family support with no waiting list.
- Use of family support advisory council, family liaisons, recreational links, parent-to-parent programs and respite.
- Approximately ninety children in out-of-district placements in residential facilities or schools targeted to be brought back home.

Development of individualized supports
- Options being pursued for people with "severe" disabilities include
    a. assisting people to rent or purchase a house and live with non-paid roommates and additional staff support;
    b. assisting people to live on their own, in a rented or purchased house, with drop-in staff support; and
    c. assisting people to share someone else's home.
- Decrease in amount of property owned by the area agency; change in expectations of vendor agencies.
- Assisting people to make choices about where they want to live and with whom.
- Financing of homeownership and regular use of Section 8.
- Planning with families to develop options, including taking on the roles of vendor and case manager.

Quality assurance
- Based on the "five accomplishments" drawn from the normalization principles—(1) community presence, (2) protection of rights and promotion of personal interests, (3) competence development, (4) status improvement, and (5) community participation.

* For the case study report on the region, see Walker, P. (1992), *From Deinstitutionalization to Supporting People in Their Own Homes in Region 6, New Hampshire.* Syracuse, NY: Syracuse University, Research and Training Center on Community Integration, Center on Human Policy.

However, state officials recognized that creating a system that worked solely on a system basis, without recognition of the people involved, was not possible. As George expressed, "It is the leadership and personalities that make it work the way that it works." Robert referred to these ethereal qualities when describing another major turning point in the state:

> We got a commitment to, and a trust of, a more integrative life in the service system. And again there were certain individuals who really made that happen, who really saw it, who felt how it could be. . . . We had come along far enough that we could take the flight of imagination and belief that was required in really seeing what a person's life could be.

Local Control: Regional Differences and Community Ties

The regional system worked in New Hampshire because it was based upon strong feelings and beliefs within the state regarding local control and the role of state government. As one longtime observer and participant shared, "I think, in New Hampshire, that idea of local control, that concept or set of feelings around it is actually real." For New Hampshire, a regional system controlled by the state would not have worked well because there is a strong conservative tendency to resist centralization. As he continued, "It was very important that local people felt as though it was a local entity that was doing it." County systems would have been difficult because they "are too small to base the system on."

The area agencies have their roots in the local communities and "they really have pretty successfully managed to mobilize their communities to get community people involved and to be identified with the community." Strategies included inviting the "movers and shakers" of the communities to be on their boards and weaving their presence into the political fabric of the community." Within the state, other administrators, parents, and disability leaders refer to regions by the first name of the director.

Local control, however, resulted in a range of regional differences in how things were done, partially dependent upon the director of the area agency. The state office encouraged this sense of local control, even with its variability, setting parameters to help agencies move together in a general direction. From the state perspective, these local ties had numerous advantages, including resource development, overcoming community opposition and meeting the court order, and protection for the administrators in the central office.

The area agencies were responsible for meeting the goals in the court order, and they did so, often over considerable community opposition.

Although two major cases on zoning issues were in the Supreme Court, Tom Bradon said, "We haven't had any resistance to a group home or a place where people live since 1986." The area agencies developed and retained formal and informal relationships with "the town fathers," the president of the bank, and other community members. These local political ties could be called upon to assist with issues on the state level.

State-Area Agency Relationships: The Tension That Makes It Work

Maintaining the tension in the relationship between the state division and the area agencies was credited as being the critical aspect that "makes it work." This tension meant that relationships often needed to be negotiated. As one state bureaucrat said, "Maybe if you know that everything needs to be negotiated, you act differently." Due to the quasi-public–quasi-private nature of the area agencies, they have many of the advantages of close policy implementation that regional authorities offer, as well as community ownership of the board of directors.

From a funding perspective, the area agencies were, and are, dependent upon the state division for their resources. ("They were ours, really we owned them. We were their funding source 100 percent or equivalent of.") Yet, they had to be private, nonprofit, and independent. As Robert shared:

> They had to have the ability to say to their communities, "No, [We are] not the state telling you to do this; [We're] the families and the business leaders and the interested parties in here telling you this is what the community needs. . . . This has proven to be an extremely powerful mechanism, powerful legislatively, politically, locally, at the state level, powerful in telling us [the state office] we need to do things differently.

The two major sources of power and control held by the state in relationship to the area agencies were "the power of the purse" and quality assurance evaluation activities. Such power enabled the state to influence both the area agency directors and their boards.

However, state administrators preferred area agencies to view the central office as much more than a funding and oversight agency, as more of a collaborative endeavor. The state office tries to provide a clear message ("we want community integration") and uses money, regulations, and "nurturing" as a support to the message. The human side of why the area agency structure works means an investment in shared responsibility for outcomes in the community and of finding ways of working together to overcome the human tendencies to blame, to throw one's weight around, or to demand one's own way.

When problems occur in the regions, instead of passing on the problem to the state office and expecting it to resolve the issue, "We all work on solutions together." Problem solving became the way work was done, not trying to transfer or to fix responsibility as solely that of the region or of the state office. A cohesiveness was maintained that allowed area agencies and the state government to feel they were part of the same effort. As Robert expressed it:

> They are ours and we were theirs, and even though they are private agencies, not state government, that made no difference. And the fact [that] that made no difference is extremely important, that sense of ownership.

Strengths and Disadvantages of the System

As with any system, area agency structures have a number of disadvantages. In addition to regional variability, as a question of fairness and equity, these include the lack of control to "order" changes, the determination of eligibility by nonprofits, and the monitoring of case management.

Officials from other states really did not believe that this area agency structure design was a good idea. Their concerns were primarily about the loss of control of the waiting list and the inability to order something to get done as one might with a state case manager or a state agency. Thus, from a systems management perspective, there were serious flaws that "made them apprehensive about if it would work or not." Because placements could not be ordered by the state into the community as it could with Laconia, a constant negotiation process was required. This meant placements now needed to be done by problem solving, looking at other resources, "sweetening the pot," and "massaging almost everybody that is at risk, almost on a daily basis" which makes it "a very difficult system to run."

The area agency structure, from the state viewpoint, has at least four other advantages than those described previously. First, state systems generally seem to be inflexible regarding adaptation to change. Second, when budget reductions occur, the tendency is always to reduce the contract side to maintain funding for state employee resources. By setting up a system that does not place the private community sector in competition with the state community sector, the occurrence of such biased competition for resources is reduced. Third, the area agency structure creates a tension between state and local levels that helps to monitor the waiting list and does not allow the system to deteriorate. In essence, this is a version of the governmental checks and balances with the area agencies. Finally, when merged with the Medicaid Home and Community-Based Services waiver program, it becomes a powerful system that allows flexibility and creativity, while still fostering stability of financial resources.

MEDICAID HOME AND COMMUNITY-BASED SERVICES WAIVER: FEDERAL FINANCING OF COMMUNITY SERVICES

I think the two real critical pieces of developing communities [were] the area agency and . . . the community care waiver. Neither one of those really worked well without the other.

George Leskin, State Administrator (1991)

Brief Overview: New Hampshire Medicaid Waiver

Simply stated, a community service system would not exist in New Hampshire without the Medicaid Home and Community-Based Services waiver program (see also Congressional Research Service [CRS], 1993, pp. 371-424). According to George Leskin, Medicaid funded $55 million of the total system, with $47 to 48 million in waiver money for services for individuals. This represented about 60 percent of the total revenues in the system, including state and federal funds, client fees, and other income. The federal and state shares were both 50 percent. (For an update on Medicaid financing by state, see Braddock et al., 1995.)

The New Hampshire waiver basically funded three kinds of services: residential or personal care, day habilitation (includes adult day activities and client support), and case management services. The rate structure was five tiered, with the range being from $35 to $191 a day. Rates were prior authorized based on a combination of the needs of the people and the way the services were organized because the most handicapped are not necessarily the most expensive per se. Cost has as much to do with the way services are organized as anything else.

Compared to other states, more of New Hampshire's services were bundled under the waiver that DMH/DS managed than in the state Medicaid plan. The state planned to add some services in 1992 which were common in other waivers—respite, family support, and architectural modifications—and which were previously paid for only through state funds.

The area agencies were the only designated providers of waiver services in their regions.

As Tom Bradon, the Medicaid waiver manager, described, the ongoing "partnership" with Medicaid in Boston had been a real strength, especially "their willingness to talk with us, to listen to what it is we want to do, and their willingness to kind of allow us to do what makes sense for the people served in the system." This communication flow was critical because formal amendments were made to the waiver almost every year to reflect changes in the costs or ways that services were provided in New Hampshire.

One of the greatest strengths of the Medicaid waiver program was that it was flexible enough to change as services, philosophies and other developments have occurred in the field. As George Leskin, a very strong proponent of the waiver, stressed:

> The issue of the waiver is really important because what the Medicaid waiver really [is] is it's a waiver of the ICF/MR Medicaid rules and regulations. . . . It is very important that we continue to keep the concept of a Medicaid waiver.

The waiver, for example, was flexible enough to allow for homes of any size to be set up, and over the years, this meant more homes for one, two, or three people, for example, as George continued:

> Many agencies that operate eight-bed models that we used to run are breaking those up or have broken those up and now have eight one-person placements. . . . And they're no longer thinking of people as a group.

Individual placements were considered to be a positive development since they accommodated more individual lifestyles, promoted more natural rhythms of the family, more flexibility for the person, and more choice in where people live. As the Medicaid waiver liaison stated:

> People live in families; people live with roommates; people live by themselves with support brought in as needed. They may live with friends, friends who may have a disability or not. Some people live in [homes of] four [or] six; we do have some eight-bed residences still. People live in apartments, condos, townhouses, homes, all kinds of places.

From at least the mid 1980s, the waiver had served people with characteristics similar to people at Laconia or New Hampshire State Hospital. It seemed to provide sufficient support and flexibility for service providers to serve anybody at any level in the community. As several people explained, the waiver was "absolutely critical in closing Laconia." (See Chapters 3 and 4.)

The major limitation of the waiver had been the restrictions placed on paying for supported employment for those who were not previously institutionalized (Smith and Gettings, 1991). Most of the other perceived weaknesses came from adapting to changes in service provision that occurred within the state in service provision (e.g., increase in reserve bed days allowable so that people could spend more time at home with their families).

Generating the New Hampshire state match to the five-year waiver renewal remained a challenge. With their last renewal, George Leskin said, "For the first time, we can pay family members to provide supports in the home. It is a big step in rethinking our entitlement to services under the Medicaid waiver in New Hampshire." In part, because of the waiver renewal, which "to us was really life and death," New Hampshire did not apply for the Community Supported Living Arrangements, instead using their state match money for the waiver program (Smith and Gettings, 1994).

Intermediate Care Facilities (ICFs) for People with Mental Retardation (MR) in New Hampshire

New Hampshire never invested greatly in the ICF/MR program compared to other states (see CRS, 1993, pp. 63-66; Lakin et al., 1991). In 1992, New Hampshire had fifty-eight ICF/MR beds at seven different locations, representing a total of $4.5 million. The certificate of need process for ICF/MRs and nursing homes had always been subject to the local planning process, with any new ICF/MRs controlled, regulated, and authorized by the Division of Mental Health and Developmental Services through the commissioner's office. As the state director explained, this meant that "private providers elsewhere could not just come in and set up business and operate in the future."

As an effort to serve people with the most severe medical needs who were institutionalized, around 1986, three units were built, one a ten-bed for people with severe medical disabilities near Dartmouth Medical School (reduced from the original plan of twenty-four) and two six-bed ICF/MRs for people with challenging behaviors. Within two years, providers began moving away from even the few ICF/MRs, examining alternatives in the community that might be better. For example, some individuals with medical needs moved into the homes of staff members, following modification of the homes and vans for accessibility.

Another institution, a pediatric facility for children in the southwestern part of the state, started by families in the 1950s, was an enrolled Medicaid provider and not under contract with the state Division of Mental Health and Developmental Services. As family supports increased to keep children at home, the provider started marketing the facility regionwide in the Northeast. The area agency has been working instead to try to show families different choices of where their children can live. As George explained:

> And last year, one of the kids, [who] . . . had been living there for ten years came home and lived with a supportive foster family. And after six months, [the child] is now moved back with her natural family, where the child hasn't been for eleven years. And the family's doing remarkably well. And the child is just blossoming and is back in public schools.

New Hampshire has continued to adapt their financing to match their goals for community life for families and their children with disabilities.

Comparing Waivers and ICF/MRs: An Administrator's Perspective

The ICF/MR funding has been preferred by some providers due to its dependability and cost reimbursement, with the Medicaid waiver being viewed as more cost-effective. Basically, with ICFs, the provider had a basic budget for the year that would not vary based on the actual number of people served (e.g., in an institution, whether there were 50, 75, or 100 people, it did not matter; you had a budget for 100). With the New Hampshire Medicaid waiver, services were provided for the agreed-upon amount, and the rates could vary by individual, whereas in the institution, the same rate applied to each person. A state official shared the following example:

> My friend Ray . . . has gone into his own apartment with some little supports, and he is very comfortable and happy doing that. But when he was at Laconia, his rate was like $200 a day, and his rate in the community now is probably $20 to $25 a day.

It was not until the waiver was approved and being implemented that "we [the state] began to see how important it was to have area agencies."

Area agencies were reimbursed by Medicaid after they performed the service, which, at times, required the capacity to borrow money. The state itself did not have the capacity to operate in this way ("an impossibility"). The area agencies were in the position of needing to carry funding or to have an agency line of credit as part of the regular process. So the area agencies provided the capacity within the system to make it work that the state agency alone could not do. As the state administrator explained, "The capacity to be flexible and to do what other businesses do . . . is really important in a community services system."

Medicaid and Active Treatment

The Medicaid ICF/MR concept of active treatment (CRS, 1993, p. 875) has proved to be an impediment and has carried over into other community programs, including areas such as Part H (early intervention with children and families). As George Leskin continued, active treatment presumes a "deficiency view of the individual" and "keeps you focused on the dependency and the deficits rather than . . . the capacities." The waivers were not as oriented toward deficits, active treatment, and therapeutic services as the ICF/MR model. They thus allowed greater ability to focus on capacities and to help the individual develop his or her competencies living in the community.

One state administrator explained, in a research study of people who left or stayed at Laconia State School conducted in 1985 for the state office of New Hampshire, "we were able to demonstrate for severely disabled people in a matched comparison sample" that the people "on the community side . . . gained more in their adaptive skills . . . than the active treatment side." In other words, even if people received less occupational, physical, and speech therapy (the foundations of active treatment) than their counterparts, and instead participated in supported employment, reasonable living situations, and recreation, they gained in their adaptive behaviors and decreased in maladaptive ones.

Active treatment was tied closely with the old "train and place" model of services and became an end in itself. As this administrator explained, if you place the person and then "do what you need to do, it is only rarely something to do with therapies, and it is more to helping people adjust, getting them the support, [and] helping employers." He shared this story about a young man who had been both at Laconia and at a mental health hospital:

> He's still at Bonanza. He still works there. On an active treatment basis, we never would have been able to work with him. . . . And we

would have tried to make sure his behaviors were appropriate before we took him to Bonanza, and he never would have made it.

Active treatment added to the escalating costs of Medicaid, with federal requirements for more staff and therapies, with a state match required by the financing mechanism. The Medicaid waivers represent, in some ways, a concrete step toward the direction of Medicaid reform, including a reduction in unnecessary, medicalized expenses and restrictiveness.

REGULATIONS: THE FEDERAL/STATE ROLES

I think that the answer to Medicaid expenditures is to continue to move in the direction of individualization, of local and family community supports, and of reducing the unnecessary restrictions around fire safety codes, other kinds of codes.

George Leskin, State of New Hampshire Administrator (1991)

The basic approach to regulation on the federal level, particularly with Medicaid, tended to be to control risk through regulations. The effect on human life can be that requirements and regulations take away the everyday risks of living and that more money is spent on issues that do not substantively improve the life quality of people with disabilities. Another problem with the tendency to use regulations as the primary mechanism to ensure or promote quality is their cost. Money is spent primarily on meeting the rules and standards, without necessarily offering any benefit to the people with disabilities who are involved in the programs, but with increased costs to the taxpayers. Sometimes the costs become so great that federal programs fall of their own weight, which can actually be to the benefit of people with disabilities. As George Leskin continued:

They try to write in so many protections for a very limited amount of money that the cost of the protections eats up the money that states agree to participate.

Such regulations result in increased resources being placed into monitoring, starting a cycle of rule development whereby creativity is slowly eroded within the systems and more and more regulatory bureaucracy develops. As a state administrator, George Leskin supported regulations that help to develop community norms, not control from the state level. More important, in this framework, regulations are considered basically a misdirected response to the problems of quality in community life. Instead of placing more specific requirements and increasing costs, sometimes other fundamental changes are necessary, such as moving away from outmoded service delivery patterns such as nursing homes. As George Leskin continued:

> The issue is not how to straighten the nursing homes out by putting more regulations on nursing homes. What we should do is stop sending people to nursing homes, provide supports in their homes and their families and support for them. . . . We pay more and more money for more professionalized services in environments that don't help people.

Ways of Thinking About Standards

Regulations cut across all areas of life wherever abuse or perceived abuse can take place. Particularly when an evident injustice has occurred, the tendency is to create a standard to try to stop it from happening again. Another way to think about standards and regulations is to use a similar philosophy and approach to that taken with families. The underlying basic assumption is that a family is, or has the potential to be a good and loving family. Standards thus serve the function of facilitating problem solving at the community and family levels instead of dictating solutions through the application of rules. It is important to develop the belief that people can be assured safety more through relationships than through regulations.

Regulations presume that the best solutions can be predetermined without intimate knowledge of particular situations. The more complex and changeable these issues become, such as with the nature of human lives, the less this assumption may hold true.

Regulations tend to focus on prohibiting certain behaviors or actions when what is often necessary is to facilitate positive actions, allowing people to "do the right thing." This perspective is based on the belief that people at the operational level have the capacity and willingness to "do the right thing" with support. Regulations are increased by the desire for consistency across regions. The New Hampshire State Legislature also tended to demand greater specificity. One example of an effort to move away from rigid standards was in the area of family support; regulations were rewritten to be more user friendly and then criticized "because they didn't have enough body to them, and too much decision making was placed on the part of the family support councils instead of telling them what they needed to do."

The issue of outdated standards is a constant problem that is practically inherent within any rapidly changing field. As George Leskin explained, "The . . . [quality assurance] people are out there trying to regulate the programs on the [existing] standards, and our programs jump beyond the standards all the time."

George called fighting bureaucracies an ongoing battle that must be fought with vigilance on a daily basis. The tendency is toward standardization and toward pushing decisions up the hierarchy. As he explained:

> So . . . one thing we continue to fight against is overregulation at the central office level and to leave decision making to the lower level of the people who are actually doing the work, who know what needs to be done. We've done an adequate job of holding our own, but the press of bureaucracy to make cookie cutters out of programs is overwhelming. . . . You simply have to fight it every day.

He assesses their efforts in New Hampshire as successful, although, as with other states, "it is an ongoing battle, and I think a major, major battle that needs to be fought in . . . [every] state."

CONCLUSION

These New Hampshire state administrators shared a number of lessons from their extensive experience in developing a community service system from its fledgling beginnings a decade ago. These included the following:

- The importance of local control, the development of a sense of community ownership, and the mobilization of community resources.
- The role that intermediary structures play in allowing the necessary flexibility to meet individual circumstances.
- The need for a changing role of government as the role of family members increases.
- The flexibility and cost-effectiveness of the Medicaid waiver in moving from institutional to community life.
- The continuing programmatic and cost issues with the implementation of the outdated concept of active treatment.
- The role of negotiation, collaboration, and checks and balances between state and regional levels.
- The effect of regulations on the life quality of individuals with disabilities and on the use of limited resources.

Whether examined from a structural, philosophical, practical, or a personal perspective, New Hampshire's experiences form a base for comparative discussion in other states that face similar issues.

Chapter 7

"People Want the Same Things We All Do": The Story of the Area Agency in Dover, New Hampshire

Julie Ann Racino

> We share a similar vision: People belong in the community—[to] live, work, play, get married, have children—and our role is to provide the support for people to do the things they want to do. It is taken for granted that they want the same things that we do.
>
> Director, Developmental Services
> for Strafford County, Incorporated

INTRODUCTION

Developmental Services for Strafford County, Incorporated (DSSC), is located in southeastern New Hampshire about an hour from the Atlantic

This chapter is based on a qualitative research site visit conducted on October 22 to 24, 1991, to document good practices, issues, and dilemmas in the state of New Hampshire. The preparation of this document was supported, in part, by the U.S. Department of Education, National Institute on Disability and Rehabilitation Research (NIDRR), under Cooperative Agreement H133B00003-90 awarded to the Center on Human Policy, Syracuse University. A partial version of this chapter appeared in *Network News* in New Zealand, 1994, 4(1), pp. 8-13. The opinions expressed herein are solely those of the author and do not necessarily reflect the position of the U.S. Department of Education; therefore, no official endorsement should be inferred.

This chapter is a modified version of Racino, J. (1992b). *People Want the Same Things We All Do: The Story of the Area Agency in Dover, New Hampshire.* Syracuse, NY: Syracuse University, Center on Human Policy, Research and Training Center on Community Integration. See Appendix B for research methodology. All names of people used in this chapter are pseudonyms.

Ocean and Boston, in a county of over 100,000 people. It is one of twelve area agencies in the strongly Republican state of New Hampshire. The county has three major cities: Dover, Rochester, and Somersworth, and is also near the University of New Hampshire and its neighboring town of Durham. Founded in 1982 when very few community services existed in the state, the agency supported 180 people with developmental disabilities in the community. Nominated as having some of the best examples of supportive living in the state, in 1991, of the sixty people supported by the agency's residential services, fifty-five were living in their own places. As the director explained, the agency's agenda is to support the "same kind of valuable things in the lives of people with disabilities—friends, family, home, and work—as all of us want."

BRIEF HISTORY

In 1982, DSSC first developed day supports for people with developmental disabilities who were living at home with their families. This was followed in August 1983 by the opening of their first group home, with five people, four from the state institution at Laconia and one from New Hampshire Hospital. From the beginning, DSSC served people with severe disabilities, which was considered by staff members to be "one of the good decisions."

In 1987 to 1988, the people in the agency started planning for the changes that would be made to achieve the agency's agenda. During this period, values-based training was also considered fundamental, with many staff attending PASS (Program Analysis of Service Systems) and PASSING (Program Analysis of Service Systems' Implementation of Normalization Goals), which are based on the principles of normalization as promulgated by Wolf Wolfensberger (1972). Within six months of the start of the planning process, the first group home was dismantled, and people with disabilities started moving into apartments and houses. As the director described:

> The direct care staff got excited. We were working with the most challenged people. People were scared at first, but they saw good things happen with folks. They needed to understand that they wouldn't lose their jobs. Everyone was empowered to be part of the plan.

In 1988, twenty-seven people moved into homes, partially due to the reduction in size of Laconia State School. Since then, there was a lot of new development of residences and day supports, and finally, staff members at the agency could take a breath. The big push to move thirty-five people out of Laconia back to this region was over, and New Hampshire had become the first state in the United States without a state institution for people with developmental disabilities. Although there was still a waiting list, no money was available for developing new services.

David Traine, the Executive Director, explained that the organization was now reflecting and thinking about its direction and at ways to reorganize to better "empower the people closer to the person they are supporting to have more authority and to take some of the bureaucracy out of people's lives."

TEACHERS IN THE COMMUNITY

Ned, Susie, James, and Bob, who are supported by the agency, are highlighted in this section, with brief descriptions of each person; the interaction context during the visit; and some of the relationships, events, activities, services, and places important in their lives. Figure 7.1 includes illustrations of their personal networks, as drawn by agency staff members.

Ned

Ned, according to one of his staff, is an enthusiastic, "warm and wonderful guy with very substantial physical handicaps." A person who enjoys people, he is forty-seven years old, a slight seventy to eighty pounds, and was reportedly becoming a "fixture" in downtown Dover, where he moved after leaving Laconia, where he had been placed at the time of his father's death. As one of the agency's staff, Sally, describes him:

> [Ned] has CP [cerebral palsy] and his muscles are very tight, not a lot of cooking ability, real social; [we] think he is very intelligent. He follows movies, baseball. He knows what the score is. We were told he is a Yankees fan. He gets excited when he knows they are ahead. He is a basic meat and potatoes man, not too into quiche.

At the time of the visit, he also used a manual wheelchair. Ned was described as basically a happy man, fairly limited in ability, who can make choices (he nods yes or no); he was learning that he can make himself happier and that he does not have to completely depend on the staff. As one staff member said, "He is choosing what to eat, wear, . . . and he never did that before."

Ned spends time in the community, shopping, going to the laundromat, and sharing lunch (including at a Mexican restaurant where he ate blender-chopped burritos and fajitas and ice cream). He is a member of a church, where he also participates in activities such as bingo and raffle ticket sales. He has gotten to know two people at church, whom he has invited over to his house for dinner. The staff tell stories about how other people miss him at church when his schedule changes. Ned also goes to the movie theater on main street, has vacationed with one of his staff, and distributes payroll at the agency office.

Ned's brother, a retired postman who lives in Milton, "pops in" to visit when he is near Ned's place, which Ned shares with his roommate Mary. Ned has a niece who lives down the road, and a mother, whom we visited, who lives in a local nursing home in a brightly decorated, shared room. She was diagnosed as having Alzheimer's disease. She enjoys visiting with Ned, who stops by to see her every other week, traveling in his accessible van with one of the staff. Ned and his mom have gone out to lunch together, and she has visited his new place.

Susie

Susie introduced me to the delights of raspberry tea as we sat talking at her kitchen table. Later, sitting on her bed upstairs, with her cherished cat, Missy, beside us, Susie proudly shared some of her photographs and a newspaper article with a picture of her and Missy. Susie, who is in her late twenties and one of eight children, was described by one of the staff as a "real neat person," "who is well loved" and who loves people and animals. Her support person, Lisa, described Susie's last birthday:

> [At] a local store . . . the woman knows her very well . . . they will always call if they are concerned about her. They love Susie to visit and hang out in the store. On her birthday, they gave her presents and sent her to the beauty shop next door, and the beauty shop gave her a free haircut and a little gift basket.

Staff members describe Susie as being "very capable," as having held many jobs in the past, and as having a lot of other involvements recently, including cooking, participating in a women's group, and attending night school to work toward her diploma. She frequently goes to the local soup kitchen to meet her network of friends there. She also knows and shares meals with a large number of people who are involved with the mental health system—with which she first came in contact at age sixteen—and other people supported by this agency. She has been in and out of state

FIGURE 7.1. Relationship Networks As Drawn by Staff Members

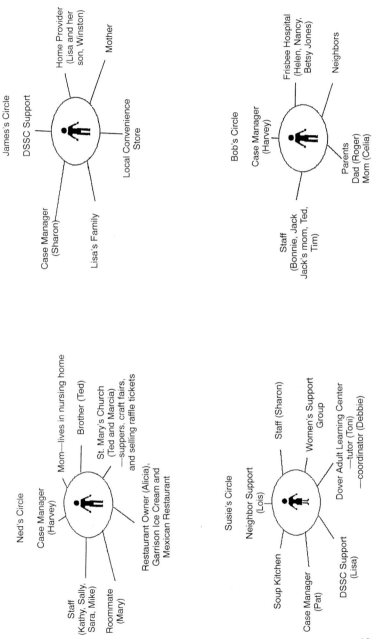

123

hospitals for brief stays, never for more than a couple of months at a time. Her ex-roommate, Melissa, still visits and stops by for coffee. Everyone in the agency knows Susie, and the staff say that she can count on them to come to meetings and advocate for her.

James

James was introduced to me by Rosie, one of the four assistant residential directors of the agency. A man in his forties or fifties, Rosie described him as "really kind of neat, very tall [six feet, too inches]; he kind of reminds me of Abraham Lincoln, kind of gray hair, distinguished looking." James had lived with Lisa, a support worker, and her son, Winston, for about two years in Milton. Milton is a small, tourist bedroom community about a forty-five minute drive from the ocean. Previously, he lived in the home of his eighty-five-year-old mother. James is intently interested in the weather and loves the ocean and the environment. His interest is lifelong—since his first hurricane in 1954 felled a tree near his family's home and his mother purchased weather gauges for him. We talked in the restaurant about Hurricane Bob, which had recently hit the East Coast, ocean surfing, and the sharp, hairpin turns of the California coast. Both Lisa and James like to travel and to visit and stay with Lisa's relatives, and they find each other to be good travel companions. They have made one trip to Florida and Alabama, where they saw the white sand beaches of the Gulf of Mexico, and another to the Mojave Desert and the casinos in Nevada. James had been in and out of psychiatric (and one general) hospitals, diagnosed as schizophrenic (e.g., hearing voices, fear of being poisoned), and tried several different living situations (staffed apartments, another family instead of with his mother). He had been out of the hospital for over a year and a half at the time of the visit.

Bob

Bob volunteers at Frisbee Memorial Hospital where he delivers the mail, a job he also did at Laconia. Bob, who has Sanfilippo's syndrome, a rare degenerative condition of the nervous system, lived at home with his family until he was eleven, before moving to Laconia where, his father explained, he "took a lot of abuse." I visited him at the hospital as he made his mail rounds, and we then shared a lunch of cold cuts, salad, and brownies at his small house in Rochester with Bonnie, one of his staff, and Roger, his father.

Support staff like Dan, who arranged for the hospital job, explained that when Bob used words such as "hello," it really had a positive effect on the hospital staff. Helen, the volunteer coordinator, and Barbara from the personnel department, came to know him as well, and as Helen said, "In the morning, he wakes up knowing [he has] a job." She explained her vision of what she hopes to accomplish through her support of Bob:

> My hope is that the 500-plus people who work at the hospital who . . . had an opportunity to see what Bob does here, has allowed them to carry that along with them outside the hospital. It has forced them to think, and hopefully, . . . people will be more responsive, more accepting, and more receptive.

Bob now lives in his own house, with staff support in a residential neighborhood in the same community as his parents. Bob has gone ice fishing and to a ballgame at the University of New Hampshire. He and Bonnie walk around the neighborhood each day, go shopping, and visit with some of the neighbors, who also came to a cookout on Bob's birthday. Three times a week Bob goes to a nearby ball field to walk around the track. He likes all kinds of food and now feels comfortable enough to take a cookie off his own kitchen counter and eat it without fear of retribution or punishment.

COMMUNITY PLACES AND RELATIONSHIPS

Developmental Services of Strafford County, Incorporated, strives to expand the network of community places and relationships in the lives of the people it supports. This can include getting to know neighbors, maintaining and reestablishing ties with family members, and meeting and knowing community members, such as store owners, customers, and others. For the past several years, it was no longer unusual for someone using a wheelchair to be on the streets, to be seen in restaurants or stores. People also might be at a regular café, with the original purpose of community presence. Now, David says, the main question is one of personal relationships. To guide staff members, he asked them to think about the question "Who calls on Saturday night?" Rosie, one of the staff members, explained:

> Our biggest step is to help people build relationships with people who are not [staff members]. . . . Some people don't even have family. And even that is something that most people take for granted, even having someone to spend Christmas with.

Supporting Connections: Staff Roles

Staff members use a range of strategies to help support the connections of people in the community. These include hosting parties and inviting the neighbors to visit, being visible (walking and greeting people in the neighborhood), teaching ways of introducing people, supporting conversation ("we were talking the other day"), building on one's own and the other person's past connections, and making other visible neighborhood efforts at building relationships. As one support worker described:

> Besides the party, we had a cleanup [on] second street, and sent out flyers. Not a lot of people came and joined us for donuts or anything, but you could see that people got out and started cleaning their lawns and stuff. We were very visible, and we talked to people, and Ned talked to people. It was nice, gave a positive atmosphere.

Connecting was viewed as a process whereby both good and bad experiences were expected. People needed to spend time with each other, see how they interacted, and how comfortable they were in the world. Sometimes the connections were "neighborly, not real close friends." Staff members were encouraged to develop their own unique relationship with each person and to find activities that they could do together with that person. As David, the director, said, "We all have different connections in our own communities, and through those different connections, you know different people and have new ideas." Another staff member explained that the workers had to remind themselves that building connections takes time. As she said:

> As service people, we think that connections will happen quickly. We need to step back and see where people are coming from. Ned is more connected than me and I have lived here for six years.

Knowing What It Means to Live Together

People with disabilities and their staff play a role in educating others about what it means to live together. Through the examples of their lives, professionals and agency staff were learning about possibilities that they had never previously envisioned. For example, David told me about a conference in Maine during which one person from that state who had visited Ned stood up from the audience and said the following:

> I went and visited a man by the name of Ned in Dover, New Hampshire, and I can tell you that there is nobody in the state of Maine

who is as disabled as Ned. And he is out in the community in his own apartment, with a roommate, with staff, and we went to the restaurant, and people knew who he was, and that doesn't happen here.

This type of leadership on the part of people with disabilities often happens in partnership or alliance with others, such as this speaker, with support workers, or with community members such as Helen, who share a vision of what coexistence means and who try in their own ways to create this in their lives and in the lives of others. Bob's father, Roger, recognizes the importance of this vision and what it means to his son and others who have repeatedly faced negative societal experiences. He responded with strength and graciousness to Helen at the hospital, stating:

> I think that is a lesson you taught within the building, to learn to associate and be a part of the lives of those with handicaps. Apparently, the people who have been here before have never been exposed to that segment of society. So now you have taught them a lesson of coexistence. That is very good.

SUPPORTING WHAT PEOPLE WANT

The assumption at this agency was that, in a general sense, people with disabilities want the same things that everyone does. Yet, although staff members strive for "individuality, not groupness or stereotypes," they also recognize that "we are all one people"; that is people share a commonness with one another that is more fundamental than surface differences such as disability labels.

Getting to Know and Trust One Another

Getting to know people and listening to what they wanted became a priority. One way this was done was by involving people with disabilities and their parents in the interviewing process. Roger, for example, said he appreciated "the courtesy of" being involved in the last interview. In Susie's interviews, she asked these questions:

> What are you going to do for me? Are you going to help me with banking? Are you going to have lunch with me? Are you going to help me with my cat food? I want to know.

The agency workers also have a reputation for listening to what parents want for their children, and what they need to satisfy their own personal sense of security and comfort. Roger recounted about his first meeting with SSC:

> The first day we met . . . they said what do you want for Bob? . . . We told them things that any parent would be concerned about. We didn't want him in an abusive situation. We wanted him to receive the care he should receive, the medical care, the dental care, just the things that any parent[s] would expect for their child.

People at the agency seemed aware that learning what people want is based on building trust and rapport. They do not assume that people with disabilities or their parents should automatically trust them, but that such relationships are a process of becoming comfortable with one another and of overcoming past negative experiences with the services system. People with disabilities needed to feel safe and to be assured that the negative experiences they have had in the past will not be repeated in the new situation or relationship. Moving into the community, as with any major change, especially one involving the unknown, can create a lot of stress and tension.

Often it was the little things that helped to build trust between people and the agency workers. For example, one dad saw a rocking chair he thought would be perfect for his son's new house. He called and was astonished when the agency said to buy the chair. Another time, the staff spontaneously called to see if Bob's parents would like to come over to supper. They came and had dinner with their son "like anyone would," but it was something that, for them, had not happened in all these years.

Supporting People: Flexibility and Change

Supporting people meant that the agency needed to be flexible and able to make changes in concert with the changes in people's lives. The underlying assumption was that the nature of human lives involves change and that human service systems must adapt to, and not direct, these changes. As the director explained:

> People's lives change, and a service system that makes sense is not determining what the change will be as much as trying to help people grow so that when they change or the circumstances change, the nature of the supports can change too.

Sometimes, what the agency needed to do to respond to what people wanted in their lives was relatively straightforward, though most agencies were not organized to do even these simple changes. For example, one woman, at various times, wanted to live in a different place or with another roommate. Similar to all of us, she changed what she wanted based on her experiences, opportunities, and life circumstances. In some organizations, she would be given the message that she could choose only once and then would need to stick by that decision. In contrast, this agency assisted her to make different decisions, even though it was cumbersome to do so within the system. As one of the agency staff described:

> When Susie came in contact with Developmental Services, she said she wanted to live in downtown Dover. The agency staff recruited a roommate and did the bulk of the apartment hunting together with her. The first apartment they found was on the third floor. When an apartment opened on the first floor, Susie and her roommate wanted to move; the agency took the time to recertify the downstairs one so they could do so. Later, Susie and her roommate decided to recruit a third roommate, a woman they knew. Then Susie wanted her own apartment [with ten hours a week of paid services].

In this agency, it was common for staff members to look to their own networks and personal resources, including in times of crisis. For example, once, when Susie was evicted from her apartment, she stayed at a staff member's home. Rachael, the staff member, described the time Susie lived with her:

> She lived with me for a month, and I got to know her very well in that month. It kind of was nice, and you don't know people until you live with them. So it really worked well. She liked living with us, but she hated Rochester, which was a town away. She decided that she definitely wanted to move back to Dover, but initially, there was no money to move her with, so we needed to wait until next month's check.

Making Mistakes

In this organization, a recognition existed that mistakes inevitably happen and that each person develops his or her own unique relationships. Everyone needed to go through a process of getting to know one another, including each staff member and the person he or she supported. Of course, this learning process was particularly hard on people with disabili-

ties who often repeated this process over again as staff come and go in
their lives. A tension existed between realizing that mistakes happen to all
of us and acknowledging that the situation may not be working out well
for some people. For staff and administrators, this meant always going
back to the questions "Who is it I work for?" and "Why is it I am here?"
and reflecting on being "true to the person you are supporting" and
learning to listen better. This remained a critical challenge to overcome.

When Staff Disagree and Values Differ

As in any organization, people would disagree with one another based
upon their own styles, opinions, and personal values. However, people
tried to remember whose life was central and whose values really mat-
tered. As one staff member explained:

> We are all different people and have different ways of doing things
> and different ideas of what is best. . . . The most important part is that
> we really listen to what the people want we are providing support to.

Sometimes figuring out what to do was a real challenge for staff, especially when a person's decisions did not seem very responsible or were
against the moral values and beliefs of the staff member. As one staff
member said:

> We need to step back and realize that we are not their parents . . . we
> need to be careful not to force our opinion . . . because we may
> alienate her . . . [and] she may not want to come back and say, "Hey
> can you help me out again?"

PERSONAL CHOICE, SELF-ADVOCACY, AND FAMILIES

This agency is a strong supporter of both families ("parents are real
important to us"), and adults with disabilities, with some adults assisted to
reconnect with family members with whom they have lost contact for
many years. Yet, most of the agency services are oriented toward adults
who do not have parental ties, with the region's family support council
consisting primarily of parents with young children.

Parents and Their Children

Since the establishment of the family support councils and the success
of families in passing family support legislation in New Hampshire, some

people in the state are viewing families as the central element of the service system (see Chapter 2). David, who represents what appears to be a minority position in the state that is also shared by the advocacy community, explained that it was important to distinguish the views of parents from those of adults with disabilities.

> We [have] got to be clear that the person we provide support to is the person with a disability. While 95 percent of the time, the family's interest and the person with a disability's interest may be exactly the same, sometimes they are not going to be, and that is exactly the issue. . . . At some point, I am not here to represent the interest of the family [parents].

In one example, presented by another staff member, parents and their adult child might disagree about whether their child (i.e., the agency's client) should come to the funeral of a relative. Although the staff would try to encourage people to talk their differences out together, and give information, such as the possible effect of a decision to attend the funeral on her relationship with her parent, ultimately, "if the person wants to do it, [he or she] will get support to do so." In the same way, the agency staff will support people to maintain ties with their parents, even if this is viewed as not in the person's best interest. As one staff member explained, "It is not our job to dissuade family . . . but it can be difficult at times."

Personal Choice and Self-Advocacy

Personal choice occurs as part of the "natural course of living," as part and parcel of every aspect of a person's life, and differs from self-advocacy. In thinking about personal choice, one issue that commonly arises is how people who have never been exposed to many options can make choices. As the director described through an analogy, people needed to have experiences to make choices. He recounted the following:

> I'll invite you over to my house tonight, and you can have the choice between Ethiopian and Peruvian food. Well, what kind of choice is that? If you don't know what Ethiopian or Peruvian food is, you have no choice at all. And a lot of people we are working with, by virtue of their institutionalization or their experience in the community, don't have any idea what their choices really are. So part of what we do is help them see and experience some . . . the world so they can actually tell they like this better. . . . That's just basic; that's fundamental.

Another aspect of personal choice in relationship to the system is how staff can help people better articulate their choices and pay closer attention to what people want. This is a difficult challenge, and people hope that avenues such as assisted communication will help this process.

In contrast, the self-advocacy movement was defined as "people collectively standing up and expressing a point of view." Self-advocacy was seen as directly related to the lack of power that people with disabilities hold in society and as a way of entering into the "public fray" and political issues involved in people's lives. This holds the possibility that people with disabilities possibly can be hurt in the process; the director was concerned about naively sending people into situations in which they would have no real power. Although some people from this agency were involved in the state's self-advocacy efforts (which is sometimes confused with citizen advocacy), a women's group also had evolved over time on the local level. Group members developed a basis for friendship and closeness and were moving toward dealing with broader issues that often fall with self-advocacy's purview (see Chapter 5).

WAYS OF ORGANIZING TO PROVIDE SUPPORT

This agency was in the process of examining ways to reorganize its resources—people, services, finances—to figure out how to determine and to provide the support that people want or how to assist people to develop the connections or relationships whereby such support would occur. The director explained this organizational process:

> Eighty percent of things are routine, so it gets people fired up. . . . Some of it is . . . figuring out how to use the talents of the people you've got. . . . We don't want the talents of people squandered or [for people] not to feel they are appreciated and their potential untapped.

Their agency change processes often involved staff groups coming together to figure out better who they were and what they had to offer. This extended to all parts of the organization, with the transportation providers also developing their own mission statement.

Staff

The director described the staff in this agency as good people who were no different than people in other parts of the country. He believed a lot of problems exist today in services because people do not know where they were going and how to go about accomplishing it. He explained:

> They [the staff] are regular folks. They are in Butte, Montana, Keokuk, Iowa—they are everywhere. We have to find them, good people who work hard, care about people, like what they are doing.

In selecting staff, emphasis was placed on a clear commitment to a core set of values regarding people with disabilities and acceptable ways of being with each other, whether people with or without disabilities. What the staff consider to be most valuable in their lives—friends, family, work, home, and so on—is also considered to be most valuable for people with disabilities. Staff were challenged to think about such issues as the meaningful and productive use of people's time; how choice and good leisure time would be defined by individual people; where the person would spend his or her time; what kinds of interests the person really had; and how staff could help people get their own homes, become connected with friends, and develop a range of relationships.

Decision Making and Problem Solving

Unlike some organizations, in which support staff were expected simply to implement the decisions of others above them, this agency was striving, though not always successfully, to respect and support the decisions of those who worked most closely with people. As one assistant residential director said:

> We all have to realize that the people who do direct care have a harder job, and you have to listen to what they are saying about people because they are in the trenches. And you also have to be willing to get your hands dirty.

Staff members were encouraged to problem solve and make decisions, using directors and others as consultants and resource people. All staff were involved in areas such as the agency's budget so they could better use their creativity and respond flexibly and spontaneously. The director strongly believed that if people throughout the organization understood how money works, then they could see what translated into supports for people with disabilities. This system or approach to budgeting also could give the flexibility for individual staff to decide at their level what somebody needs on Tuesday instead of on Wednesday.

Personal Commitment and Networks

Personal commitment was fostered between people, and it was not uncommon for support staff to share holidays or vacations with the people they supported. People celebrate together, especially birthdays, which were considered an often neglected personal holiday in the lives of the people supported by the agency. For example, when one man did not know his birthday and the information was irretrievable, he chose a date to create a past that he could carry into the future. People were also encouraged to use their own personal networks to locate staff, roommates, and others who might become involved in people's lives. As in all relationships, some of the best ones "happen" or were "flukes," with people sometimes being friends of an agency staff member.

Roommates, Neighbors, Staff, and Their Roles

This agency was beginning to examine issues such as the roles and relationships of neighbors and roommates who may also be paid in some way by the agency. As one staff member explained, the relationships workers were trying to promote were different from that of paid staff:

> We are trying to support a more normal relationship than a paid relationship, even though in reality, they are giving a service and they are getting something in exchange, but it is not quite the same. So the way that we support that is quite different. We try to encourage, not govern as we would staff, not regulate, not as much agency involvement.

In looking for roommates or neighbors, the agency workers particularly were wary of people who simply might want to do this for a free apartment, searching instead for someone who would invest the time that was needed. Paid roommates (people who share the same apartment or house) and paid neighbors (who may live in an adjoining flat) generally received room and board for providing some kind of support to the individual with a disability. A written roommate agreement was unique for each situation. For example, Ned's roommate sleeps over seven nights a week and has free rent and food and a stipend of $300 a month. According to the agreement, the roommate needed to be available from 10:00 p.m. until 8:30 a.m., and had responsibilities in the evening and nighttime, such as getting Ned out in case of a fire or responding to other emergencies. Michelle, who was a student, was involved in Ned's life and went out to lunch with him. She is "considered part of the whole house," would bring her friends over, and she shared the place with her pets, a bird and a goldfish. Yet, the agency asked Michelle not to keep one of her animals. People continue to struggle with the tension in these emerging roles, which at the time of this visit more resembled those of staff than of typical roommates or neighbors.

The agency was asking the question "Whose home is it?" The concept of shared households, with varying kinds of relationships among house-mates, still seemed new. Sometimes, a staff member said a person with a disability was "living alone" when they actually had a roommate. Also, many roommates were short-term arrangements that resembled boarder situations. The first choice of people supported by the agency generally seemed to reflect an agency bias toward two people living together, one with and another without disabilities.

Living in a house or an apartment with one other person can have both negative and positive implications. Though the agency sought to support connections, this was still a very small part of most people's day. David shared some of the positive aspects:

> We certainly have seen time and time again, as we have moved people out of those congregate settings to their own place, that people have just blossomed. You don't need to worry that someone will steal your corn flakes. You can have quiet if you want quiet, or yell.

The agency was also attempting to address some practical questions. For example, with the Internal Revenue Service (IRS), for purposes of taxes, was it stretching the definition of foster care too far to have a lease in the person's name? How did labor view these arrangements? Are support staff considered to be independent contractors? The agency tried to act responsibly by keeping current and obtaining legal opinions, but many of these issues remained unclear or in flux.

The Problem of Valued and Paid Work

David held that the decision about whether to work, have a volunteer job, and/or participate in other community activities should be guided by the individual person. Acknowledging that all else being equal, work can increase status, promote contacts with others, enhance one's personal sense of value, and be a source of contribution, he believed "we" needed to keep remembering "Whose question is it?" However, a number of people supported by the agency have little, if any, involvement in paid, integrated work. For some people, this was viewed as appropriate because options such as adult day services offer other opportunities to work on relationships and other objectives. Yet, other people were experiencing tremendous difficulty in finding and keeping jobs, though they would like to work. People had very few options for work or other integrated activities during their days, with agency staff providing services in the home and at work.

The State Role

The state support the agency had was critical in the day-to-day reality of the director. This support included an atmosphere in the state whereby "one could speak up if one believed something was not right." David, who has traveled and trained people in other states, believed New Hampshire's state leaders made decisions in the context of an overarching set of values about people and that many of the people who worked at the state level were "very decent human beings." These included the state director who really cared about people and who was a good politician, which was needed at the state level. The most critical person from the agency's vantage point was the field representative, who was the liaison between the area agency and the state office. David said the field representative knew the people in the region and was a "good filter of information . . . done within a very strong commitment to see to it that we get better at providing supports to people."

Todd, the "Medicaid whiz kid" at the state central office, figured out how to make the fiscal situation work, not just financially, but from the personal viewpoints of the people involved. For example, when they were "under the gun" to close Laconia, Todd called to see how many of the remaining people could move to this region. When David said they wanted to meet the remaining people, Todd reportedly replied:

> Yeah. That is great. That is something I'd hope someone would say about me if I'd been institutionalized for fifty years, that they'd at least meet me before they make plans.

Costs: Moving to More Individualized Services

The agency staff felt that they were creative in keeping costs down, though some individual living situations were expensive. The residential director explained that they compared the financial costs of running the Durham group home five years ago with the costs associated with where people lived at the time of the visit. The agency was spending, on average, the same amount of money in the new smaller situations, which were better suited to people, even without inflation being taken into account.

The director explained it was important to compare the average costs, not simply the expense of a single arrangement, and that it was not more costly to have the better situations. Sometimes, the cost of an individual situation may seem to be more expensive because of how costs are allocated across cost centers. In the past, it was easier to justify community costs by comparing these costs to the exorbitant costs for poor quality living in an institution. In the future, David said, when institutions no longer exist, the cost issue will be examined in relationship to other costs in society.

CONCLUSION

As one of the younger staff explained, her generation was looking for "frontier" issues that they could "fight for." In many ways, this agency brought together people who were seeking a new way of being together with others, including with people with disabilities. They were involved in a process of learning what it meant to "support what it is people want in their lives" and to "support" people to develop relationships and become part of community life. As the director concluded, although it may not be possible to do great things through services, certainly their experience in Region 9 in New Hampshire showed that decent things could occur in people's lives.

PART III:
MOVING TOWARD UNIVERSAL
ACCESS TO SUPPORT—
POLICY IS PERSONAL

Introduction

Julie Ann Racino
Simi Litvak

Since the 1970s, attendant services has been a primary organizing theme for the independent living movement, with people with physical and other disabilities often living at home without access to employment, in-home services for basic needs, and opportunities to participate outside of the home. In the 1990s, attendant services was shifted as a concept to personal assistance services (PAS) through international organizing efforts, including the International Personal Assistance Symposium (see Table A). Termed the next frontier after passage of the landmark Americans with Disabilities Act (1990), personal assistance services (see Table B) became reflected in diverse forms in laws and programs throughout the United States (see Table C) and the world.

However, particularly in the lives of people with significant disabilities, consumer and user-directed options of personal assistance services (PAS) were elusive in day-to-day life. The New Models Research Project was designed to explore best practices with diverse groups, with this section of the book highlighting these practices in the areas of psychiatric disability, mental retardation and physical disabilities, brain injuries, and youth with disabilities.

PSYCHIATRIC DISABILITY

The psychiatric disability service structures in the United States have been well funded, yet highly criticized for a strong institutional and medical bias (World Institute on Disability, 1993, p. 39). As evidenced in the chapters in Parts III and IV, during the interim period, the reform of childrens' services in mental health became a high priority, with family perspectives resulting in national community systems' strengthening their efforts.

See Appendix A for research methodology for Chapters 8 through 11.

TABLE A. Resolution on Personal Assistance Services

RESOLUTION

WE, PEOPLE WITH DISABILITIES AND OUR ALLIES, have come together from across the United States and around the world from September 29—October 1, 1991 in Oakland, California at the symposium entitled EMPOWERMENT STRATEGIES FOR THE DEVELOPMENT OF A PERSONAL ASSISTANCE SERVICES SYSTEM.

This conference has focused on personal assistance services as an essential factor in independent living, which itself encompasses the whole area of human activities, including but not limited to housing, transportation, community access, education, employment, economic security, family life and interpersonal relationships of choice, leisure, and political influence.

Recognizing our unique expertise derived from our experience, we are taking the initiative in the development of policies that directly affect all people with disabilities.

People with disabilities are entitled to be enabled to achieve the highest possible level of personal functioning and independence through appropriate education, health care, social services and assistive technology, including, as necessary, the assistance of other people.

We firmly uphold our basic human and civil rights to full and equal participation in society as called for in the Americans with Disabilities Act and the United Nations Universal Declaration of Human Rights.

We consider independent living and the availability of support services to be critical to the exercise of our full human and civil rights, responsibilities, and privileges.

To this end, we condemn forced segregation and institutionalization as direct violations of our human rights. Government policy and funding should not perpetuate the forced segregation, isolation, or institutionalization of people with disabilities of any age. The Americans with Disabilities Act was passed into law to promote the equalization of opportunity. The passage of comprehensive federal personal assistance legislation is essential to realizing the historic promise of the Act.

The recommendations of the United Nations World Programme of Action (s 115) specifically state that "Member states should encourage the provision of support services to enable disabled people to live as independently as possible in the community and in so doing should ensure that persons with a disability have the opportunity to develop and manage these services for themselves.

In support of the international movement of disabled people in Disabled Peoples' International, which has a special commitment to setting up a network of initiatives for personal assistance services as part of the implementation of the equalization of opportunities, we call on governments and policy makers to assure greater and more equitable access to personal assistance services based on the following principles.

1. Personal assistance services are a human and civil right. These services shall serve people of all ages, from infancy throughout a person's lifetime, when the person's functional limitation(s) shall necessitate the services. This right is irrespective of disability, personal health, income, marital and family status, and without discrimination on the basis of race, national origin, cultural background, religion, gender, sexual preference, or geography.

2. All people with disabilities (and their self-designated or legal representatives, if applicable) shall be informed about their rights and options related to personal assistance services in accessible format, and appropriate languages. All levels of personal assistance services should respect the privacy and confidentiality of the user.

3. Personal assistance users shall be able to choose from a variety of personal assistance services models that together offer the choice of various degrees of user control. User control, in our view, can be exercised by all people regardless of their ability to give legally informed consent or their need for support in decision making or communication.

4. Services shall enable the users to exercise their rights and to participate in every aspect of sociocultural life, including, but not limited to home, school, work, cultural and spiritual activities, leisure, travel, and political life. These services shall enable disabled people, without penalty, if they so choose, to establish a personal, family, and community life and fulfill all the responsibilities associated with those aspects of life.

5. No individual shall be forced into or kept in an institutionalized setting because of lack of resources, high cost, substandard, or nonexistent services or the refusal and/or denial of any or all services.

6. These services must be available for up to seven days a week, for as many as needed during the twenty-four-hour period of the day, on long-term, short-term, and emergency basis. These services shall include, but are not limited to, assistance with personal bodily functions; communicative, household, mobility, work, emotional, cognitive, personal, and financial affairs; community participation; parenting; leisure, and other related needs. The user's point of view must be paramount in the design and delivery of services. Users must be able to choose or refuse services.

7. Government funding shall be an individual entitlement independent of marital status and shall not be a disincentive to employment.

8. Government funding must include competitive wages (based on consumer cost experience within the private sector) and employment benefits for assistants and related administrative and management expenses.

9. Payments to the user shall not be treated as disposable, taxable income and shall not make the user ineligible for other statutory benefits or services.

10. Sufficient governmental funding shall be made available to ensure adequate support, outreach, recruitment, counseling, and training for the user and the assistant. Government efforts shall ensure that a pool

TABLE A *(continued)*

of qualified, competent assistants shall be available for users to access through a variety of personal assistance services models, including, but not limited to, individual providers and full services agencies.

11.The user should be free to select and/or hire as personal assistants whomever she/he chooses, including family members.

12. Children needing personal assistance services shall be offered such services as part of their right to inclusive education as well. Such education and personal assistance services shall include age-appropriate opportunity to learn to use and control personal assistance services effectively.

13. There shall be a uniform appeals procedure which is independent of funders, providers, and assessors that is affected in an expeditious manner and allows the applicant/user to receive advocacy services and legal counsel at the expense of the statutory authority.

14. In furtherance of all of the above, users must be formally and decisively involved and represented at all levels of policymaking through ongoing communication and outreach in planning, implementation, design, and development of personal assistance services.

Rehabilitation and disability-related organizations, as well as individuals, are encouraged to formally adopt and endorse this Resolution. Send your letters of endorsement to the World Institute on Disability at 510 16th St., Suite 100, Oakland, CA 94612-1500. Voice and TDD 510/763-4100, FAX 510/763-4109.■

Source: World Institute on Disability (1991c). *Resolution on Personal Assistance Services.* Oakland, CA: Author. Reprinted from *Rehabilitation Gazette,* 33(2), June 1993, p. 9, with permission of Gazette International Networking Institute, 4207 Lindell Blvd., #110, Saint Louis, MO 63108-2915.

Supported Housing

Supported housing, with an independent living orientation (Harp, 1989) and an emphasis on consumer preference and housing of choice, moved in this period to systems reform efforts by state governments (see Carling, 1993).

Case Management

The voluminous literature on case management (World Institute on Disability, 1993, p. 39) continued to increase during this period, with children's mental health reform still not reflecting the perspectives of adult psychiatric survivors. Case management remained a major concern of the

TABLE B. Personal Assistance Services

Personal assistance services (PAS) are tasks performed for a person who has a disability by another person that aim at maintaining well-being, personal appearance, comfort, safety, and interactions within community and society as a whole. In other words, personal assistance tasks are those tasks which the individual who has a disability would normally do for himself or herself if the person had no disability. These tasks include (1) personal maintenance and hygiene activities such as dressing, grooming, feeding, bathing, respiration and toilet functions, including bowel, bladder, catheter, and menstrual tasks; (2) mobility tasks such as getting into and out of bed, wheelchair, or tub and transportation in the community; (3) household maintenance tasks such as cleaning, shopping, meal preparation, laundering, and long-term heavy cleaning and repairs; (4) infant- and child-related tasks such as bathing, diapering, and feeding; (5) cognitive life management activities such as money management, planning, and decision making; (6) security-related services, such as daily monitoring by phone; and (7) communication services such as interpreting for people with hearing or speech disabilities and reading for people with visual disabilities. Between 9 and 11 million Americans, about one in every twenty people, require some assistance to accomplish normal, everyday life tasks.

Source: Litvak, S., Zukas, H., and Heumann, J. (1987). *Attending to America: Personal Assistance for Independent Living.* Berkeley, CA: World Institute on Disability.

self-help movement, especially the controlling aspects of case management (see Chapter 8) and its effects within homes.

Personal Assistance Services

Lorelee Stewart (1991) has written about how she uses a personal assistant and the negotiation she did that enabled her to receive PAS through the Massachusetts' Personal Care Option (see Chapter 8). New research on PAS was funded during this period at Boston University, Center for Psychiatric Rehabilitation, with a PAS report on Massachusetts from the National Association of State Directors of Developmental Disabilities Services (Smith, G., 1994).

Nonprofessional Personal Assistance

As described in the initial proposal by the World Institute on Disability, only recently were community supports developed separately from "liv-

TABLE C. Personal Assistance Services' Guiding Principles of the Consortium of Citizens with Disabilities

---

Personal assistance services should be designed to

- be guided and directed by the choices, preferences, and expressed interests and desires of the individual;
- increase the individual's control over life based on the choice of acceptable options that minimize reliance on others in making decisions and in performing everyday activities (as called for by the National Council on Disability);
- enable PAS users to select, direct, and employ their own paid personal assistants, if desired;
- enable PAS users to contract with an agency for these services, if desired;
- foster the increased independence, productivity, and integration of these individuals into the community;
- be easily accessible and readily available to all eligible persons where and when desired and needed;
- meet individual needs irrespective of labels;
- allow payment to family members for the extraordinary personal assistance they provide;
- be provided in any setting, including in or out of the person's home;
- be based on an individual service plan; and
- offer PAS users of all ages the opportunity and support needed to assume greater freedom, responsibility, and choice throughout life.

Source: Consortium of Citizens with Disabilities (1991). *Recommended Federal Policy Directions for Personal Assistance Services for Americans with Disabilities.* Washington, DC: Personal Assistance Task Force, Consortium of Citizens with Disabilities, p. 3.

ing facilities (see Chamberlin, 1978, for consumer-run homes). Most of the concerns in these interviews and the literature, however, continued to reflect concerns of paid assistance by parents, especially in instances of abuse, and the need to develop assistance independent of the traditional service structures.

COMBINED PHYSICAL AND COGNITIVE DISABILITIES

In 1986, a paucity of materials on non-facility-based services, such as personal assistance, supported living, or support services appeared in the mental retardation and developmental disabilities literature (Taylor, Racino, and Knoll, 1985). However, since that time, community living for people with the most significant disabilities, including people who have medical needs, has taken on new directions.

Community Living: Children and Adults with Health, Physical, and Mental Retardation/Developmental Disabilities

A review article based on work in Maryland, as part of national technical assistance, highlighted best practices and current status in community living for children and adults with medical and/or physical needs (Shoultz and Racino, 1988). This followed a best practices book, inclusive of people with multiple disabilities, in Kentucky, Wisconsin, and Michigan, with field tests held in Connecticut, New Hampshire, and Wisconsin (Taylor et al., 1987a).

Personal Assistance Services

PAS began to appear in the mental retardation literature in the mid-1980s, mainly in unpublished materials on organizations (e.g., Johnson, 1985, in Wisconsin), user direction and training (e.g., Ulciny and Jones, 1988) and policy development (e.g., National Association of Developmental Disabilities Councils, 1990). The independent living sector moved to national surveys on services of the centers (e.g., Means and Bolton, 1992), including cognitive disabilities (Jones et al., 1988) and policy reports (Nosek, 1991).

Personal Assistance Services and Self-Advocacy

As described in Chapter 9, personal assistance services was discussed in national and international forums (World Institute on Disability, 1991b), including by the emerging national self-advocacy organization (e.g., University of Minnesota, 1990; Cone, 1998; Shoultz and Ward, 1996), and placed into new conceptual frameworks (e.g., O'Brien, 1992).

Support Services

Instead of PAS, the field of mental retardation and developmental disabilities experienced a proliferation of literature primarily in supported living, employment, recreation, and other forms of support in community life. These frameworks may or may not use personal assistance services

(Racino, 1995b) when describing similar functions to broadened PAS models (Consortium of Citizens with Disabilities, 1992). Accounts of these approaches by people with disabilities and their parents reemerged (e.g., J. Kennedy, 1993), together with new studies by the ARC on self-determination (Wehmeyer, Kelchner, and Richards, 1995), and studies of PAS within the context of the Americans with Disabilities Act (ADA).

Lifestyle Planning

Seminal work with people with health and medical needs remained as functional life planning (Green-McGowan, 1987), an individual planning process. Community membership involvements that described PAS were developing during this period (e.g., Ludlum, 1991, Communitas, Connecticut). New articles emerged as an outgrowth of person-centered approaches in schools, community living, and employment and were tied, in part, to agency change to be more responsive and flexible to people's needs (see Chapter 16, From Person-Centered to Better Quality Lives; Racino, 1995a).

People with Multiple Disabilities

People with significant and multiple disabilities, as represented by organizations such as TASH (The Association of Persons with Severe Handicaps), may have hearing, speech, and visual impairments, at times in addition to mental retardation. Facilitated communication (e.g., Biklen et al., 1992) in the 1990s was a major effort in assisting people to communicate who may not have had such opportunities in the past.

BRAIN INJURIES

Extensive literature reviews on the effects of brain injury on the individual and his or her family and the need for services and support were completed through the 1990s (e.g., Williams and Kay, 1991), with ongoing research indexes of new studies (e.g., Arokiasamy, McMorrow, and Moss, 1994).

Community Living

The impetus for policy research in community living was fostered by the movement of people with brain injuries back to their states (e.g., in

New York), with work on national best practices occurring simultaneously (e.g., Reynolds and Rosen, 1994; Wright, 1993). Community (re)integration (Condeluci, 1991) and rehabilitation medicine both included PAS, in apartment models and user-directed forms, respectively. Housing and support approaches with adults with significant cognitive disabilities remained controversial (Racino and Williams, 1994), with independent living centers seeking to play an even more active role in cases of brain injury.

Research and Personal Assistance Services

Brain injury research remained medicalized, with substantial overlap with health research (e.g., adolescent health and decision making). The literature includes one of the clearest descriptions of user-directed PAS within this context (Christiansen, Schwartz, and Barnes, 1993).

Support Services

However, there is an emerging nonmedical family support movement (see also family perspectives, Singer and Nixon, 1990), as well as research (Kruetzer et al., 1989) and national think tanks (Thomas and Menz, 1990) on employment. Studies on the lives and perspectives of people with brain injuries remain sparse (Bergland and Thomas, 1991), with accounts of people with brain injuries with PAS newer to the literature (Watson, 1991).

YOUTH WITH DISABILITIES

The disability literature is replete with extensive research on caregiver burden, threats to family survival, and the need for supports (informal and formal) to shore up the family's capacity to care for family members of all ages and disabilities at home (World Institute on Disability, 1993).

Family Support

In family support, together with the emergent family movements and family-centered approaches to care, personal assistance services usually are in the forms of home care and related services. Reform movements of systems have centered on a movement toward families (see for example, Covert, 1992, and Chapters 2 and 6 in Part II; and Chapters 12, 14, and 15 in Part IV). Reversing the concept of burden and the movement toward regular approaches to youth growth and development are still only marginally reflected in PAS.

Personal Assistance

However, as confirmed by Megan Kirshbaum (1996), a leading child-rearing and disability expert, little information was available on the benefits of personal assistance for young people with disabilities (Litvak, Zukas and Heumann, 1987, 14-16). Litvak, Zukas, and Heumann (1987) argued that the use of nonfamily, paid providers to foster independence in disabled children had hardly been considered. Sascha Bittner (1991) writes eloquently of the frustrations in depending upon her parents for assistance and the lack of support for her to attend extracurricular activities as did everyone else. Chapter 11 describes the results of interviews with adults with disabilities regarding these options, including with adults living in Minnesota. Youth information access, policy options, regular development, and major institutional areas for change (employment, recreation, housing) are described in Racino (1997d).

RESEARCH QUESTIONS

The following chapters report, in part, on the New Models Research Project, which was designed to explore the following questions:

1. What are the differences and similarities in service and support need between diverse populations?
2. Why do some groups use the existing system more than others? What are the systems barriers to wider access?
3. Are fears regarding safety well founded? Are there ways to decrease the risks of independent living without also eliminating individual choice and control over one's life?

Racino (1995b) presents an overview of the initial review of the field status with these groups and PAS. Since 1991, when the interviews were completed (and reported, in part, in the subsequent chapters), field developments have continued to occur across the United States. These have included

* new public analyses of PAS systems designed originally for people with physical disabilities (J. Kennedy, 1993);

- the use of intermediary organizations for consumer-directed PAS (Flanagan and Green, 1997);
- consumer-directed models in home care (Doty, Kasper, and Litvak, 1996; Sabatino and Litvak, 1995);
- studies and evaluations of PAS from the developmental disabilities systems (Walker et al., 1996; World Institute on Disability, 1993);
- public policy analyses of PAS and community integration by leaders in the independent living movement (Nosek and Howland, 1993); and
- more explicit inclusion of PAS in supported housing designs in mental health (Carling, 1995).

We hope the reader will learn from the perspectives of the consumer experts who have experienced PAS and have hope for more positive futures for the generations to come.

Chapter 8

Psychiatric Survivors, the International Self-Help Movement, and User-Directed Personal Assistance Services

Julie Ann Racino

INTRODUCTION

As one of the rallying cries of people with disabilities, personal assistance services (PAS) has been espoused as the major way for the Americans with Disabilities Act (ADA) (Chamberlin, 1992; Haimon, 1991) to become a reality in community, social, spiritual, educational, economic, and political life (Consortium of Citizens with Disabilities, 1991; Litvak, Zukas and Heumann, 1987). This chapter describes the results of consumer expert interviews with adults with psychiatric disabilities, and/or psychiatric survivors in the United States, on their leadership in informing public policy and practice as part of this international movement.

PERSONAL ASSISTANCE SERVICES

The mental health field itself has some eloquent writers who have described user-directed assistance as an individualized support (J. Chamberlin, 1990), as embedded within the independent living movement (Deegan, 1992) and as reflecting the principles of consumer control and

This chapter is a modified version of Racino, J. (1995c). "Personal Assistance Services: Psychiatric Survivors and People with Psychiatric Disabilities." In *Toward Universal Access to Support: An Edited Collection on Personal Assistance Services.* Syracuse, NY, and Boston, MA: Community and Policy Studies. The detailed quotations in Chapters 8 through 11 are from interviews for this research study. See Appendix A for research methodology.

cross-disability (Stewart, 1991). However, these perspectives are often isolated in the self-help literature and have not yet been acknowledged in relationship to major systems approaches (e.g., case management models) or in systems change in states, particularly with children with mental health needs and their families.

Personal assistance services (PAS) as understood and applied in the field of psychiatric disabilities was in its early stages of development in the 1990s, with reportedly a few service practice examples in Massachusetts, California, and Hawaii. Although the idea of personal assistance services was viewed as holding promise for people with psychiatric disabilities, conceptualizations of funded PAS were formulated primarily in terms of physical assistance, making other forms of assistance appearing to be an afterthought. Psychiatric survivors and/or people with psychiatric disabilities also would be unlikely to have had exposure to existing models of PAS for other population groups. As one leader in the psychiatric survivor movement explained:

> We need to educate the community of people with psych[iatric] disabilities that this is an option they can choose. This is an option they can fight for. This is an alternative to hospitalization and other kinds of treatment or things like case management.

For these informants, the most promising aspect of a personal assistance model is the feature of user control of the services. ("PAS is user-controlled. It is based upon what the person themselves wants. It is just all the things we have been talking about in the survivor movement.") Without this feature, the model or approaches could end up resembling other mental health services, which is not a desired outcome because the mental health system is primarily interested in ensuring compliance and in compliance outcomes.

EXPECTED OUTCOMES OF PAS

The expected outcomes (see Cook, 1992, on outcome assessment in psychiatric rehabilitation; Farkas and Anthony, 1987; Nosek, 1992; DeJong and Hughes, 1982; DeJong, Branch, and Corcoran, 1984, for outcomes in independent living) of a user-controlled model of personal assistance services (i.e., definition of and control of services) could be revolutionary. People with psychiatric disabilities, by definition and assumption, are often considered to be incapable of directing their own lives and making decisions about their own health care ("Probably 99 and

99/100th percent of the people who are considered such are not"). Enhancing control, particularly in medicalized situations, was a high priority, as explained by one PAS leader:

> And for anybody whose life is becoming medicalized, the most valuable thing you have is control over your own life, and anything that can be done for any individual enhance [his or her] ability to control [his or her] own life, is a high priority on my list, and I bet on the list of anybody whose life is becoming medicalized.

Arguing for this option, potential outcomes of PAS were better quality of lives, sometimes referred to as independent functioning, independence, increased ability to function outside an independent living situation, or ability to be self-determining in relation to one's own life and what one is trying to achieve in one's life. On the personal level, people could feel better about themselves, enjoy life in the community, engage in activities they could not do before, and experience alleviation of symptoms that previously interfered with life pursuits. PAS could result in better accommodations in housing, jobs, freedom from sheltered living situations, and increased opportunities outside the home or apartment. An overarching outcome could be improved life quality, based upon the person's own definition.

Personal assistance services could also result in reduced costs compared to more costly hospitalizations ("If it works, for me the best outcome would be that the person does not end up back using high cost, very high cost mental health services.") One of the most needed outcomes was to help keep people "out of jail, off bridges, and out of the system," through a fundable, distinct system. Thus, PAS might prevent the trauma, victimization, and other effects of hospitalization. A consumer versus provider outcome-based approach to personal assistance services could be individualized, based upon a person's individual goals in contracting for PCA services, highlighting the person's freedom to make decisions.

PERSONAL EXPERIENCES AND PAS DEVELOPMENT

Briefly, all the people who shared their views regarding personal assistance services have roots within the psychiatric survivor and/or self-help movements and can be considered to be international leaders (e.g., Chamberlin and Unzicker, 1991; Deegan, 1988). Several informants discussed their experiences, surviving the system, breaking through their personal isolation, organizing with other people, and coming out; for example:

I was diagnosed, incarcerated, drugged, isolated and given shock treatments. . . . I was fairly disabled by the treatments I received and, after several years, met other people who had been through the system and were speaking up and fighting back. . . . I started working with other people in 1978.

Holding an environmental, political, social, and/or spiritual view of people's problems instead of medical views (Deegan, 1992), the informants had varying degrees of familiarity with the independent living movement (i.e., cross-disability movement of people with disabilities, which was led by people with physical disabilities) and with its capacities and willingness to include the interests and wishes of people with psychiatric disabilities. For example, as one informant described:

My professional experience and my involvement with the consumer movement are very intertwined with each other. I have worked as a service provider in independent living centers . . . and helped to develop a benefits advocacy component that was providing independent living services to people with mental disabilities.

As part of a political self-help movement, these leaders are conscious of the powerful role of language, with the use of the term cognitive disabilities not generally considered acceptable. This is, in part, because the disability may be defined as affecting abstract reasoning and functional problems in controlling emotions (see P. Carling, personal communication, December 12, 1994). The terms people with psychiatric disabilities and psychiatric survivors both reflect different perceptions of how people view themselves or others, and vary in meaning from people with psychiatric histories to people who are involved with the mental health delivery system. For people not involved in the service system, the terms consumers, service users, and service recipients are inaccurate. People who have not made it through their experiences may be viewed as victims and others with similar experiences may not have been "caught" by the service system.

The Relevance of Abuse, Trauma, and Victimization

As an activist adult constituency, the informants had less familiarity with developments in children's services (and vice versa for the leaders in children's mental health; Friesen, 1993; Duchonowski and Friedman, 1990), other than their own experiences. A strong literature exists on the experiences of psychiatric survivors of the service systems and the connections with other movements toward better life quality (Chamberlin, J., 1990).

Knowledge about the person's own experiences, inclusive of the process of disablement by treatments, stigmatization, and feelings of victimization and trauma provide context for potential pitfalls in the ways in which services are constructed. Treatment (which may or may not be differentiated from service) may be seen as arbitrary and punitive, with diagnosis, incarceration, drugs, isolation, restraint, shock treatment, experimentation, and/or seclusion. Other types of treatment, such as behavior management, recreation, or occupational therapy may be viewed as meaningless or demeaning. Even if hospitalization was entered into voluntarily when no other options were available (e.g., as a relatively safe place during a time of crisis), people can experience a loss of rights as part of their treatment process. A current user of PAS described her hospital experience:

> It is a very strange situation because you go into the hospital; one minute, you had all the rights in the world, and the next minute, you don't have any rights. Now all your rights are called privileges, which you need to gain by doing what was considered to be appropriate behavior by the staff of the hospital, which could be anything.

This type of control and a loss of basic rights to personal autonomy can extend into the community, to all aspects of life, without room for self-direction or privacy. For instance, intensive case management (see Dvoskin and Steadman, 1994; Ebert, 1990), considered to be among the progressive community practices, was termed by one informant as a form of outpatient commitment (Applebaum, 1986; Miller and Fiddleman, 1984). As another survivor explained:

> If you are a client, the Department of Mental Health, it absolutely infiltrates about every corner, every aspect of your life. Mental health does your food shopping; mental health does your money management. Mental health does your life. Mental health says whether or not you can get married. Mental health has absolute, enormous control, and when I talk with people from other disability groups, they are just amazed at the control.

As children, several informants experienced abuse in the family, and one informant believed such abuse to be widespread enough to be taken into account as a significant factor in development of a conceptual model for people with psychiatric disabilities (see Carling, 1995), particularly with the use of family members as personal assistants.

SYSTEMS DESIGN: ASSUMPTIONS AND BARRIERS

Ingrained assumptions and ways of thinking about psychiatric disability and how the institutional and community service systems work were shared by the informants (see also, Estroff, 1981, for an ethnography of the system). To the extent they were described, people viewed their issues or problems in functional terms, such as controlling emotions or participating in job, home, social activities, and community life, and as exacerbated by stigmatization and discrimination (Crossmaker and Merry, 1990). Unlike other fields, psychiatry has both right and wrong counterpoints, instead of common, shared standards.

Individualization, Not Diagnoses

Several informants strongly believed that diagnoses were not particularly relevant in determining who would use personal assistance services (Litvak, Zukas, and Heumann, 1987, pp. 16-17). First, even people who have the same diagnosis might have different kinds of functional needs. Second, even if the diagnoses are the same, different people may prefer diverse kinds of personal assistance services based upon their views of what might be helpful. As the director of a then newly funded research project at Boston University described (1995c):

> People with psychiatric diagnoses—it manifests itself in so many different ways depending upon what it is that people have trouble with. It is not just a question of what is your diagnosis. One person could be depressed and conceptualize needing PAS for one thing and another person could be depressed and have a very different conceptualization of what would be helpful.

Third, use of diagnoses with personal assistance services begins to medicalize this process. People want to be viewed not as members of a categorical disability group (though acknowledging, for some people, their identity as a survivor) but as individuals with their own ways of thinking about their lives.

A suggested approach was to work with an individual based on his or her lifestyle and not on the needs of a population of people from a categorical disability group. Because of the environmental impact, however, people with diverse disabilities often have similar experiences, such as discrimination, treatment, and poverty (see Chamberlin, J., 1990).

Independent Living Centers and People with Psychiatric Disabilities

At the time of the study, at least two independent living centers (ILCs) in the United States had directors who were psychiatric survivors and known by the informants. The informants held differing views on the extent to which the ILCs and the movement were addressing the concerns of people with psychiatric disabilities, with some of these views being highly public (Deegan, 1992; Harp, 1990; Harp, 1993). A California-based ILC was one of the first to include people with psychiatric disabilities, but cross-disability issues arose, including competing priorities for funding, space, and resources; the extent to which people with psychiatric disabilities were hired as employees; and the hierarchy of disabilities (Yucker, 1983). Strengths of the ILCs noted in relationship to people with psychiatric disabilities were their increasing cross-disability base, their expertise with PAS, and a collective mind-set perceived to be more open and less stigmatizing, particularly compared to mental health.

Case Management and PAS in Mental Health

The U.S. conception of case management, a major concern of psychiatric survivors, was described as emphasizing control instead of empowerment, overmonitoring and overruling people, practicing intensive case management of people's lives, giving advice, and as having a focus on illness and psychiatric drugs. Of particular concern with PAS were any requirements of case management to obtain other services. As described by one leader:

> If the kind of services is really going to be maximizing client choice, then the person should not be compelled to accept any service component.

Another concern is that PAS could become a professionally provided service, very similar to other community mental health services (see Ridgway, 1988). In the extreme, PAS itself could also become required, extending privacy and rights invasions into homes and communities:

> I would hate to see PCAs or PAS become an institution of one . . . where people are forced to have a PCA . . . where they follow them around and call the police or call their psychiatrist. And it is just all medical model right in your own home.

The primary distinctions between PAS and existing community mental health services include the following: who defines the problem and assistance (i.e., what someone else wants for you and what you want); cognitive life activities (e.g., money management) currently done without consent for people with psychiatric disabilities (instead of under their direction or through negotiation); the level of intrusiveness in people's lives (versus personal control of the kind and degree of worker involvement); and the professional nature of existing community services (versus the employer-employee relationship of PAS).

Supportive Housing/Living and PAS

Other than case management, the informants did not spontaneously discuss the relationship between PAS and other mental health community living arrangements (Bachrach, 1994), which were seen as very dissimilar. However, a few perspectives are highlighted for those involved in the relatively new developments of supported housing (see, for example, Braisby et al., 1988; Carling, 1993; Knisley and Fleming, 1993; Tanzman, 1993).

PAS was viewed by one informant as a subset of supported housing, as overlapping with psychiatric rehabilitation (Dion and Anthony, 1987), and as part of existing community services, including peer counseling and advocacy with public benefits (Shreve, 1991). However, she expressed reluctance to compare things that are not really similar. Another informant described supportive living as an option for people who might not otherwise live in the community, which would involve a social worker coming to the house to see how everything was going with the personal care assistants (PCAs). She saw supportive living as different from PAS because of the number of hours available. Another informant described sheltered living situations in relationship to PAS and seemed to see PAS as part of a range or continuum of mental health community services (in contrast, see Taylor et al., 1987a; Taylor, 1988, for call for nonrestrictive environments).

Consumer-Run Drop-in Centers and PAS

Opinions varied in terms of the potential role of consumer-run, advocacy and support drop-in centers (see Carling, 1995) as sites for the delivery of PAS. Issues ranged from locating cross-disability PAS services at these centers, to concerns that the drop-in centers were too closely linked to the mental health system to locate PAS at these sites, and, finally, that drop-in centers should not offer PAS because they are not service oriented.

TASKS AND ROLES OF PERSONAL ASSISTANTS

Personal assistance services can be conceptualized in many different ways. In terms of the types of tasks, one informant suggested that all service types fall primarily in the three areas of physical, emotional, and cognitive (Stewart, 1991; description in Racino, 1995c). Other types of tasks from the working PAS definition (see "Introduction" to Part III) seen as applicable to people with psychiatric disabilities include infant and child rearing, which may involve work with other members of the family. Yet, if limitations are not placed on what types of tasks a personal assistant performs, tasks such as gardening or changing tires could be included.

How Tasks Are Defined

The ways in which tasks are defined and who decides how the services will be provided are critical elements typically neglected in service design. For example, providing security through a monitoring process is very different from a person you know calling you during the day to see how you are doing. Although the task and functions may be similar in both situations, the person's experience, sense of self-control, and sense of self-esteem may be very different. Personal assistance services does not mean control, treatment or supervision of the person, *but assistance based on needs as defined by the person.*

On a practical level, to obtain assistance in the current system, one PAS leader from Massachusetts described how she needed to translate legitimate emotional needs into a framework based on physical tasks (see Table 8.1). For example, she used overnight attendants because of "sedating medication" and "terrible night terrors" and, at times, needed help walking to the bathroom to avoid falling. Emotional support was essential for basic day-to-day living and translated into concrete activities with which a person could or could not be involved. For example, she explained:

> There were times when I had crippling depression and I couldn't mobilize myself to leave my apartment, couldn't mobilize myself to clean my apartment or cook for myself or do a lot of things that a person needs to do to keep [herself] going . . .

Needing to translate psychological distress into physical terms was considered an existing service design and regulatory barrier to access to current PAS services by people with psychiatric disabilities.

Roles of Personal Assistants

The informants supported a user-controlled model of personal assistance services, which places the person with a psychiatric disability in the role of employer and the personal assistant(s) as his or her employee(s).

TABLE 8.1. One State Example—Personal Assistance and Psychiatric Survivors: Making the System Work in Massachusetts

The best-known example in the psychiatric area of personal assistance services (PAS) was in Massachusetts, where one of the informants had successfully accessed the existing PAS system and modified it to meet her needs. Some perspectives of how this system works, in relationship to assessment, allocation of hours, and interviewing with people with psychiatric disabilities, are described below based upon her experiences.

Assessment process. The process in this state included assessment by two professionals, with the criteria based primarily on the needs of people with physical disabilities. As she explained, [the assessment process involves use of a questionnaire]. "In other words, what they are looking at is what they call hands-on support, so the ot [occupational therapist] comes to my house [for example] and asks how much weight I can lift [what transfers I use and how often I shave my legs]." Continued use of professional assessments was viewed as a given if governmental funding was involved. The lack of worker knowledge about PCAs for people with psychiatric disabilities and also the eligibility criteria were viewed as needing to be changed for the services to become accessible for people with psychiatric disabilities.

Allocation of hours. The allocation of hours through the Medicaid-funded program was a problem in that funding could not be used at the work site. She had been able to obtain "more than thirty-five hours a week" of PCAs after an appeal. She needed to supplement wages to obtain good PCAs. She was able to use the hours as she wished within the home, including for overnight attendants.

Interviewing process. In this state, the person could interview her or his own potential assistant(s) and also include other people, such as other [currently employed] PCAs in the process [of choosing a new one]. Initially denied the right to hire and fire her own attendants, even though she did these same functions at the independent living center where she served as Executive Director, she located an agency on the other side of the state who would work with her.

Source: Stewart, L. (1991). For Racino, J. (1995).*Toward Universal Access to Support: An Edited Collection on Personal Assistance Services.* Syracuse, NY and Boston, MA: Community and Policy Studies.

Note: Words in brackets are clarifications, April 1998.

As these leaders described, the personal assistant would be a nonprofessional who was *not* a therapist, savior, baby-sitter, case manager, overseer, supervisor, behavior manager, or drug enforcement agent. Suggested roles for the personal assistant were as a bridge, a navigator, an advocate, an intermediary, a facilitator, or a negotiator. Compared to roles with people with physical disabilities, PCAs in the psychiatric disability field would need to have greater individualization and flexibility.

The personal assistant was viewed as needing to act as an assistant to the person with a psychiatric disability with what the person wants done. One informant argued that having others do things for you could in fact define privilege, not disability. The PCA role was not solely task related, since the relationship can be an intimate one (Adler, 1993), and at times, simply the presence of the person may be desired. For example, just knowing someone is available and supportive may ease problems; a person may only be needed once or twice, if the availability is assured and *if* it is desired.

The personal characteristics of assistants were viewed as important. Although specific preferences may vary from person to person, human characteristics such as patience, tolerance, noncontrolling behavior, warmth, caring, good sense of boundaries, day-to-day operational understanding of rights, commitment to an empowering and teaching model, willingness to learn new skills, and an understanding of power imbalances were considered valuable assets.

In describing the tasks and roles of personal assistants, the informants also held strong beliefs about what PCAs *should not* do. In particular, the biggest expressed fear was that people could be forced to have a PCA, which would become a framework of monitoring or oppression and rob people of decision making. Another perceived danger was for PAS to become defined as a form of treatment, which could legitimate oversight by case managers, with an actual loss of personal freedom, a feeling of personal manipulation, with people feeling pushed into doing things that they cannot do. Unlike the traditional service worker functions, several informants believed that the role of a personal assistant should not include teaching and training because those being helped might become dependent, wanting the PCA to do things for them or manipulating the system (e.g., cannot clean house versus do not want to) in ways that may be perceived as unfair.

Further areas for investigation on the roles of personal assistants include treatment versus personal assistance, emergency PAS with recipient-run crisis teams, and payeeships (see Racino, 1995c). Two major concerns were behavioral issues, including their relationship with (the "slippery slope" of) involuntary commitment, and people already involved with the mental health system (due to "internalized oppression") regarding PCAs as therapists, no matter how their roles are formally defined. Although some of these issues reflect old debates, (see the voluminous literature on commitment, for example, Blanch, 1992), they need to be revisited in the context of developing conceptual and practical models of personal assistance services.

Relationships: Friends and Families

At least six areas related to relationships with people's own families and friends need further exploration: (1) survivors' efforts to counteract the perception of being a burden (Cook et al., 1994); (2) having others with dissimilar or even counterviews representing their own (e.g., national parent organizations); (3) the need for people to rely on families for support when no other options are available, even when the family relationship may be part of the problem (e.g., in an abusive situation); (4) the effect on friendships, including the nature of the power balance, the setting of boundaries, rules, and authority, and paid relationships; (5) the use of personal assistance services for children as an alternative to residential foster care (see Lindsey, 1991; Friedman, 1988, on foster care); and (6) parents' overprotectiveness of their children with disabilities.

STRATEGIES AND ACCOMMODATIONS

In terms of specific types of strategies that might be applied by people with psychiatric disabilities or psychiatric survivors, the clearest example was the *use of advance directives* (also Grodin, 1993) *and other forms of self-help strategies.* The incorporation of PAS into work (see Andrews et al., 1992; and reasonable accommodations, Colligan, 1986; Mancuso, 1993) and the inclusion of advocacy and support components into the PAS model were just beginning to be considered.

Use of Advance Directives

In decision making, a person with a psychiatric disability could set up advance directives (High, 1991), situational applications, or crisis plans with his or her personal assistant. This could include strategies for how he or she would like to have specific situations handled, such as self-injurious behaviors. By articulating these directives to the personal assistant beforehand, the person would be able to maintain a degree of self-control during times when he or she may not be able to clearly direct others on how to handle the situation.

Incorporating Self-Help Strategies

People described their own self-help strategies, ranging from "working with voices" to dealing with self-injury, depression, or suicidal actions. People shared different ways in which they dealt with their symptoms to function better in daily life. For example, as one woman described:

> People, like myself, very often get flooded by voices that are dis-tress[ful] [and] begin to have a very difficult time screening out. We lose the ability to distinguish figure and ground in terms of auditory perception. . . . So when I am hearing voices that are extremely distressing that becomes part of the scenario. So when I am not hearing voices I like to be able to work on developing the skills of pushing auditory stimulation into the background.

Another person described nontraditional, nonpsychiatric practices, which included forms of relaxation such as massages and hot tubs, which "not only got me out of the original stuff that made me feel crazy to begin with, but also the worst part of it—the revictimization and retraumatization that I experienced in mental health." Although people may define their own self-help strategies, sometimes people "need a partner in terms of implement-ing these strategies."

PAS, Accommodations, and Work

Personal assistance services for people with psychiatric disabilities were perceived, in part, as an issue of fairness in accommodations. One major issue was whether PCAs, as a form of accommodation, should be paid for in whole or in part by the employer. One perception was that PAS at the workplace was an Americans with Disabilities Act issue, with trans-portation and flexible time two key work accommodations that were dis-cussed as part of that movement (see Racino with Whittico, 1998). The use of personal assistants for activities such as travel (e.g., international con-sulting) and conferences was considered essential for the performance of some jobs. However, one informant had difficulty picturing what PAS at work would mean, since he perceived overcoming devaluation and feel-ings of worthlessness as the primary issues people faced, explaining that for some people, "the job might be the source of the problem." Supported employment was already an existing option (Anthony and Blanch, 1987;

Wehman et al., 1991) for some people, and the great variability in job types and individual differences were cited as reasons why it was difficult to describe PCA roles in employment.

Other Types of Options: Making PAS Work

An advocacy and peer support component, connected with personal assistance services, might have several different functions, including preventing undesired entry into institutional psychiatric services (Ebert, 1990). Without such a mechanism, PAS may not be accepted as a viable option by some people. People may need support the first time "things get strange," and mechanisms need to be in place to refer people away from the institutions and to keep people out of the mental health system.

Proposed community approaches to personal assistance services included the use of community consumer-counseling services for money management and a role similar to that of a hotel concierge. In the latter, the fear was expressed that this comparison could be misperceived by the public (i.e., as not a real need or as wasteful of public funding). However, use of these community options, with possible expanded roles of community organizations, may be one way to move away from the use of mental health and social service systems.

DECISION MAKING AND CONSUMER CONTROL

Self-determination contrasts with treatment in a traditional mental health sphere, which may be a hierarchical construct in which a professional or a team of professionals "gets to decide what is in your best interests." PAS differs from these mental health services in that such services allow control to remain in the hands of the people who are seeking assistance "in ways they choose and want to be assisted." This feature would distinguish PAS from other existing community services, allowing people to have control over who comes into their home and to determine aspects of the job the PCAs perform. As one PAS user explained:

> Personal assistance services allows me to interview people and bring people I feel comfortable with into my home to do things that I tell them that I need. And if they don't do that, I can get rid of them. . . . With personal care assistants, I can stay in my own home. I can sleep in my own bed. I can eat the food I want to eat.

Personal autonomy and control can help people maintain their personal health and stability. For example, as one person said, "Giving people control actually helps them to be more relaxed and [not] feel pushed, and you know, and they probably won't act out as much."

Assumptions Regarding Competency

People with psychiatric disabilities are viewed, by virtue of their diagnosis, as incompetent at handling their own affairs and, thus, may be deemed unable to direct their own PAS. This core assumption has contributed to the development of an existing community services system in which people are "managed"; they are given implicit messages that they do not know what is best for them (Chamberlin and Rogers, 1990; Ridgway, 1988). As one informant explained, recognition of self-determination exists up to a point, then "clinical judgment substitutes for the consumers' best interest" (see also, on clinical judgment, Biklen, 1988). This leaves little room for bad choices or the opportunity to fail, even in non-life-threatening areas such as choosing what to eat. What were called bad decisions were often simply those decisions with which others disagreed. Similar to treatment of adolescents, much literature exists on best interests and clinical judgment, primarily from the professional and legal viewpoints (e.g., Kapp, 1994; Perlin, 1994; Schwartz, 1989).

User Control Components

People in all sorts of different disability groups have all varying levels of motivation to gain control back over their lives.

In terms of features promoting user control and self-determination, the main components suggested were (1) to be able to choose who comes into your home and to fire assistants who do not meet your expectations; (2) user decisions regarding what services they want and how these services would be provided; (3) for the user to also define how situations should be handled during times when they might not be viewed as capable of making those kinds of decisions; (4) a system of advocacy and other safeguards to keep people from becoming involved with the system; and (5) management options available through consumer-run organizations. Informants also suggested other roles for people with psychiatric disabilities in the development of PAS, such as experts in model design, individual providers of PAS (PCAs) to other people with psychiatric disabilities (see in contrast, use as case management aides, Sherman and Porter, 1991), trainers of one's own employees and group sensitivity, and organizational providers (e.g., consumer/survivor-run organizations), and board members.

Assistance with Decision Making

Due to the assumptions regarding the capacities of people with psychiatric disabilities, informants varied on their philosophical stance toward who could or could not self-direct their own PAS. While supporting as much independence as possible in directing one's own life, according to some informants, some people may need training and support in order to be considered competent. Two primary implementation approaches were mentioned as ways to assist people who might need some help in decision making: surrogacy (i.e., decision making performed by another, such as a parent, relative, or agency representative) and the use of a psychiatric living will. Other options to consider in decision making are the use of limited guardianships, the *definition of personal assistance services as other than treatment*, the ways in which questions are phrased in obtaining information, and the availability of training, information, support, and advocacy (so people can effectively counter claims of incompetency and challenge the ways they are "managed") (see Racino, 1995c).

Other Coordination Models

One perceived need was the dissemination of various coordination and management models as they currently exist (Egley, 1994) to compare PAS related to people with psychiatric disabilities to other models. Two additional mechanisms were the potential use of clearinghouses or registries and the need for people "behind the scenes" to make PAS work (e.g., cutting paychecks, keeping track of sick days, and making arrangements for events, such as the departure of a personal assistant).

Preservation of Rights

> We all have a right to make bad decisions too, even if those decisions mean . . . we don't take our medications or don't eat the proper kinds of food. . . . All those kinds of decisions people have a right to make even if they are bad decisions.

People may be denied active participation in their own treatment. ("We want the opportunity to question our medications which anyone would who is on mind-altering medications.") They may also be at risk of involuntary commitment (Morgan, 1990; Schwartz, 1989), and this potential risk could extend to actions taken by the personal assistant if advance directives are not followed.

PRACTICAL ASPECTS OF PAS

Practical aspects of assistance include universal access, training of personal assistants, credentialing, and wages and benefits; Table 8.2 highlights financial concerns (Racino, 1995c).

Universal Access

One informant explained that she believes there is a "desire to include those who have not been included," and that people with diverse disabilities

TABLE 8.2. Financial Concerns with Personal Assistance Services

- The argument that personal assistance services would be less costly and more beneficial than the use of hospitalization
- The political and financial barriers of moving funding from nursing homes to personal assistance services
- The need to make Medicaid funding more accessible to people with psychiatric disabilities based on their needs, including supporting people at work
- The perceived need to develop arguments to counteract fears about the potential high expense of PAS, especially twenty-four-hour-a-day, seven-days-a-week availability
- The possible need to prioritize the use of money based upon its use to preserve life or to support activities such as work
- The incorporation of PAS within Plans to Achieve Self-Sufficiency (PASS) as one financing mechanism
- The problem of the medicalization of services (including areas such as worker certification, clinical judgment, and individual financing) through the tie to Medicaid funding
- Lack of availability of money for pilot projects through independent living centers or designated for personal assistance services for people with psychiatric disabilities
- The lack of funding to pay for services without becoming part of the mental health system, including diagnoses and so forth
- The need for accountability if third-party payments are involved, including the potential for abuse of user-controlled personal assistance services
- The need for adequate funding amounts to cover other costs such as unemployment, FICA, IRS, and wages.

Source: Racino, J. (1995c). *Toward Universal Access to Support: An Edited Collection on Personal Assistance Services.* Syracuse, NY, and Boston, MA: Community and Policy Studies.

have similar fundamental concerns. Universal access was viewed as access by all people with disabilities or as access for all people who needed personal assistance services whether or not they had a disability. One person expressed the fear that if universal accessibility was not in place, one group would lose out by possibly receiving inferior services. Another leader specifically mentioned that no exclusion from PAS should be made on the basis of family members in the household, disability, or age.

The concept of *consumer-controlled services* makes sense and is a perfect fit with people in the psychiatric survivor movement. Yet, reportedly, no working PAS system was addressing state-by-state needs in the United States for children, youth, or adults with psychiatric disabilities.

Strategic planning, a real "thinking through" of issues, ranging from safeguards to involuntary commitment to development for all people, was needed, together with systematic knowledge generation. Although several leaders expressed a desire for a model that works for all people with disabilities, care must be taken so that PAS does not become another form of professionally directed care in the community.

Chapter 9

Self-Advocacy,
the Independent Living Movement,
and Personal Assistance Services

Julie Ann Racino

INTRODUCTION

Personal assistance services (PAS) are politically part of an international movement of people of all abilities, ages, incomes, ethnicities, and cultures (American Association on Mental Retardation, nd,b; Litvak, Zukas, and Heumann, 1987; Nosek, 1992; see Table 9.1). In its user-controlled or directed forms, PAS tends to be associated with independent living centers (Wong and Millard, 1992), whose predominant users are people with physical disabilities with increased usage by and programs for people with diverse disabilities (e.g., Jones et al., 1988; Sigelman and Parham, 1981).

However, in some places in the United States, home care or health agencies (Eustis, Kane, and Fischer, 1993) and those in the fields of mental health, mental retardation, and brain injuries (see Chapter 8, 10, and 11) have moved in these directions with support services. This chapter reports on the results of interviews with service users of PAS and selected advisors, parents, educators, and facilitators.

This chapter is a modified version of Racino, J. (1995c). "Personal Assistance Services: People with Mental Retardation and Physical Disabilities." In *Toward Universal Access to Support: An Edited Collection on Personal Assistance Services.* Syracuse, NY, and Boston, MA: Community and Policy Studies.

TABLE 9.1. PAS for People with Cognitive Disabilities: Personal Perspectives

---

Beverly Evans

Attendants are supposed to help with cooking, cleaning, personal care, lifting, transportation, helping read your mail, facilitation, all this other stuff—housekeeping, shopping, doctors' appointments, dentists, taking you if you have to go someplace—they're supposed to be taking you places.

Martha E. Ford

I realize now that Jud (my brother) had quite an extensive cadre of informal assistants who have helped him to function within the family unit and the community. Jud was regularly seen around town in the company of one of us, doing things that people typically do—going to the barbershop, post office, grocery store, or church; going to the drugstore for a coke; or as teenagers, riding around listening to rock and roll.

Connie Martinez

I was asked to be involved in the DD Council (State Council on Developmental Disabilities in California). . . . I was involved in independent living . . . already, seeing a lot of things I would like to see changed. I was involved in People First, so I was ready to change certain things—in my dreams and my hopes.

Jeffrey L. Strully and Cindy Strully

Shawntell (our daughter) is a person who is truly gifted. However, she needs a lot of assistance in order to have a decent quality of life. This assistance and support comes from three levels: family involvement, friends, and an integration facilitator. . . . What we envision for Shawntell and what she envisions for herself is life filled with rich diversity, fun, friends, and exciting adventures.

Source: Weissman, J., Kennedy, J., and Litvak, S. (1991). *Personal Perspectives on Personal Assistance Services.* Oakland, CA: Research and Training Center (RTC) on Policy in Independent Living, World Institute on Disability, InfoUse, and Western Public Health Consortium, pp. 49, 27, 45, 15, respectively.

UNIVERSAL ACCESS TO PAS

Everyone who needs and wants personal assistance services should be able to have it. Personal assistance services are "a need not a privilege . . . a need, a definite need, I couldn't do without it."

Universal access to PAS is one way of "trying to include everyone in society," including in homes ("living in the least restrictive society"), on the job and in the classroom ("right" to education). Barriers continued to include "fear of prohibitive cost," the need to educate the general public as to why services are a necessity, not an extra or luxury, and service barriers such as inadequate wages for demanding work for personal assistants who perform demanding work.

People who have been typically excluded from PAS are: people "with mental illness" who do not have access to any or minimal supports and services, people with visual impairments, and people who have "typically not been afforded supportive living opportunities in many areas of the country. "These may include people who may not be able to "walk or talk or anything" (see Taylor et al., 1987). Outreach to minorities was also "vitally important," together with involving the family "as much as you can, which is essential with close-knit communities (e.g., the Latino community).

Access Based Upon Need

In these interviews, there was an underlying theme of access based upon need for personal assistance services (see Racino, 1995c, p. 5). The need might be perceived as any of the following:

- *A human need, common to everyone*
- *A medical, professionally endorsed need*
- *A form of prevention for people at risk*
- *A felt need by people with and without disabilities*
- *A right, not a privilege*

Access for People of All Ages, Capacities, and Ethnicities

Personal assistance services is often described as being for people of all ages, disabilities, ethnicities, and cultures (Heumann, 1993; Tate and Chadderdon, 1992). The question of access (DeJong and Lifchez, 1983) can be viewed as primarily one of *nondiscrimination* (i.e., not being excluded from access opportunities that are available to others). One activist clearly described how the discrimination issues of minorities parallel the experiences of people with disabilities, with access considered in terms of *assimilation*. This activist described his People First Group in Missouri:

> As a matter of fact, right now we have two African Americans in our People First Group, and they fit right in, so to speak. Nobody discriminates against them, or anything, because we have all been through discrimination in one way or another, and so we don't discriminate against anybody.

Another person explained that a total of thirty-six states and countries were represented at the 1994 International People First Conference. However, he continued that in terms of service access, particular groups of people (e.g., "Indians," "Spanish") are still perceived as having difficulty with involvement of people with disabilities.

Ages

Consistent with the philosophy of the independent living movement (e.g., Frieden and Nosek, 1985; Budde and Bachelder, 1986; Michaels, 1989; DeJong, Batavia, and McKnew, 1992), one leader explained how personal assistance services should be available to people of all ages, including children ("because to me you are never too young to have those supports"), adolescents, and elders (e.g., "if they have Alzheimer's or something else) as well as adults. Personal assistance services for children or youth were generally described as being provided by the parents (see Nosek and Howland, 1993).

INFORMATION ACCESS TO PAS

Access to information about PAS and choices as to whether or not to use the services are a matter of civil rights of adults—rights that should not be interfered with by service coordinators or parents to object. However, joint decision making tends to be supported for adults living in their parents' home. Assumptions for exclusion of information access involve concerns that the person will not "understand what the personal assistant is there for," or the safety of the person, particularly in controversial areas such as sexual activity and access and training in the use of condoms.

Information access is perceived as important because it forms the basis for people making decisions about what they need, and is a part of the right to think freely ("everyone should have the right to think about things that they need help with or things they don't need help with"). To be accessible, information must be understandable, and available in other forms (e.g., large print), and preferably through the public media.

Information Access by Children and Youth

Parents have diverse ways of raising their children; some parents "encourage their disabled child to do what they want, how they want, where they want . . . and others protect, protect." As a leading self-advocate from Tennessee explained:

> You could talk to the parents as a parent. And talk to the son as their son, but treat him as a person and ask him what he wants. But, the parents are still going to be his parents. He's still got rules and regulations in his house. But when he's old enough and he wants to know more, I think he should still do it without the parents even knowing that he's doing it.

This stance is partially reflected in the recognition that children and youth do things with their peers when growing up that may not be approved by their parents (see Chapter 11). As one self-advocate explained:

> They are going to do what we did when growing up. . . . They're going to drink a beer. They're going to do something they want to be part of the crowd. . . . I want them to be treated just like anyone else.

However, parents of children with disabilities also will take diverse stances, including on issues such as what information should be accessible to their children.

COMMUNITY ACCESS

In terms of generic community access, the primary perspective on this approach involved comparing the institution with the community access ("Instead of giving money to the institution, they should give it to the community"). Strategies might involve moving money from institutions to the community, having greater access in community settings to going to community places (e.g., going shopping or to the movies), and having people move out of institutions. One person described the issue of PAS and access to the Americans with Disabilities Act (ADA), noting that accessibility involved more than changes in buildings. Community access was also described in terms of physical changes in the way cities, towns, or communities approach areas such as their public works. For example, as described in Berkeley (Racino, 1993):

> Here in California, they have noisemakers or streetlights or some kind of thing that would help people with disabilities who have a visual impairment, or whatever, identify what it means to walk across the street or don't walk or stop or go or whatever.

Another self-advocate, who lived part of his life in an institution, explained:

> If the community starts opening up their doors and giving people a chance to show them that they are people, [they would find out] . . . they don't have to be afraid of them.

Community approaches to PAS include the use of panels (parent, teacher, assistant), task forces, and small community organizations with representatives from all involved areas.

VIEWS OF MENTAL RETARDATION

It is important to understand that none of the people who were asked considered themselves to be mentally retarded or to have mental retardation (see Bogdan and Taylor, 1982; Edgerton, 1979). Instead, people talked about being labeled as having mental retardation and what practical meaning had in their lives. The label was connected with being institutionalized, of being seen as not having potential, as being slow (e.g., at tying shoes), and of not having opportunities to learn (e.g., "reading skills") and to be out in the community ("I just want to see people who do get labeled out in the community."). One person explained how he held a very different view of himself than the ways the state labeled or saw him:

> The state says that I am mentally retarded. But I don't consider my[self] to be. I'm slow in doing what I do, but I am darn proud of what I do.

Acceptable Language

In response to what language would be acceptable in describing approaches to personal assistance services, one self-advocate explained that people needed to stop using the word mental retardation, using instead something similar to "person with a disability." He expressed how when a person is labeled as retarded, she or he is not treated like a person with a disability, and this weighs on a person's mind throughout his or her life. As he explained:

People that do that make me really. . . . I don't want to say angry, but they disappoint me because they don't treat me like a person with just a disability.

RELATIONSHIP WITH SELF-ADVOCACY

Partially due to the selection process, most of the people interviewed were involved with organized self-advocacy groups or a particular movement (see also Chapter 5). Several people described themselves in terms of their self-advocacy roles (e.g., self-advocacy coordinator). Self-advocacy groups are to be run by people with disabilities, so people will have an opportunity to learn to speak up for themselves and to work on different issues such as transportation, personal attendants (DeJong and Wenker, 1983; Ludlum, Beeman, and Ducharme, 1991), and friendships. Self-advocacy groups are organized on the local, state, national (Alexandria, Virginia, 1994), and international levels (1994 meeting in Toronto, Canada). (For international update on self-advocacy, see Dybwad and Bersani, 1996.) Self-advocacy provides the following opportunities:

- Confront discrimination, address limitations on what people are allowed to do, and counteract disrespect
- Act as a role model for others and assist other people to become part of the community—get them a regular job, get them ready to be in a group home, and show them that they can be a person first
- Actively express and act on a commitment to work for the betterment of life for other people with and without disabilities as well as for oneself

MEANING OF PERSONAL ASSISTANCE SERVICES

Personal assistance can have a variety of meanings, because everyone has their own way of thinking about what personal assistance is all about. This could include the traditional definition of a personal care attendant as someone (see Litvak, Zukas, and Brown, 1991) who would take care of needs that "I couldn't take care of on my own . . . and help me do things that I can't do."

Personal assistance services is still a new idea from the perspective of people with mental retardation (see Table 9.1), who thought it was only for those with physical disabilities, (see DeJong and Lifchez, 1983, on environmental access). However, with expanded approaches, PAS is also "for people who need cognitive support, like I do, and for people that are hearing impaired" (e.g., the sign interpreter, sign language).

PAS As an Alternative to Institutions and Facilities

For some people, personal assistance services holds the promise of an alternative to their own experiences with institutionalization, that they may have had as a child when their parents died. Yet, some people may be perceived as being too disabled to use personal assistance services, as one research informant described a person she knows who might use PAS:

> She needs round-the-clock care, so to speak, and they [her parents] need a nurse to come in, a therapist to come in and help them and all that, and someone like that, in a way, would be too severe to have personal assistance services because she's not all that mobile. . . . I don't believe she can be placed in a wheelchair, even.

In contrast, PAS may be seen as a supplement to existing twenty-four-hour agency (comprehensive) support systems.

PAS As Designed by Service Users

PAS could be increasingly defined by the service users, with an initial expansion suggested by staff, advocates, and parents to include helping people to become part of their community and to facilitate friendships and services beyond those provided by specific agencies (e.g., Lutfiyya, 1992). Personal assistance services has also been conceptualized, in the field of mental retardation, as a subcategory (extension) of supportive living or community living, with people having the opportunity to choose, hire, and fire their own assistants, to choose people to be part of their support services and their lives, and to spend time with people outside of paid time (see Center on Human Policy, 1989a; Johnson, 1985; O'Brien, 1992; Racino, 1991e; Racino with Whittico, 1998). Table 9.2 describes a self-determination project on personal assistance services in New Hampshire, with national surveys (Wehmeyer and Metzler, 1995) and decision-making studies (Kishi et al., 1988) during this period.

As described in these interviews, personal assistance tasks include therapies and exercises, personal hygiene, interpretation, financial management, office work, home activities, community activities and errands, jobs, household management, adult education and volunteer work, relationship facilitation, safety, transportation, cognitive support, and management (see Consortium of Citizens with Disabilities, 1991).

TABLE 9.2. Demonstration Project on Personal Assistance Services

New Hampshire Self-Determination Project
In 1993, the Robert Wood Johnson (RWJ) Foundation awarded a three-year grant to Monadnock Developmental Services, Inc. (MDS), to design and implement a demonstration project that develops a service delivery system, including the provision of PAS, whereby the consumer and his or her support network (e.g., circles of support) were truly in charge of their own needs. . . . The primary objective of the project was to test whether the methods of self-determination applied will decrease per capita spending and increase the quality of life for those participating in the project. The self-determination project has three major components: • Each consumer with severe, chronic disabilities (mental retardation, epilepsy, dual diagnosis, cerebral palsy) is given the opportunity to control the planning (on an annual and as-needed basis) of their service needs with the assistance of the family members and friends he or she chooses. This group is often referred to as the consumer's "Circle of Support." • Each consumer in the demonstration controls a certain amount of Medicaid and state dollars (e.g., their individualized budget), which he or she has the authority to spend on all residential, employment, and personal needs as he or she and the Circle see fit. • Needed services (including PAS) are purchased through a variety of brokering methods. Each consumer is able to contract for any and all services through discrete contracts.

Source: Flanagan, S. and Green, P. (1997). *Consumer-Directed Personal Assistance Services: Key Operational Issues for State CD-PAS Programs Using Intermediary Service Organizations.* Cambridge, MA: The Medstat Group, Appendix V, pp. 46-47.

SUPPORT AND DECISION MAKING

Decision making (e.g., "right to have a say") was described as both a right in relationship to people's own lives and to services and as part of human dignity, happiness, and freedom from coercion (e.g., "we have feelings . . . we have our own ideas"). People deserve the right to have more say in what type of support and help they want, without being punished. One informant described the history of choice in services in his life:

> Before . . . [it was] just presumed . . . just thought that's what we
> want. Like it was forced upon us, and so that's why I feel that we
> should have more of a say in what they get or receive for support and
> help.

As in institutional settings and with young children, adults reported that
they needed to "do what the group home tells you. You get up when they
tell you. You go to bed when they tell you."

Personal assistance services (PAS) offered the hope of moving from
controlling environments ("The kind of assistance that I need is not being
told what to do . . . and I don't like the way they are taking care of me.")
Obtaining services or help does not mean that a person is denied the right
of making his or her own decisions. For example:

> No, I would still have my decisions. I would just have someone to
> help me budget my money better so I could put some money aside so
> I could go on vacation.

Distinctions were made between people who were perceived as able or
unable to make their own decisions and people who have or have not been
taught to make decisions (see Guess, Benson, and Siegel-Causey, 1985,
for a seminal work that was intended to counteract the beliefs that persons
with severe disabilities are not capable of making choices in their own best
interest).

PERSONAL ASSISTANCE SERVICES AND EMPLOYMENT

Four major points were made by the primary informants regarding the
development of personal assistance services in relation to employment
situations. First, some people still work in workshops, which were described as places for people with disabilities. Personal care and hygiene
(e.g., bathing) are part of what is discussed in "workshops." Second, a
personal care attendant may be perceived as only needed in the home
setting, partially because that is how the payment scheme is sometimes set
up (see, for example, California IHSS—in-home support services—and
the federal Community Supported Living Arrangements; Allen, Shea &
Associates and Forrest, 1993; Vivona and Kaplan, 1990). Third, in competitive jobs, the need or request for personal assistance services can be
perceived as an incapacity to meet the requirements of the job (see also
Chapter 8). As one research informant explained:

> To me, if a person comes to get support for a job, I don't think they
> would be hired in the first place because most businesses expect you
> to know everything and to do everything, from what I understand.

Fourth, support staff may assist people with volunteer work at community sites, in finding another job, or in advocating for employment. In the supplemental interviews, issues regarding assistive devices, transportation, and in-home supports for the job were raised, together with the roles of job coaches and personal assistants. Supported employment (Albin et al., 1993; Brooke, Barcus, and Inge, 1992; Wehman and Kregel, 1990) was not mentioned by name, only through references instead to the job coach model.

VULNERABILITY AND ABUSE: PERSONAL ASSISTANTS

In developing models of personal assistance services, another area of consideration is the possibility of abuse, including from personal assistants, staff, and parents (see Sobsey, 1994; Ulciny et al., 1990). For example, assistants or attendants may "bring drugs into the house," might "stay out all night," might "steal" from the person, could "abuse" the person verbally or physically, could hover over the person ("they look down on me" in my wheelchair), or may leave the person alone ("might not show up for work").

While these actions could occur anywhere, "a person with a disability" may not be taken seriously if he or she says something is wrong, and may feel the need to keep these feelings inside. People who take medications may also be perceived, for example, as being "drunk" when it could mean that "he could be tired or something like that." "People may also panic about abuse"; actions taken in response to complaints can include silencing of the disabled person and staff accused of abuse are rehired to work with other people with disabilities.

Personal assistants may not provide the services for which they are paid. If the situation does not work out to the satisfaction of the service user, he or she may be able to switch agencies or hire a new person. As one person described:

> Well, they would come in and tell me they're going to sit down and watch TV, which they did, and I put my foot down. And I just told them I'm the boss, and they didn't like it.

PRACTICAL ISSUES OF PERSONAL ASSISTANCE SERVICES

A tremendous demand exists for community services (see Hayden and DePaepe, 1994), such as personal assistance services, with one informant reporting over 1,000 people on waiting lists in Connecticut. Personal assistance services are often described in terms of two major forms of service delivery: first, the independent living model, with hiring, training, and firing of the personal assistant by the service users and, at times, independent living center support (see Racino, 1993b, for description of the Berkeley Center for Independent Living), and second, agency models whereby the agency is the primary employer, making decisions related to management of the assistants. Practical issues in the personal assistance debate are highlighted in Table 9.3.

Parents As Personal Assistants

Parents are considered to be the primary providers of personal assistance for their children (see Table 9.1 for diverse perspectives on PAS; see Turnbull and Rutherford, 1985, on independence), with "extraordinary" assistance, due to the child's disability, often the subject of debate on service payments. As children and youth, the primary informants either obtained assistance from family members or lived in out-of-home placements or institutionalized settings away from their families. When they became adults, one mother continued to provide assistance, and one spouse would provide backup, especially at night.

Viewpoints regarding the payment of family members varied based on traditional rationales: (1) the competency of the family, (2) the decisions made by each family, and (3) the responsibility to care for your own children and siblings. Minimal distinctions were made during this period between underage children and adults living in or out of the home, or the relationships with parents who were advocating for post-twenty-one family support payments. As one informant described, in family situations, "there's always a need for more supports for the family, to get away and have time for themselves and have time with their other children, and to show that they're important too, and not just this one person, just because he needs extra time or special care."

Agency Models of Personal Assistance Services

Some people use an agency model of personal assistance services, with assistants being supplied by the agency. In agency models, the agency may assist or handle the financing, select and train the assistants, and handle the paperwork. These models may resemble traditional approaches to in-home nursing services by home health care agencies, or they may function more as support organizations (see Michael Kennedy, 1993, for another approach used in Central New York).

TABLE 9.3. Practical Issues in the Personal Assistance Debate

- Whether therapies and nursing services should be considered as medical services or be subsumed as part of nonprofessional personal assistance services
- Whether personal assistants should be teachers/skill instructors, provide personal assistance services only if the person cannot do those functions himself or herself, and/or work at the direction of the service users
- The nature of help, including whether people will be required to prove they can perform skills before being permitted to then do things on their own
- The nature of help, whether it is for people with disabilities or everyone, and who should decide how the support or assistance gets done
- Whether personal assistance on the job should be more traditionally defined (e.g., personal care) and separated from other employment issues
- Whether personal assistance can be incorporated within the context of everyday community places and events (e.g., beauty shops)
- Whether and, if so, how, to incorporate areas of emotional support in personal assistance in nonstigmatizing, less prejudicial ways
- Whether personal assistants who work with people with psychiatric disabilities need to be qualified
- The nature of the relationship with the personal assistant, including respecting a person's wishes;
- The distinctions between seeking support one needs and wants and teaching/providing living supports
- The issue of readiness for being on one's own, levels of independence, and degree of assistance
- The meaning and use of cognitive support
- Infant and child care issues, including assistance for parents who work and the continued treatment of adults with disabilities as children
- Personal relationships, circle of friends, and sexuality, including decision making, physical assistance with sexual activities, and relevance of where people live

Source: Racino, J. (1995c). *Toward Universal Access to Support: An Edited Collection on Personal Assistance Services.* Syracuse, NY, and Boston MA: Community and Policy Studies.

In these interviews, personal assistants were the name given to staff who appeared to be employed by a mental retardation agency, within the context of a group home or facility (see Litvak, Zukas, and Heumann, 1987, p. 16). In agency models of assistance, one informant explained that a change had been occurring from *standardized to person-oriented pro-*

grams that reflected the person's *individual needs* (see Racino et al., 1993).

> Before it seemed like all the programs were one size fits all, so to speak. It didn't fit the person. So the person was expected to fit the program. But, you know, with the small person-oriented program, the program fits the person. Because everybody has their own individual needs and wants that might be different from somebody else's. Like our metabolism, it's all unique to that person.

Assistance can be provided within the context of families and group home settings, and for some people, moving out on their own is still a goal. People can be viewed as either able or unable to live on their own, based upon whether they can learn the skills that are necessary to live independently (see Taylor et al., 1986, for critique with people with severe disabilities). The kind of assistance people might need, however, might be different from what the same person might need in another living situation. As a person who has been trained in PAS, but who currently lives at home, described his situation:

> Since I'm living at home, I don't need help that much, and to me, I want to live out on my own in a real bad way. Get away from my parents, because I feel that it would be better in the long run for me. . . . Well, the only support and help I need on that would be how to operate a washer and dryer, and dishwasher, because I can cook for the most part. . . . I would [also] need money management.

Training

One self-advocate from Missouri specifically obtained training on personal assistance services and had previous SRV (social role valorization; Wolfensberger, 1983) and PASSING (Program Analysis of Service Systems) training, developed by Wolf Wolfensberger of Syracuse University (Wolfensberger, 1972). The latter is a form of program evaluation of human services used in countries such as the United States, Canada, and Great Britain.

Other types of training raised as potentially relevant included the following content areas:

- *Disability awareness* ("teach people what it's like being disabled, or what it feels like being discriminated against")
- *Sexuality, relationships, and marriage* ("if they want to get married, let them get married")

- *Why people need to be in the community* ("You know I was in an institution for eleven years in my life and it was hell")
- *Mainstreaming and needs* ("that these are people too")
- *Abuse and community safety* ("They don't tell them what is going on in the community, what to watch out for")
- *Medications* (staff "would have to be med certified")

Training was needed not only for personal assistants but for advisors, staff and directors in group homes, the people they serve in group homes, people living in institutions, teenagers and adults, as well as communities and neighborhoods. Some training could be done by People First, by other attendants who have experience in this area, and by professionals such as the police, lawyers, and the Justice Department).

Some people may wish to train their own assistants (the independent living model) (Ulciny and Jones, 1988), whereas other people may prefer that the assistants have basic training prior to working with/for them. As one person described:

> Before they work with me, I would like them to be trained because if they are not trained, then it makes it harder for me. . . . I would like them to know a little bit about me before they come to my house.

Nature of the Relationship with Assistants

People may have different expectations of what the nature of their relationship will be with the personal assistant. Some people prefer an employee-employer relationship, whereas others may expect the person to share friendship or to be part of their family. As one person described this relationship:

> Some attendants, they're just employer-employee. They don't go beyond the friendship, and some attendants do that, even though we have to rely on them the rest of our lives. Some attendants are like family.

Assistants who view the relationship as one of employment may have other demands and expectations about the conditions in which they will work, including relationships with their own friends. Several people with disabilities expressed a strong preference for having the option to select and fire their own assistants, for example:

> I would prefer to do that because when you're working for the state, you automatically have to take whoever they give you . . . if they screw up and everything, then you fire that person . . . but you have to have a good reason.

Another informant explained that an assistant/attendant would have to "like the job and be committed to it; otherwise, it won't last too long." Another person affirmed that if it were not for his attendant, "I'd probably be in a nursing home."

Service Availability

The primary principles of service availability named by several informants included availability of personal assistants depending upon individual needs ("should be available when somebody needs them"), in times of emergency ("Respite" might be one option to function "almost like a backup person"), on a twenty-four-hour basis if needed ("usually a person doesn't need anybody when they are asleep, unless something should happen to them"), and based upon personal choice ("Right now the state tells you how long you can stay at a party").

Quality of Services

In regard to the review of satisfaction and quality of services monitoring (De Paiva and Lowe, 1986), suggestions included the use of volunteer community monitoring teams to act as watchdogs, to get to know the person and act as independent voices and the inclusion of other people in particular circles, for example, with people who do not speak. Quality of service approaches include those for residential services and community living, citizen and self-advocacy, non-facility-based services, and evaluation by service users. Also, one person stated it was important to see that people did not take advantage of the assistance system when they did not need it.

Two perspectives stated by people in two different states (who use different forms of assistance) were that the agency-based system was too controlled by "the state" and the opposite that the state should take more control in monitoring for potential abuse. (For more information on quality of services, see, for example, Towell, 1988, in the United Kingdom; Eustis, Kane, and Fischer, 1993, on home care; and Bradley and Bersani, 1990).

Financing of Personal Assistance Services

One person explained that the biggest barrier to the expansion of personal assistance services was still money. Two people noted that the state "only pays for what they have to pay for" and "won't pay for it if they don't think you need it." Some people would prefer to receive the money for assistance directly instead of having the state give money to the agency or having the agency act as their payee:

> I would like to get the money from the state that Med Center gets, $19 an hour, and instead of the state giving to Med Center, I would pay Andy myself.

This position was echoed by another informant who explained:

> Give me the money so I can pay my own PCA and have people that I want. . . . I would want to pay my own people . . . because the agency—I'm not knocking the agency at all, but I feel that if I pay the person, the person would have to come in and take care of me when I set up the time for him.

With the California in-home support services program, one informant stated that "personal assistant[s] should be paid for everything that they do . . . . They should get paid to feed me, to put the spoon in my mouth. Or they should get paid [for] taking me on a trip, like to Disneyland, or something." The same person described how attendants did not get paid if they stayed overnight. Another person believed, however, that "if they do need it [PAS], they should pay a little something for it. I'm lucky. I don't pay for any of it; the state pays for me." Disincentives in funding remained in relationship to marriage as well as the potential loss of benefits upon employment.

CONCLUSION

This chapter is one step in the identification and development of models of personal assistance services for, by, of, and/or with people with mental retardation and physical disabilities. Existing models and approaches, whether personal assistance services or supportive living, are operational at the state and local levels, and further development continues to occur. Significant policy implications for PAS in the field of mental retardation and developmental disabilities include

- the 1992 American Association on Mental Retardation definition of mental retardation, which reflects the concept of "support" in its multidimensional approach;
- the relationship between home care, interventions, and health policy;
- the continued expansion of service coordination with new approaches, including cash subsidies and vouchers; and
- the issue of control of PAS by service users, consumer choice and employment policy, and agency versus family financial resources.

Chapter 10

Children, Youth, and Adults with Brain Injuries: Implications for Personal Assistance Services

Julie Ann Racino

During my third year [at West Point], I was involved in a near-tragic accident where I received an open head injury. . . . I was in [a] coma in a locked-in state . . . that's where you are conscious, but you can't communicate. That particular period was the most horrifying I ever had in my life . . . not knowing if I was going to be able to come back. . . . [In] 1987, [I became] pretty active in head injury circles . . . and after a time, started a survivors' task force . . . and created a group of friends who are survivors . . . some of who[m] need personal assistance, and still others who will need it the rest of their lives.

INTRODUCTION

Personal assistance services has been viewed as one way of translating the Americans with Disabilities Act into a reality, with people with disabilities gaining employment and interacting in political, social, economic, community, and spiritual life. In the field of brain injuries, PAS often has a medical and rehabilitation focus that is distinct from cross-disability health care reform and movements toward universal access (e.g., inclusion of people with the most significant disabilities). In the field of developmental

This chapter is a modified version of Racino, J. (1995c). "Personal Assistance Services (PAS): Children and Youth with Disabilities." In *Toward Universal Access to Support: An Edited Collection on Personal Assistance Services.* Syracuse, NY, and Boston, MA: Community and Policy Studies. See Appendix A for research methodology.

disabilities (which sometimes subsumes brain injury), the movement toward a support and empowerment framework, distinct yet overlapping with independent living, has also affected the field of brain injuries.

MOVING TOWARD INTEGRATED APPROACHES TO PAS: BRAIN INJURY AS A SUBFIELD OF DISABILITY

Fourteen major thematic areas were identified to assist in the movement toward integrated approaches to PAS (Racino, 1995c). These are: guiding principles related to PAS; writings identified as authored by survivors; nature of the disability of brain injuries; status of the research and practice in community life; practical forms of assistance; community living and services development; recreation, employment, housing, and education; definition and uses of personal assistants; definition and solutions to cognitive issues; nature of social and emotional support; physical disabilities and substance abuse in brain injury; children's issues in brain injury; relationships in family life; and policy and systemic issues.

Guiding Principles Related to PAS

Independent living (DeJong, 1979) and its service component of user-directed PAS have as guiding principles a commitment to personal autonomy, the support of diverse community lifestyles, and access by people of all ages and abilities. The philosophical tenets that are the essential underpinnings of user-directed PAS or self-directed care, are reflected sporadically in the brain injury literature, with less emphasis on community membership, an emerging dimension in the field of disability that appears in relation to independent living in forms such as community assessments. The research has a quality of life orientation, inclusive of principle-based outcomes (e.g., noninstitutional) and clinical outcomes as rated by survivors, without mentioning life quality as defined by each person (see Bergland and Thomas, 1991, for a wholistic approach to outcomes). Table 10.1 contains guiding principles from a regional coalition in Central New York that included representation by the independent living sector.

Cross-Disability and People of All Ages

However, common connections were generally not being drawn across disability fields in supports (see, in contrast, emerging work in behavioral supports by the Research and Training Center on Non-Aversive Behavioral Interventions, University of Oregon [Horner et al., 1990]). Cross-disability analysis has occurred primarily in relation to employment (Weh-

TABLE 10.1. Central New York Traumatic Brain Injury Coalition Guiding Principles

---

Opportunity: Recognition of the potential of all human beings to develop and improve and offering settings and supports to accomplish those goals.

Equity: Fairness in the distribution of resources.

Access: Ability to gain entrance to services and supports that enhance the expression of the whole person.

Individuality: Support and empowerment to make choices.

Productivity: Any activity that is meaningful to the individual.

Inclusion: An affirmative position to the public to provide opportunities for all people to participate in all aspects of community life.

Involvement: Inclusion from the perspective of service design, recognizing that a person can be integrated without being included.

Source: Central New York Traumatic Brain Injury Coalition (1994). *Mission Statement.* Syracuse, NY: Author.

man et al., 1991; Wehman et al., 1993) and alcohol and substance abuse (e.g., Kreutzer and Harris, 1990: Kreutzer et al., 1989). As in other fields, adolescence was viewed as a neglected research area (with a national center on youth with disabilities established across all areas of disability). Pediatric clinical and family support approaches have not yet been reconceptualized to support quality of life in the community.

Professionals and Survivors

Although primarily written from a medical, clinical, and/or professional stance, excellent accounts by adult survivors and their parents have appeared in professional journals and papers, as well as new essays on PAS (Biscup, 1990; Gwin, 1994) and a book describing Jim Brady (Dickenson, 1987). Qualitative research studies that recount the perspectives of survivors or their parents from a quality-of-life, holistic perspective have begun to enter the brain injury literature.

Nature of the Disability

The nature of brain injuries (see Table 10.2) was highlighted as very distinct from that of other disabilities, with the following four primary areas targeted for further cross-disability development in communities.

TABLE 10.2. Facts on Disabilities—Traumatic Brain Injury

• A head injury is a traumatic insult to the brain. The injury is not always visible but may cause physical, intellectual, emotional, social, and vocational changes. No two injuries are alike.
• There are 1,000,000 incidences of head injury per year nationally. In Wisconsin, there are 10,000 incidences per year.
• In 1980, nine of ten people who sustained head injuries died. In 1990, nine of ten survived.
• Forty-two percent of all head injuries are caused by motor vehicle and motorcycle accidents. Alcohol use is often a contributing factor.
• Two-thirds of people with TBI received their injury when they were younger than thirty years of age. Although many return to independent living and competitive employment on their own, most require extensive support services.

Source: Vocational Consulting Services (1994). *Facts on Disabilities.* Madison, Wisconsin: Author.

Lack of Holistic Integration

The picture that generally emerges of people with brain injuries in the professional research literature is one of multiple deficits (including emotional, behavioral, cognitive, medical, and physical disabilities), with relatively little holistic integration (across life areas, as a whole person). (In contrast, see Condeluci, Ferris, and Bogdan, 1992.)

Uniqueness of Injuries

People with brain injuries are viewed as unique individuals, but generally on the basis of the uniqueness of his or her injury (see informant interview from Racino, 1995c, on the individualistic nature of head injury). This picture contrasts with approaches that view people as varying widely from one another by virtue of their individual preferences, lifestyles, and personalities.

Acute, Life-and-Death Nature of the Injury

For some people, their immediate medical issues must take precedence over longer-term concerns, which may involve, or in some cases require, community support services. However, this involvement, relative to community support, increases the role that medical personnel play, marking a different relationship with families, survivors, paraprofessionals, and community support personnel after the medical crises are over.

Roles of Cognition, Emotions, and Behaviors

The brain injury literature contains clinical, rehabilitative, and medical emphases on emotional and behavioral problems, and how cognition is understood to relate to daily life functions. A gap among the medical, rehabilitation, independent living, and support methods reflects sharp discontinuities in approaches to community life for the same individual. Environmental (e.g., getting around) and practical (e.g., job loss) concerns may instead be interpreted as personality, relationship, and community problems of the individual. (See a political-feminist analysis by Morris, an author from Great Britain who suffers from a spinal cord injury, on attributions to personality in her 1991 article that describes housing and personal assistance services.)

Status of Practice in Community Life

Research in community living for, by, and with people with brain injuries has remained relatively unexplored on basic, key dimensions, with practice literature focusing on independent living and community support (Jacobs, Blatnick, and Sandborst, 1990; Johnson, 1985; Condeluci, 1991).

Clinical "Real World" Studies

According to this literature, even from a clinical (versus community, rehabilitative, support, or independent living) perspective, there has been no systematic study of deficits in behavior (or positive experiences) or in "real world" functioning in children and adolescents with traumatic brain injury (TBI) (Fay et al., 1993). From a rehabilitative framework, a paucity of literature on childhood intervention practices and nontherapeutic approaches to support in brain injury exists. Emerging issues, such as the comparisons between the growing family support movements and early intervention practices, remained primarily deficit based with the exception of emerging policy studies (e.g., Reynolds and Rosen, 1994; Wright, 1993).

Continuum-Based Specialization versus Family and Individualized Support

Workers in the brain injury field, with strong ties to the insurance industry, attempted to organize a continuum of services, for example, from the acute hospitals and specialized residential treatment facilities to community living. Community living tended to be framed as concerned with specialization (e.g., specialized group homes for people with brain injuries) and individual functioning in daily living. This contrasted with support for families to raise their children at home (see Williams and Kay, 1991) and regular housing with support services for full and meaningful lives. In New York, children were sent out-of-state for placements, and finally, in the 1990s, as part of a national movement, they returned to their home communities with services support (see Table 10.3).

Qualitative Studies of Community Life

Relatively few analyses of individual responses to living with a brain injury, especially in-depth studies, existed, and the perceptions of the person with the injury and that person's experience were often discounted. Research studies of other aspects of community life, such as the relationship between survivors with brain injuries and the organizations and workers funded to assist them, were virtually nonexistent; research studies comparing people with brain injuries, other disabilities, and people without disabilities were in progress at the time of this writing.

Practical Forms of Assistance

In brain injury, cognitive remediation (Gordon, Hibbard, and Kreutzer, 1989; Ben-Yishay and Diller, 1993) has been both a theoretical and a rehabilitation concept regarding practical assistance. Two common ways of thinking about competent functioning in daily life activities are to remediate the deficit or problem (restorative approaches) or to use alternative coping strategies (compensatory approaches). Compensatory strategies (similar in part to functional substitution) can be approached from a teaching and training perspective (e.g., self-awareness as prerequisite) or as a process of patient discovery (e.g., the patient may discover alternate strategies for accomplishing tasks). Other training approaches are habilitative in nature and include the use of assistive devices, environmental modifications (rearranging or modifying existing living space, designing new components in living space), and the use of personal care attendants (Christiansen, Schwartz, and Barnes, 1993). In communities, the movement has been toward respecting the strengths and contributions of the person with a disability, supporting the development of competent, accepting, and caring communities, and facilitating supportive relationships with family, friends, and people in daily life.

TABLE 10.3. Medicaid Home and Community-Based Services Waiver Program for Individuals with Traumatic Brain Injury

Medicaid State Plan Services and Supports	
clinic	pharmaceuticals
physician/dentist	medical transportation
hospital	medical supplies and equipment
therapies	eyeglasses
home health—includes	hearing aids
personal care	
other	
Other State- and Federal-Funded Services	
VESID	HEAP
housing subsidies/	mental health
subsidized housing	substance abuse services
education benefits	other
Waiver Services	
service coordination	structured day program
independent living skills	substance abuse programs
training and development	intensive behavioral programs
community integration	therapeutic foster care
counseling	transitional living programs
home and community support	environmental modifications
services	respite care
special medical equipment	transportation
and supplies	

Source: New York State Department of Health and New York State Department of Social Services. (1993). *Home and Community-Based Medicaid Services Waiver for Individuals with Traumatic Brain Injury.* Albany, NY: Author.

Note: VESID = Office of Vocational and Educational Services for Individuals with Disabilities; HEAP = Heating Energy Assistance Program.

Community Living: Family Support and Person-Centered Services

Patterns of service development tended to reflect disability versus normal growth and development of children, youth, adults, and elders (Racino, 1997d). Children and youth perspectives were not yet well represented, including in family support (often interpreted as parent or caregiver support versus supporting regular patterns of family life, such as recreational interests of the adolescent). The concept of flexible and indi- vidualized services was only recently described in brain injury, with the primary approaches still tending to be therapeutic, educational, or self- help. A person-centered, nonclinical approach was highlighted in a brief description of life planning (Racino and Williams, 1994).

Status of Practice in Community Life: Recreation, Housing, Employment, and Education

Employment, friendships and relationships, education, and housing and support are briefly highlighted in the following material, since personal assistance services affects participation in all environments throughout the life course. However, personal care systems were initially organized around home life and in-home services (Doty, Kasper, and Litvak, 1996), with participation in the community, including economic, social, political, and employment activities, viewed as secondary. These roots are reflected in how funding is organized, the qualifications of staff, the regulation of these services by government, eligibility and assessment criteria, and the services' capacity to respond to the needs and interests of the service users.

Employment

From a community integration perspective, some of the stronger pro- fessional practice literature remains in vocational rehabilitation (Golden, Smith, and Golden, 1993; Skord and Miranti, 1994), including systematic efforts to investigate the use of community and supported employment for people with brain injuries and its implications for public policy (Goodall, Lawyer, and Wehman, 1994; Thomas and Menz, 1990). Although many people with head injuries return to their previous employment, others may need or want special support, such as flexible hours and payments, train- ing to assist with specific issues such as memory, support from co-work- ers, a liaison with rehabilitation workers, and environmental modifications (Crisp, 1992). Some of these special supports could be available to all employees through the use of flextime and the creation of workplaces that are accepting of diversity, in line with the changing workforce.

Similar to people with other significant disabilities, the relatively high rate of unemployment following traumatic brain injury strongly suggests that traditional approaches to vocational rehabilitation and community reintegration have been entirely inadequate. The literature reports numer- ous personal barriers to hiring and job retention (e.g., cognitive/communication; program and user outcomes (Wehman et al., 1993); emotional and sociobehavioral control), with attention to the nature and features of the work settings and the personal concerns of people with traumatic brain injuries, such as the stigmatization of having job coaches at work sites (Wehman et al., 1991).

Friendships and Relationships

People with traumatic brain injuries and their families have reported that their disability led to changes in their relationships and expressed dismay at the reactions of other people, including friends. In one qualitative study (Bergland and Thomas, 1991), 75 percent of the individuals and their parents reported difficulty in establishing and maintaining new friendships and also noted reduced opportunities for social exchange. It was considered common for people with brain injuries to feel uncomfortable around people with other disabilities. This expressed attitude was attributed, in part, to the retention of their preinjury self-concept (Thomas and Menz, 1990), a concept currently being disputed partially because of its blaming nature. Emerging literature outside the brain injury field has been examining social relationships (see Cooley, Glang, and Voss, 1997, for qualitative research in brain injury); the relationships between formal and informal support, including with friends; the effect of governmental payments on family and friendships; and friendships between people with and without disabilities.

Education

From the perspective of the provider sector, resources were prepared that focused on the roles of schools, the needs of students within the school setting, and the roles of school assessments (e.g., Virginia Department of Education, 1992; Western Regional Resource Center, 1993). These tended to again emphasize deficits, structured teaching techniques, and specializations. For children, ameliorating deficits and the effect of brain injury on school performance were two areas of research, with less emphasis on aspects of integration, inclusion, and prevention approaches (other than prevention of the head or brain injury itself, for example, through the use of helmets, or drug and alcohol use prevention).

Housing and Support

As compared to both developmental and psychiatric disabilities, regular housing and support was a neglected area in brain injury (Betts, 1994; Racino and Williams, 1994), with a continued concentration on program models. A separate review, conducted in 1993, identified principles for housing and support (Research and Training Center [RTC] on Accessible Housing, 1993, in Racino, 1997d) and for community development (community development as a way of thinking; capacity building as a goal; the state role as supporting local efforts; and user-driven outcomes). The review resulted in a new schema for the categorization of community support and services, reflecting field status at that time (Racino, 1993c).

Definition and Uses of Personal Attendants

In relationship to the definition and uses of personal assistants, aides, or attendants (known in the movement as PCAs), four areas were highlighted regarding future development for people with significant disabilities.

Self-Directed Care and User-Directed Models

Self-directed care models were described in brain injury rehabilitation, as well as the use of personal assistants or personal attendants. For example, "Part of the rehabilitation process for people who are going to require attendant care is that they learn to recruit, hire, supervise, and if necessary, terminate personal care attendants" (Christiansen, Schwartz, and Barnes, 1993, p. 195). In user-directed personal assistance, this process is controlled by the person with a brain or head injury; it is not a professionally directed process.

Broadened Definition of PAS

Personal assistants may be employed for a variety of life tasks rather than solely for physical tasks, though people with brain injuries may also need physical assistance "An important and difficult aspect of working with a care attendant is to be able to define all of the self-care and daily living tasks which will require assistance" (see also Watson, 1991). For the international personal assistance services symposium held in Oakland, California, Sherri Watson, a survivor of brain injuries, described potential areas of assistance *for her* to include emotions, memory, daily structure, fitness/physical needs (e.g., joining a health spa), transportation (driving to programs), organization, and decision making. Personal assistance definitions may be gender, class, and culture biased.

Comparison with Existing Roles

Sherri Watson (1991) viewed personal assistants as a substitute for case managers, including in the performance of such tasks as "cuing," structuring and organizing the day, and offering reminders, such as an administrative assistant might do. She also explained how it would be difficult to train personal assistants in areas such as emotions, though this would be an essential part of their role. Similar to coaches, a personal assistant, in a work setting, could help assess the situation afterward and engage in activities such as role-plays. Another similar role is that of life coach (Jones et al., 1991), though this approach does give substantial control to the professional in terms of determining fading or transfer of control functions. Personal assistants are directed by the person with a brain injury and were not described in relationship to education or recreation.

Comparison with Self-Care Tasks

A broadened definition of PAS corresponds with how self-care tasks are defined (i.e., those daily and routine activities necessary for living), with life quality as one of the standards. These tasks can include personal care and instrumental activities of "food preparation, laundry, housekeeping, shopping, the ability to use the telephone, use of transportation, medication use, and financial management" (Christiansen, Schwartz, and Barnes, 1993, p. 178), child care, leisure, and recreation. However, the nature of who decides what will be done and how these tasks are accomplished may be substantially different in self-care than in PAS, which places greater control in the hands of the service user.

Definition and Solutions to Cognitive Issues

One of the most complex issues in relationship to any person with significant cognitive (term used by the Consortium of Citizens with Disabilities and the World Institute on Disability) impairments is the practical translation of the self-determination principles, as promoted by the independent living movement, into the natural course of living. The field of brain injury developed as part of the disability field's medical and clinical disciplines, including multiple complex ways of understanding and presenting issues of cognition. Cognitive support is one of the terms used in relationship to people with mental retardation, psychiatric disabilities, elders who may have Alzheimer's disease, and people with AIDS who may later on experience dementia, as well as with people with brain injuries.

Cognitive Issues in Brain Injuries

Cognitive problems resulting from brain injuries were described in great detail. Whyte and Rosenthal (1993), for example, have cataloged many types of cognitive issues that may face individuals with brain injuries, and these are reflected in the community provider training materials. Other significant cognitive issues that affect decision making and support models are objects of research: relationship with self-concept; predictions of independence; perception of control and relationship to well-being; relationship between cognitive deficits and everyday living skills; self-concept and independence; limited role in choice of provider; role of uncertainty in medical decision making; study of cognitive processes; generalization; categorization of cognition by practitioners; reported concerns by professionals; issues of concern to people with disabilities and their families; relationship with self-care training (capacity to manage); use of computers as a training tool; communication disabilities (language and speech); and the relationship between cognitive functioning and behavior.

Cognitive Rehabilitation and Remediation

In the field of brain injury, "cognitive rehabilitation strategies have been developed to improve independent living, intellectual, and vocational skills of persons with brain dysfunction" (Kreutzer et al., 1989, p. 30). These efforts have followed the development of clinical techniques oriented toward improving physiological functioning and performance of daily living skills. However, the theoretical and research base for cognitive remediation techniques and strategies is still considered to be in the validation process for field use (Ben-Yishay and Diller, 1993, p. 204) with both adults and children.

Common Issues in Decision Making

Particularly with people who may be viewed as needing and/or wanting some assistance in decision making or with cognitive tasks, several concerns are relevant to PAS. These include self-awareness (including the perceived discrepancy between how the person views his or her capacities and how others do); being realistic (defined by others as letting go of the future one had hoped for); ownership of cognitive issues by medical professionals (e.g., competency to train and manage assistants) and ethical considerations; expertise and the need for reframing of cognitive functioning to day-to-day language; decision making free from coercion and manipulation; legal competency to handle a person's own affairs, including medical, financial, vocational, and other decisions; life and death decisions by family members and the appointment of a conservator or guardian; and status of assessment and use by service providers and educators in determinations about support needs.

Nature of Social and Emotional Support

One definition of social support (Cobb, 1976) is the belief on the part of individuals that they are emotionally supported or involved with others.

Support includes at least six dimensions: actions, values, personal experiences or feelings, relationships with others, standards and expectations, and goals and accomplishments (Racino and O'Connor, 1994). Perceived issues and definitions related to the development of user-directed PAS approaches were at least threefold. First, the goal and focus regarding emotional and behavioral issues were often framed in terms of managing these problems with a strand of work on professionally guided self-management. Second, problems tended to be clinically defined, which created pictures of people who are needy, not likely to be good companions, and may even present safety risks to themselves and others around them. Third, few accounts described emotional and behavioral concerns from the personal viewpoints of brain injury survivors (e.g., silliness as a mutual stress reliever), within a full life context, or with positive interpretative contrasts, with accounts primarily from professional or parental viewpoints.

Physical Disabilities

The importance of physical problems (e.g., seizures, hypertension, bowel and bladder dysfunction) has been minimized in some sets of literature. Yet, there was some concern that "individuals with TBI who experience significant sensory and motor impairments are most likely to experience psychological distress" (Antonak, Livneh, and Antonak, 1993, p. 90). At least three areas should be considered regarding physical disabilities, ongoing medical needs, and their relationship to PAS development: the continuing relationships with multidisciplinary medical professionals, which influence ordinary people to view situations in clinical ways; the performance, learning and teaching strategies of daily living skills and/or the use of assistive devices; and the interrelationship between the clinical needs and other impairments, such as cognitive disabilities.

Alcohol and Substance Abuse

Dual diagnosis (in brain injury) is used to refer to people who are believed to have alcohol and/or substance abuse problems; this differs from the usage of the term in mental health and in mental retardation. The systems, theories, organizations, strategies, and treatment approaches regarding substance and alcohol abuse are distinct from those governing the field of brain injury (and other disability) services. Second, substance and/or alcohol abuse may be closely tied with lifestyle issues before and/or after the injury and become central to questions of self-determination, including questions of safety, risk, and clinical/professional judgments.

Pediatric Issues in Brain Injury

Pediatric clinical research remains distinct from family and educational research; however, overlap exists with studies on family functioning following injury, decreased performance in schools, and the social adjustment and relationships of children, all areas for which relatively little information is available (Rivara et al., 1994).

Lack of Systematic Study Regarding Children and Adolescent Issues

Although head injuries are one of the most common forms of childhood injuries, leading researchers in traumatic brain injury hold that comparatively little systematic study has been conducted regarding the effects on children and adolescents as compared to adults. Parents may offer support to their young and adult children; as such, the injury can be viewed as affecting the entire family system, also leading to need for research and assistance in family support (Williams and Kay, 1991; Williams, 1996).

Description and Interpretation of Children's Behaviors

Children's behaviors following brain injury may be described as psychiatric issues, issues of social competence, behavior problems, or emotional maladjustment. The children's behaviors may be interpreted in a motivational framework as being willfully resistant and inappropriate (Burke et al., 1989); these types of frameworks are prevalent in mental health and are in opposition to frameworks that highlight strengths, contributions, and the environmental, social, and communicative roles of behaviors.

Pediatric Cognitive Remediation

Pediatric cognitive remediation (Crowley and Miles, 1991), which was in its early stages and distinct from early intervention, has tended to be focused on basic academic skill building and increasing self-awareness. Self-awareness may be part of what is termed (by others) disability consciousness in independent living and acceptance of the disability as part of who the person is. In contrast, the holistic study of the relationship between the challenges of living with a brain injury (e.g., attending school, maintaining a healthy self-concept) and the in-home and community approaches to improving the life quality of the child and his or her family have not been as well developed.

Relationships in Family Life

A growing body of research in brain injury exists on marriage, sexuality, and spousal and family relationships, including the perspectives of siblings (Complair, Kreutzer, and Doherty, 1991; Rosenthal and Young, 1988). Much emphasis was placed on family caregiving and coping, including the high stress and isolation experienced by family members, the changed expectations in spousal roles and the effects on children (e.g., Linn, Allen, and Willer 1994). This is similar to feminist approaches that emphasize the burden of caregiving and caregiver perspectives, instead of the perspectives of the service user or survivor. Family issues have received some attention from the perspectives of family members, both as reported directly by family members (Pieper, nd) and as presented by researchers (Singer and Nixon, 1990).

Concept of Family Responsibility and Burden

Reflected in the literature is the belief that family members should be the first line of physical, social, and emotional assistance for both children *and* adults with a brain injury. This parallels common societal attitudes in the United States (and countries such as Great Britain) that formal services should be accessed only when the informal system is unable to meet the person's needs. Although the support of family members has been considered critical to the rehabilitation process, the assumption has translated into the *expectation* that parental families be the first choice in living arrangements for children *and* adults. The primary framework is to continue to view the person with a disability as a burden, with burden of care measured in stress and behaviors that affect the family (Bragg, Klockars, and Berninger, 1992).

Nontherapeutic Family Support

Relatively little information is available on the national family support and preservation movements that have assumed national importance in the field of developmental disabilities (Williams and Kay, 1991; for context in the mid-1990s, see Williams, 1996). However, a recent effort was made to conceptually introduce nontherapeutic concepts of family support into the brain injury field. These concepts included family subsidies; family-centered services such as support workers, support groups, chore assistance, and in-home training to deal with crises and behaviors; and the provision of durable goods that may be related to medical condition (as presented) or to family need. Implementation of such services has occurred in many states (Wright, 1993). Personal assistance has continued to be equated with in-home services as one kind of family support service, with the workers generally responsible to the parents, in contrast to forms of youth (to adulthood) assistance.

SYSTEMIC AND POLICY CONCERNS IN PAS

The literature review on personal assistance services and brain injury included public policy concerns and the funding of long-term support services (e.g., DeBuono and Glass, 1985; Keefe, 1994; Goodall et al., 1991; Noble et al., 1990; Willer, Linn, and Allen, 1994; Veldheer, 1990). A primary funding source is the use of the home and community-based Medicaid service waivers, which vary from state to state, and can be applied for specifically in the area of traumatic brain injury (see also Racino and Williams, 1994).

One major national review of support services in brain injury, inclusive of community colleges, home living, and employment, with implications for health services, was conducted by William Reynolds (1991) of the New York State Department of Health. Funded by the Milbank Foundation, the findings were adapted for use by the National Council of State Legislators (Wright, 1993). Many of these practices are included within the funding structure of the New York State Department of Health (New York State Department of Health Traumatic Brain Injury Program, 1997) to support people with brain injuries returning from out of state placements. Table 10.3 displays examples of funded categories of services.

CONCLUSION: PERSONAL ASSISTANCE SERVICES AND FUTURE CONTRIBUTIONS

Children, youth, and adults with brain injury are returning to their home communities in some states where previously people might have been sent out-of-state, away from family and friends. Personal assistance and support services are aspects of fostering community and service capacities. This review of PAS in the field of brain injury contributes to understanding:

- the nature of cognitive, emotional, and behavioral support (particularly the lack of self-directed strategies), which holds commonalities across disability groups;
- the relationship between personal assistance services and habilitation (e.g., the training and hiring of assistants by service users versus the habilitation of people with brain injuries by workers) to support greater control by service users of their own destinies;
- the need for more holistic approaches and studies of the lives and perspectives of people with and without brain injuries in the context of community life;

- the critical nature of perceived family responsibility with adults (which may force adults to live in parental homes against their will); and
- the distinctions between self-directed care and personal assistance services, with the latter more clearly articulated by psychiatric survivors as defined by service users.

PAS offers hope for the future, with opportunities for changes in community organizations, businesses, and institutions (e.g., educational, religious, political, medical) serving and interacting with youth, their families and friends, and adults of all ages.

Chapter 11

Youth and Community Life: Perspectives of Adults with Disabilities on Personal Assistance Services

Julie Ann Racino

INTRODUCTION

Personal assistance services grew out of a social movement by adults with disabilities to control their own destinies (see Chapter 9), and only secondarily did it move toward developing approaches with young people and families. The latter, the province primarily of parent leaders, had as one of its priorities the development of community services (in some fields started in basements and family homes); second was the reduction of professional stigma and blame on families, and the last, a movement toward family support in its diverse forms (Agosta, Smith, and Deatherage, 1991; Arnold and Case, 1993; Koroloff et al., 1996; Weiss, 1989).

In contrast to the family movement, this chapter draws upon interviews with informants with disabilities ("consumer experts"), some of whom are parents, living primarily in Minnesota and California (see Table 11.1), which are considered the leading states in personal assistance services for youth with disabilities. Supplemental national interviews were conducted with other informants (e.g., National Center for Youth with Disabilities, University of Minnesota [NCYD, 1992] on the development of youth models of personal assistance services (see Table 11.2).

This chapter is a modified version from Racino, J. (1995c). "Personal Assistance Services: Youth with Disabilities." In *Toward Universal Access to Support: An Edited Collection on Personal Assistance Services.* Syracuse, NY, and Boston, MA: Community and Policy Studies.

TABLE 11.1. Research Informants: Youth with Disabilities and Personal Assistance Services

Graduate of the University of Berkeley, with a social science degree, who interned at the World Institute on Disability and was categorized as "severely impaired" by California's IHSS (in-home support services) program.

Community college student working on a mechanical engineering degree who has cerebral palsy, chronic asthma, and wears a hearing aid.

Student at Moorehead State University in Michigan who is the father of a teenager, an All American Scholar, and on an ADA (American with Disabilities Act) committee. He also broke his neck at age twenty-three.

Finance auditor for Honeywell who has a hotel administration degree from Suffolk State University in Massachusetts. He has muscular dystrophy and uses a wheelchair.

Student in management at St. Paul's Technical College, Minnesota, who works at Toys "R" Us and was diagnosed as having muscular dystrophy as a teenager.

A self-advocate and ARC/MNASH (Minnesota Association for Retarded Citizens/Association of Persons with Severe Handicaps) board member who lives in a group home for seven and works in a sheltered workshop in Minnesota.

A twenty-year-old member of ADAPT (American Disabled for Attendant Programs Today) who is an activist for attendant care, has a physical and learning disability, and resides in Berkeley, California.

An ADAPT (political disability activist) organizer who knows and uses PAS (personal assistance services).

Source: Racino, J. (1995c). "Personal Assistance Services: Youth with Disabilities." In *Toward Universal Access to Support: An Edited Collection on Personal Assistance Services.* Syracuse, NY, and Boston, MA: Community and Policy Studies.

Personal assistance services, most well known in the field of physical disability and political action, with its policy formulations in federal disability legislation (see Americans with Disabilities Act, 1990), has come face to face with transition to adulthood for youth with disabilities (e.g., Blum et al., 1993; Ferguson and Ferguson, 1993; Hanley-Maxwell, Whitney-Thomas, and Pogoloff, 1995; Kregel et al., 1986; Wehman, 1996), including support in homes, employment, leisure, and spiritual and community life (e.g., Nisbet, Rogan, and Hagner, 1989; Racino and O'Connor, 1994).

TABLE 11.2. Youth Model of Personal Assistance Services As Proposed by Informants

---

- *Use of a peer age and gender model.* Such a model would support social interaction with peers and provide peer-to-peer support ("A peer model. . . . They should probably have assistance from persons who are close to their own age and probably of their own sex, and those with some enthusiasm, [as peer support] will more likely create opportunities for social interactions.")

- *Use of a model based upon the nature of children and youth.* Such a model would be cognizant of social, legal, and developmental factors that would support the empowerment of children and youth and the natural involvement of personal assistants in day-to-day life. These significant factors are the "instability of youth," the role of parental involvement and consent, the perceived ability or inability of children to define what they want and what they want the personal assistant to do, and the natural growth of youngsters from a very early age.

- *Use of a family-based model.* The proposed model from Ann Turnbull of the Beach Center on Families and Disability is inclusive of the nature of power relationships (e.g., hierarchical or egalitarian), the use of paid providers (and its relationship with informal supports), the role of a personal assistant as a social relationship facilitator, the self-determination component, and traditional components of daily living/personal care (A. Turnbull, 1991, personal communication).

- *PAS and schools.* A personal assistance model also would need to involve PAS in schools. Factors raised were inclusion in home schools, issues of funding coordination and constraints, who should provide it, assistance to both the family and the student, assistance within and outside of school, roles of teachers' aides, and the role of the student in assistance services.

- *A model that addresses the concerns of people with disabilities, including labeling.* People are concerned about being labeled "with mental retardation," and with having services and programs that describe service users or potential service users in that way; lends support to community approaches to personal assistance services.

Source: Adapted from Racino, J. (1995c). "Personal Assistance Services: Youth with Disabilities." In *Toward Universal Access to Support: An Edited Collection on Personal Assistance Services.* Syracuse, NY and Boston, MA: Community and Policy Studies.

UNIVERSAL ACCESS

Universal access is based, in part, upon beliefs about the relationship of human beings to society and the ways in which societal acceptance and "rights" are understood. Universal access refers to how "everyone" should be treated with the right to live as they want. As one informant explained:

> True definition of PAS promises that every man, woman, and child in the United States is entitled to services that support their living in a community of their own choosing . . . the diversity of our population calls for a flexible design of PAS.

Universal access has diverse meanings, and access by everyone was not a goal of all informants. Some people felt strongly that no one should be institutionalized ("They shouldn't be in institutions, no matter what."), whereas others explained that sometimes, although in a limited number of cases, a person might "have to be institutionalized." People with AIDS, chronic fatigue, psychiatric disabilities, and environmental illnesses may use personal assistance; however, sometimes this option was limited based upon categorical disability (e.g., physical), need for assistance, capacity for integrated living, or capacity and willingness to pay for personal assistance or other support services ("We cannot afford to pay for everything for everyone.").

Universal access may be interpreted to include people of all incomes (see Litvak, Zukas, and Heumann, 1987, pp. 104-105), cultures, and ethnicities ("Everybody has an equal right to access and to knowing what is out there."), with health services for youth a global concern (Bowes et al., 1995; Friedman, 1993). This means that people should not be impoverished to obtain services ("My family has to remain poor in order to get services.") (Center on Human Policy, 1989a). Multiculturalism, which has been conceptualized as inclusive of disability (see Chapter 1), was a perceived barrier to universal access. Language (Bittner, 1993), resources, and lack of exposure to information were stated barriers to minority service access.

BENEFITS OF PAS

> It [PAS] would allow people with disabilities and senior citizens to live at home longer, instead of being stuck in a nursing home-type setting.

Personal assistance services offers a number of benefits to children, youth (Bittner, 1991), and adults with disabilities; people seeking employment as or who are providers of personal assistance; and society at large (e.g., taxpayers). The potential benefits of personal assistance services in societal terms include the following:

- Promoting adult independence (e.g., jobs, societal contributions) through the use of attendants by children (see also Sinnema, 1988)
- Improved quality of life for people with disabilities ("to live independently," "live at home longer, and "start working and become productive")
- Increased opportunities for employment (as PCAs)
- Increased contributions to society by disabled people ("we as disabled people have a lot to give back to the United States")
- More cost-effective to society (by allowing people to live at home longer, have "more control over their care," and "go out and start working.")

On a personal level, PAS can enable youth to move from abusive family situations; to get involved in the community; to participate in youth activities independent of family; to develop relationships with other teens; to go to school, plan a career, and locate a job; to feel emotionally supported, safe, and not abandoned; and to reduce time spent on some tasks, to make available time for other activities, such as school or work. PAS can assist a person by doing things that he or she cannot do on his or her own.

INFORMATION ACCESS BY CHILDREN AND YOUTH WITH DISABILITIES

Everyone regardless of age or ability has a right to know about PAS. After all, the objective of PAS is to give the entire disabled community in the United States an opportunity to achieve independence.

Information access by children and youth with disabilities shares common and distinct features compared to information access by adults or elders with disabilities and adults who have legal guardians. Children and youth need to have an opportunity to know that the "program" or "services" exist, and "consumers" have a "right" to "shop around" for the program (that) best satisfies their needs." Information access is a safeguard, for example, against a guardian taking advantage of the person. As one informant noted, "Just because someone's a legal guardian doesn't mean that [he or she is] going to do everything in the best interest of the person." Access is based, in part, upon how people view children's "right to know" potentially controversial information (e.g., similar to teaching sex education in schools). As one research informant described:

> Children have a right to gain that knowledge. I mean, we teach reading, writing, and arithmetic. We also teach sex education, but that's a hot-button issue with some parents.

PAS information could be made available to those who may want it through other programs specifically serving the disabled, such as high schools, colleges, universities, and hospitals (e.g., Benshoff, Kroeger, and Scalia, 1990). For outreach to ethnic groups "who may have a harder time knowing what's going on out there," people who are credible and of the same ethnic background might be helpful. Information content suggested by the informants were access to information on how to work (the) human service system ("I wish I had known about the whole service system . . . how to work with the social workers."), how to live with a disability, and on rights and the disabled movement as the basis for choice and prevention of out-of-home placement ("I didn't know what my rights were . . . I really didn't know anything about the disabled movement when I was growing up.").

PERSONAL ASSISTANCE SERVICES TASKS FOR CHILDREN AND YOUTH

Many personal assistance tasks (see Table B "Introduction," Part III), although applicable to children and youth, have often been defined within the framework for adults. For children and youth, parents may do all the things that a personal assistant does, from lifting to dressing to respiratory therapy and cooking. Parents' responsibilities change as the children grow older and may shift between the parents or caregivers (e.g., mother providing more assistance in lifting and bathing when the daughter was younger and father assisting when she got "bigger" and he was available) or between parents and their children (e.g., son cooking when mother was at work). Whether family members would like a personal assistant to come into their home may also vary with the age of the child, with more acceptance as the child becomes older (and, in some cases, heavier).

Sometimes personal assistance tasks can get done more easily through informal relationships with the personal assistant, family, or friends instead of through formal negotiation or agreements with agencies or the service system. Sometimes a person may need assistance for only short periods of time with tasks that he or she is unable to do for himself or herself. Without backup arrangements for personal assistance (including telephone emergency assistance), a person can end up being left even unable to move out of bed.

Types of personal assistance mentioned by the informants, with all having a copy of the working definition (Litvak, Zukas, and Heumann, 1987), included (1) personal care (e.g., menstruation); (2) meal preparation; (3) safety (e.g., getting out of bed in an emergency); (4) money management; (5) cleaning, shopping, housekeeping, laundry, and long-term heavy cleaning and repairs; (6) speech and interpretation (e.g., for telephone calls for prescription renewal and information; interpreting as an ongoing social, job, and personal need); (7) medical treatments (e.g., from a registered respiratory therapist or nurse; also stretching exercises or massages); (8) transportation (e.g., driving cars, starting vehicles, washing cars or vans, travel for business); and (9) raising a family. Other forms of assistance are described in the following sections, including cognitive and emotional support and PAS in schools, employment, and community recreation.

THE MEANING OF COGNITIVE AND EMOTIONAL SUPPORT

Sometimes people may not want or need physical assistance with tasks, but may need to know how to do something (such as laundry) or need to feel that they are able to do something. Another person stated that people with AIDS may have needs for cognitive support related to dementia (see also PAS and AIDS, Weissman, Kennedy, and Litvak, 1991). Emotional support (see Chapter 8; on social support, see Vilhjalmsson, 1994) can be a form of personal assistance, which may be offered, provided, or shared in different ways. Emotional support can be viewed as particularly important for youth: ("maybe not what everyone needs or wants"), as a way to talk through problems ("It helps to have somebody else there to talk to."), as a way to accept one's disability ("My youth was a trying time . . . I didn't accept my disability . . . until I was thirty years old."), as an information role for personal assistants ("giving the patient all the information"), and as something that is not always needed ("Needs change and there may be a time when some of that might have been much more helpful").

PERSONAL ASSISTANCE IN SCHOOLS

Several different ways of thinking about assistance in the context of education (Biklen, 1992; Dryfoos, 1991; Jackson et al., 1993) and in

schools were raised in these interviews as people reflected on their childhood experiences. These included personal care as part of the student's
school program (i.e., teaching personal hygiene and care instead of other
educational options); regular assistance from the teacher to the students
("Any assistance I had would have been from a teacher, helping me with
my coat on or off, or whatever."); assistance from students to other students (such as pushing another in a manual wheelchair); one-on-one aides;
and assistive technology or equipment, such as an electric wheelchair for
more independence.

At least one informant mentioned the need for PAS in schools during
elementary and secondary school, during college years, in school/residen-
cy programs, for adult education (reading, writing, career changes), and
during extracurricular school activities (e.g., instead of calling parents to
be available on field trips, a paid personal attendant might be used). Two
women had used the school/residency program at University of California
at Berkeley, and one of the women filed legal action against the school for
lack of attendant care for extracurricular activities.

Some informants did not have an opportunity to learn to read or write as
children ("I went to a segregated school when I was little, so there was no
emphasis on reading and writing."). These experiences have impacted
negatively on their work options as adults ("I'm stuck doing things that I
don't want to do. As far as the day program, I think I am a lot smarter than
that."). The four areas of assistance needed by children and youth that
were mentioned focused on tutoring, homework, reading, and note taking
("The biggest thing I use for school is notetakers.") in high school and in
college (see also supported education in Chapter 8). Simply being aware
of PAS options is "a really big thing," so children will not become "completely dependent upon" their parents. PAS can be considered to be a
"right to be just as independent as their nondisabled peers," "to hire an
assistant versus relying on their parents," and to have a break from their
parents ("When parents do it all the time, you get sick of them.").

CAREER AND EMPLOYMENT

PAS was viewed as a way to help people contribute as taxpayers,
instead of drawing on society's resources (see the nation's goals of productivity and their relevance to people with severe and multiple disabilities, Ferguson and Ferguson, 1986). The same societal money could be
spent instead on assisting a person to make an income and to pay taxes,
with better personal life outcomes (stronger relationships, more activities,
higher life quality), at less cost than society would need to spend to care

for a person who did not work. Two options for PAS at work are to redelegate job duties to accommodate the job functions a person can perform (e.g., accommodation, job modification, and job sharing) and to provide assistance for daily living functions, such as using the bathroom or eating lunch (Racino with Whittico, 1998). Other types of work assistance could include assistance with meetings, letter writing, grant writing, interpreting, and business travel, or whatever else is needed.

One independent living center (see Nosek, Roth, and Zhu, 1990, for national survey) had a career planning project "designed to give the client the choice of deciding his or her own career plan" and to be "flexible according to what the client needs" to get a "job where she wants." Work disincentives (e.g., loss of benefits) make it "very difficult to get out and really hit the workforce." Independence makes it more likely that a person will seek and find jobs for himself or herself. PAS should be available for volunteer work, too, because "people need something to do in the daytime or during the day." (For perspectives on the meaning of work, see Freedman and Fesko, 1996.)

RELATIONSHIPS, COMMUNITY, AND RECREATION IN THE PAS CONTEXT

The nature of adolescence or youth (Takanish, 1990; Coleman, 1980) involves the development of social life with other youth (having "fun," "getting involved in the community") and, often, the expansion of interests into new unexplored areas (see also, on recreation, Litvak, Zukas, and Heumann, 1987, p. 15). A teenager may start to date, vacation separate from his or her family, develop interest in sports, participate in group social functions (e.g., dances, football games), and spend time with friends in shopping malls, at the movies, in restaurants, and at dances.

Teenagers develop their own lifestyles, which they may take into adulthood (Clark and Foster-Johnson, 1996; Crittiden, 1990; Erikson, 1965; Friedenberg, 1959; Kittrie, 1971; Miller, 1994). For some youth, this may involve an active, independent lifestyle, with outdoor sports such as motorcycle racing, water skiing, and downhill skiing, while other youth may prefer an indoor sport such as roller skating (Kelley and Frieden, 1989). Personal assistants may also be "there to help them if they need it."

Young people may also start taking vacations with friends who may or may not be able to offer some forms of assistance. As one adult informant expressed about his own situation, "I haven't done a lot of that because it's not really easy to do that. First of all, I have to have a friend willing to do that."

Some activities or events in which teenagers may participate are group social functions that may involve a social circle of peers. As one father described:

> If they're going to go to dances . . . to football games . . . to social functions . . . they are interacting with the people that are around and they've got a social circle of peers. Eventually, I would think that they would not need to take a personal attendant with them . . . pretty soon it's things that friends do together.

A young person may need to figure out the role of his or her personal assistant ("I can't imagine a first date and you're wondering about taking a personal care assistant with you."). For some young adults, without personal assistance (e.g., assistance going to the bathroom), some social options might not be possible (e.g., going out to the movies or dinner). Not every young adult will want a personal assistant along, and each person will need to figure out how to handle dining out, for example. The same father, quoted previously, described his own way of asking for assistance in restaurants:

> For me, a lot of times it is easier to go out to eat than it is to eat at home just because it is too hard to cook . . . if I'm having steak, I can't cut up the meat, but what I've found is that most people, when you do go some place, if you're bold enough to ask, they're usually really receptive about helping out.

Adolescents spend time with other youth and may informally ask someone to assist them. Adolescents can go out with friends without having to depend on a personal care assistant. However, the youth may still want his or her PCA to go along.

PERSONAL ASSISTANCE, FAMILY SUPPORT, AND YOUTH

> My family, when I was young, if they would have been able to have someone come in and do what I needed done, it would have been a lot better off for everyone because it would have taken some of the pressure off them.

Family support continues to be viewed and practiced primarily as parental support, with the concept based, in part, on a view of the child as a "burden" (Nolan, Grant, and Ellis, 1990). As one young man explained, some parents might need respite, relief, or a "break from being a parent" because their child needs constant care. With this respite (Salisbury, 1990), "everyone" could "be better off . . . because it would have taken the pressure off them." One man, who was injured later in life, described his own biggest obstacle in finding assistance:

> What I was looking for with personal care assistants was, you know, I'm probably about 6'2", 200 lbs, and I need some help getting out of bed in the morning. . . . That was probably one of the biggest obstacles that I've had was just finding people that are physically able to do those kinds of things.

Personal Assistance As a Youth Service

Another way of thinking would be to see personal assistance as a relief or service for the child or teenager (As one parent said, "I know that for her it gets to be a big relief to have them come in. . . . I think any family can become overbearing for a teenager."). Respite can offer youth the freedom to participate in life independently, away from family ("As the youth got older, it may allow them more freedom . . . to do more things if they had someone else come in rather than a family member."). This is a different way of thinking about personal assistance services than as a family support to relieve the parents or caregivers of the burden of their child. Describing his experiences later in life, one man recounted the following:

> All of a sudden I was going to take off across the country, and some of my family was in a real panic because they were like, "You can't do that." I said, "Why not?" [They replied,] "It's not the same for you as it is for anybody else." Well, I think that generally people have got to be allowed the independence and the opportunity to find out what they can and can't do.
>
> I was up on the north shore of Lake Superior . . . that's the first time I have ever been up there since I'd broken my neck. So I used to hike all the cross-country ski trails and the snowshoe trails and things like that, which is exactly what I did after I was in a wheelchair. . . . I ended up dumping my wheelchair into a rut coming down the side of the mountain. . . . It was kind of funny because I had pictures when I got back home . . . that was a 300-mile drive with a broken arm.

PAS for youth can be framed in the context of an independent living perspective with PAS as a "part of everyday life." For some youth, they may experience more independence "living with family than outside of family," while other youth and adults may find more independence outside the family (e.g., with a live-in PCA).

The following are other issues affecting youth: having too many services; finding own level of independence; others having too much control over their lives (e.g., "no opportunity to make mistakes"); finding the line between restrictiveness and support; the experience of forced independence by being left alone; and family concerns about risks for the children and youth, often leading to overprotectiveness (see also Chapters 8, 9, and 10).

Adolescents or youth may not be asked how they feel and may feel unable to be assertive. Youth may have their own goals regarding where they want to live and who they want to work with as they grow older. Children and youth may access personal assistance in contrast to parents' accessing it for the children and youth.

Personal Assistance to Address Abusive Family Situations

Some youth may want to move out of home "on their own" due to abuse in home situations ("I feel very strongly if there is this kind of situation . . . [youth] ought to be allowed to do [leave home].") (See Child Welfare League of America, 1993, for youth leaving out-of-home care). Having this option does not mean that "all youth in America with disabilities would all of a sudden wake up and say 'We may have the right to move out of our parents' home, so let's do that.'"

Youth Relationships with Personal Assistants

> I don't know any youth with [a] disability that hasn't done something they probably shouldn't have done. And it really becomes difficult because a lot of parents are going to see the personal care attendant as somebody . . . [who is] supposed to be responsible to them.

In the context of the nature of adolescence, youth need to maintain relationships with the people who work with them and with their own parents and guardians ("Certainly if they can't get along with their parents, it is not going to work."). Though parents may believe the personal care attendant is responsible to them, the teenager may feel more comfortable talking privately with his or her assistant. For example, one PCA described the situation with one young woman who had a severe head injury:

> She's got a communication board, and she can use that some. And she can kind of raise one arm to answer yes-and-no questions. . . . There are a lot of things that I know that just really bother her that she can't communicate to her parents and she'll tell her personal care assistant.

The situation becomes even more complicated when the teenager or adolescent is, or wishes to be, involved in some behavior or action which is either illegal or which the parent finds to be an immoral, unethical, or premature decision. These activities may go unnoticed or be more easily ignored with youth without disabilities, whereas an adolescent accompanied by an assistant or attendant faces a very different situation. One father described a potential scenario:

> If they find out that their kid gets along just great with their attendant, but every time their parent leaves they find they are smoking pot behind the barn [see also Kandel, 1986], [they] probably need some way to pull the reins back on it, if they are doing things that might be potentially hurting them.

Several critical points were made regarding the nature of the relationship with personal assistants. First, attendant care is real work and a job, not a favor. Second, sometimes the personal assistants or attendants may want to "do something" when the child, youth, or adult would "rather be alone or with someone else." Third, friendships may develop as part of the working relationships, especially if camaraderie exists or if one or both people tend to be friendly by nature ('If it's going to work out, you end up being friends at least to some extent."). Fourth, it can be hard to ask for assistance, even when one's personal assistant is paid ("I have a hard time asking people for assistance if I don't know them well.").

Parents and Siblings As Personal Assistants

> It depends upon whether the parents need to have someone assisting the individual because they are out doing their job. Because if they can't do their job because they have to care for an individual with a disability, then why not pay that individual's care attendant?

Parents are often expected to continue to provide assistance to their teenagers, including when they participate in activities and situations in which youth without disabilities might typically do with other teenagers. Sometimes caring by parents is a natural part of people's relationships, given their circumstances. For example, one informant explained, "Whenever I go anywhere, like on a family vacation or something, I still do that with my family and they take care of my treatment." Yet, parents or other family members providing personal assistance services may become a barrier to teenage peer relationships. As another informant described, "If they are going out with their parents, . . . they are much less likely to get hooked up with those kinds of people [whom] they could do things with later." Parental assistance may foster youth dependency (e.g., "If I wanted to go out to a movie, I would have to call mom and dad."). Parents may also be expected to be the emergency providers of PAS, even for adult children who are living away from home. Yet, other family members may also step in during times of crisis; for example:

> After my divorce . . . I lived with my brother at this time for about a year. . . . Although my brother was able to give me the care that was needed . . . well, he helped me out pretty good, but it got to be kind of a burden on him and the rest of the family at the time because they had to assist me with my needs.

Relatives and Friends As Personal Assistants

Sometimes youth, adults with disabilities, and/or their families might prefer that a friend or relative provide personal assistance services. For example, as one woman described:

> I am fortunate enough, and I do stress fortunate enough, that the people that work as personal care attendants of me—one is my sister, and I'm very close to her, and another, actually I met her through this agency, and we've [been] together now for several years and have become close friends.

Another person explained that being able to pay friends makes it less like charity work and makes him feel more independent. Some people distinguish between youth and adult living circumstances when deciding what their positions are on whether payments should be made to family members to provide assistance to their child.

Adolescents As Personal Assistants to Other Adolescents

Some informants believe that adolescents (teenagers or youth) might prefer personal assistants who are similar in age because of the possibility of similar interests in activities, more natural integration into relationships with other teens with or without disabilities (see Table 11.2), and the possibility of developing less of a caretaking or "babysitting" relationship. One father described a situation involving teens wanting to go out and play basketball. As he explained:

> If . . . you've got someone who is sixteen or seventeen years old, they're in a wheelchair, they need some help, but they'd like to play basketball. . . . If you're hiring somebody who is eighteen years old, and they're working with somebody that's sixteen, seventeen, or eighteen years old, they're probably going to want to do it for the sake of doing it . . . more just mutual interest.

Such a paid assistant relationship could result in more independence for the youth and new relationships, for example, with neighbors, rather than having "somebody out there working with them to do recreational activities." The father continued:

> And all of a sudden they'll find themselves not playing basketball with a personal care attendant, rather with the neighbor kid down the street.

PRACTICAL ASPECTS
OF PERSONAL ASSISTANCE SERVICES

> As long as I don't have to deal directly with the agency, and I'm dealing with the people, I haven't had a lot of problems with getting those things done. But I'm not sure they fit within the structure of the system. With families and friends, [I am] also able to get things done instead of hiring somebody who was just strictly following procedures.

The practical aspects of personal assistance services range from the types of service modes, settings and PAS; scheduling and emergency backup services; selection, hiring, training, and termination; wages for assistants; monitoring/quality; and financing. Several aspects are highlighted in this section (Racino, 1995c).

Modes of Assistance

The informants described assistance based upon different types of involvement, collaboration, and control. Several of them described different modes of personal assistance services that already exist: *independent provider* ("I get funds from them. I am entitled to to find my own attendant, interview them, and hire them and I am responsible to train them."); *family provider* (a family member or relative cares for the disabled individual and the individual is paid by the agency); and *managed care* ("when the agency takes over the clients' life").

Settings and PAS

According to the informants, PAS can be provided or offered in different types of settings, including group homes (where people may not have chosen to live) and apartment buildings (e.g., Section 8 places with twenty-four-hour live-in attendants and personal assistants accessible by cord or beeper; for research study on Section 8 housing allowance, see Newman, 1994). PAS may be organized in different ways, for example, with agencies covering "a wide variety of disability groups").

Scheduling and Emergency Backup Services

Scheduling with the personal assistant or staff member may be handled through informal and/or formal arrangements, not necessarily at the convenience of the service user (e.g., "You call and you wait until they are available to help you"; "One of the biggest problems I had was getting the treatment to fit my schedule instead of accommodating *their* work schedule."). Flexibility for an agency may require more funding to "hire another staff person to work a different shift . . . to have somebody on call all the time." Various backup and/or emergency service arrangements are sometimes arranged informally (e.g., "generally somebody available that is more than willing to stop by or give me a hand with whatever I need") or through formal types of arrangements (e.g., city emergency backup; temporary organization for twenty-four-hour backup services; telephone approval for backup assistant).

Financing

> I like to think that I might be able to be self-supporting, but if I can't do that and will always need to rely on services, to have those services not get the funding that they need, will have a great impact on my lifestyle.

Whether services obtain funding impacts on the lifestyles of individual people who require those services. Primary financial areas raised were the following:

- Interpreting as an ongoing expense for all waking hours;
- Decisions on reimbursable service coverage (e.g., the need for twenty-four-hour assistance; or whether specific tasks such as gardening or snow shoveling are allowable);
- Low wages, limitations on benefits (e.g., health care), and lack of a career ladder for personal care assistants;
- Arguments on the cost-effectiveness of giving money directly to the person instead of an agency ("going through a private organization instead of paying an individual or the attendant directly probably costs $6,000 to $8,000 more");
- The disproportionate payments to the agency instead of the assistant ("personal assistants get less than half the money paid to the provider organization");
- Making too much money to qualify for benefits ("if you make too much money, you don't get the services");
- Limitations on property tax in order to retain homeownership;
- Restrictions on savings, including for homes and vehicles;
- Need for similar standards in different settings;
- Creation of security about retaining services; and
- Income and asset exclusions and their effects on hiring a personal assistant (raise the income and asset levels).

Payment to Parents and Family Members

One of the barriers to financing PAS with youth and children is the perception of parental responsibility for caregiving functions. Some people believe parents who give up a job or career to perform such functions with or for their child (e.g., as an interpreter) should be reimbursed or paid for the services they perform. Others believe the child's feelings should be considered in determining whether a parent or an outside personal assistant should be paid for providing personal assistance (see England et al., 1990).

Although most state and local governments are reluctant to pay family providers or attendants, some informants said parents should be paid to provide assistance to their children at home, but also have someone else come in to give the parents a break (see Litvak, Zukas, and Heumann, 1987, p. 112, on eligibility of family providers). Even when family members are eligible for assistance, restrictions (e.g., certification of family members) may apply. One informant suggested that payments to families of youth living at home could be based upon the age of the child, the capacity of the youth to make choices, and/or decisions of both the family and adolescent.

CONCLUSION

While some of these concerns vary over time and by program, state, and categorical disability, many are long-standing issues with PAS from the late 1970s when the initial programs were being developed in New York. In relationship to federal programs, policy decisions are often reflected in legislation, with some decisions made at the state and local levels. The perspectives in this chapter continue to be underrepresented in the burgeoning family support literature, with universal access and community approaches by any definition, still a dream in the lives of some people with and without disabilities.

PART IV:
HOUSING, FAMILIES, AND COMMUNITY
SUPPORT—POLICY EVALUATION,
RESEARCH, AND ANALYSIS

Introduction

James A. Knoll

The chapters in this section bring you, the reader, face to face with an inescapable reality of change: *I have to start thinking and acting in a different manner.* The "I" here is "you," the likely reader of this book: the university professor or researcher, the evaluation consultant, the state policy analyst, the administrator, or the graduate student in the areas of human services and public policy. Throughout this text, and perhaps most clearly in the following section, we confront the reality that a rhetoric of support and empowerment has meaning that reaches beyond the day-to-day interactions of the direct service worker or the redirection of funding streams. Certainly, many in our society have acknowledged, in this post-ADA era, that prejudices toward people with disabilities need to be laid to rest and that, as in all other arenas in which we confront human diversity, we all, as citizens, need to examine our own attitudes. I assume this level of change. The implications of these chapters go beyond this to a fundamental reexamination of how some of the very professions and organizations that have contributed to this broader social change must themselves come to terms with a new reality.

What was unimaginable just a few years ago is happening today. The battle to do away with the large, isolated, sterile institution as a model of service for people with disabilities is on the verge of being won. Although some states contend there will always be a need for relatively traditional institutions, the trend is clear. It seems apparent that sometime early in the next century, the institution, the asylum, the developmental center, or the state school for the mentally retarded will all become historical artifacts—footnotes in the social history of the United States, icons for the ability of human services to be neither human nor of service.

So, the war is over—the Berlin Wall is down; people with developmental disabilities are in the community—now we can relax. Right?

Wrong! By clearing away the monolith of the institution, we have finally reached the point at which we can focus on the real challenges confronting people with disabilities and their families, friends, and allies. As each successive chapter has underscored, the real battle is about presence, participation, competence, choice, and contribution—full inclusion of people with disabilities as valued members of our communities. We now come face to face with the way service systems respond to families and their children with disabilities and to adults with disabilities as they make decisions about where and how they wish to live.

Can we come to terms with the simple fact that "home" is not the same thing as a "homelike environment," an "alternate residential unit," or an "SIP (supported independence program)"? Can we finally bury the myth of "special places for special people" along with the monolith of the institution? Are we able to deal with the realization that support for families cannot be defined in terms of narrow, predefined service options such as fourteen days of respite a year, parent counseling, or "sibshops"? Do we realize that person-centered and family-centered are not just new models for doing "I ___ Ps" but are invitations to creatively design, *from the ground up,* what *this* family or *this* person needs? Will we be able as policymakers, administrators, researchers, educators, service providers, and neighbors to realize that community support of people with disabilities entails an essential change in thinking and acting that makes the movement from the institution to the community seem simple by comparison?

I begin this introduction by raising the specter of the institution because, for all the progress we have made, most of our service models, funding structures, quality assurance mechanisms, evaluation strategies, public policies, and ways of thinking related to people with disabilities are derived from the institutional model, with all its inherent emphasis on deficits, incompetence, and the need for professional decision making and control. We have only begun to shake off these shackles and realize that community membership requires totally new ways of planning, funding, and supporting people.

The material in this text shows that the issue of choice and control is central to the transformation confronting us: Who's in charge? None of us deny the reality of people's disabilities—we are here because we are very aware of them. We want to be sure that the need for assistance and support that is so much a part of the life of people with disabilities does not overshadow their entire existence. We know that there is nothing inherent in raising a child with a disability that should require families to complete myriad forms and await endless approvals to have their determination about the needs of their child and family affirmed by a bureaucrat or a service provider. A diagnosis of a disability and the need for support in certain aspects of life does not nullify the rights of adults to make decisions about how they wish to live. The challenge we confront is designing supports that respect and affirm the home, the family, and the choice of each individual.

SUPPORTING FAMILIES

With the hard-won right to a free, appropriate public education, supported by the documented effectiveness of early intervention, and galvanized by their own experience, grassroots parents' organizations have, since about 1980, been pressuring policymakers to shift funds and priorities. They have insisted that *all* children have a right to grow up in a real home with a family. They have fought for family-focused services to become the first priority in a state's developmental disabilities budget. As this family support movement has coalesced, a core of policies and practice has emerged that begins to sketch the outline of a true community system of service.

The emerging family-centered approach has been central in defining the new way of thinking and acting on the part of administrators and providers. It takes as its cornerstone the understanding that families need to exercise choice and control over decisions that affect their daily lives. Parents need to be affirmed in the depth of knowledge that they have about their children and family. Professionals are most effective when they abandon a judgmental diagnostic model of service and join in partnership with families to address the challenges they confront. When the community—including public, private, formal, and informal resources—joins with families of children with disabilities to mobilize resources and build connections, half the battle is won. With these priorities, the bonds between the person, family, and community are never broken. Inclusion and community membership are not questions because they are a daily reality.

The ultimate family support is available when parents can begin to rest assured that their son or daughter has settled into a stable secure adult lifestyle. Unfortunately, in this crucial area, most service systems provoke anxiety rather than offer security. When a person needs assistance in daily life, the best most systems can offer is a place on a waiting list for a group home "slot." This, in itself, is a cruel charade, since movement off the waiting list usually occurs not because the son or daughter has reached the top of the list but because of a crisis in the family. Families that hope for a smooth transition into adult life for their child and a change in their lifestyle as their children leave home instead find their adult child with a disability continuing to live with them until they die or become incapacitated.

In Chapter 12, the value of case studies as a critical window into the reality of how systems interact with families is explored. This theme is further developed in Chapter 14, in which the tension between rhetoric and reality is directly confronted. Both these chapters leave us with a deeper understanding of the distance systems and individual professionals have to go to truly understand and operationalize family support. Chapter 14 bridges the gap between a focus on children within families and the needs of adults by examining the complex range of issues that emerge when foster care is used as a model of individualized services for people in need of supports in daily life. Here, as in other chapters, the need for a clear sense of direction, with a focus on membership, and community building to guide a system of supports and avoid the pitfalls of a deficit-driven model are underscored. It is only through research methods that actually touch the realities of daily life that these critical concerns can be examined.

SUPPORTING ADULTS

Adults with developmental disabilities—as do other adults—want a piece of the American dream. They want a *home* of their own. Home is your space, where you are in charge—where you can be yourself, not who someone else wants you to be. Home is the place the United States Constitution protects from governmental intrusion. Setting up housekeeping—moving out—these are transitions that mark the onset of adulthood. Unfortunately, the majority of the professional literature and the popular media continue to create the myth that people with developmental disabilities *require* housing in something called homelike environments.

Such thinking continues to define the housing needs of people with disabilities in terms of facilities and betrays the depth of the institutional mind-set in our culture. An industry has developed that is based on non-disabled people making a living—and sometimes a substantial profit—controlling the lives of adults with disabilities. What remains constant is the simple fact that this industry continues to be firmly rooted in the defining characteristic of institutional care—paid staff managing the lives of people who have, by their placement, been designated as being dependent.

The good news contained in the case studies in this text is that an increasing number of organizations are struggling with the meaning of concepts such as choice, control, quality of life, personal satisfaction, and community membership. They often use applied participatory research techniques to engage themselves in the process of learning how to achieve their mission (see, for example, O'Brien and Lyle-O'Brien, 1992). Central to this process is the willingness to enter into a dialogue with people with disabilities and with communities. To summarize much that is found in these case studies, we can look at the work of John O'Brien and Connie Lyle-O'Brien (1991). They have talked to many individuals engaged in this creative dialogue. They find these new relationships occur within learning organizations that are marked by the following characteristics: (1) commitment to vision; (2) acceptance of ambiguity; (3) active raising of questions; (4) trying new ways to look at and do things; (5) introspection on self and own life support; (6) support for asking for help; (7) personal involvement with the people they assist; (8) acceptance of working outside usual program boundaries and routine; (9) reaching out to involve new people in their work; (10) negotiating for what they believe people really want and need; and (11) taking time to reflect and to invest in learning new things.

Chapter 13 explores how case study research provides a valuable vehicle for understanding the struggles inherent in moving a state system from a deficit-driven, facility-based model to a truly person-centered approach to providing individual supports. The use of case study methodology as a critical tool in examining, understanding, and evaluating this process of change at the local organization levels is explored in Chapter 16.

PROFESSIONAL ROLES

This new level of engagement, this new alliance with people with disabilities, requires that individual professionals working in the field really listen to the people. Then we can hear "I want an education, a home, a job, friends, a family." Goals that were written off as unrealistic expectations were only unrealistic within the context of our limited, and limiting, frame of reference. We quickly need to learn two very important lessons: (1) our carefully managed, normalized environments are one of the major limitations on the people we said we were committed to helping, and (2) individuals with disabilities have a different view of what is truly support.

The change can be particularly striking for individuals trained to be professional helpers by assessing and teaching them, designing individualized plans and programs for them, and modifying their behavior. Once beyond the professional steps, beyond the limits of the traditional way of thinking, they find their roles redefined as assisting people to achieve the most natural—and varied—human goals. They now find themselves trying to figure out what it means to work *for* people with disabilities. The term client is no longer a meaningless euphemism that thinly disguises that the people so identified are commodities traded in the human service market. They are called on to become responsive to their customers. The profound nature of this change in consciousness leads to a redefinition of priorities. No longer do we concentrate on identifying deficits; we concentrate on identifying individual and collective strengths. Unrealistic expectations based on diagnostic categories are abandoned in favor of exploring personal hopes, dreams, and goals. Minimal expectations in terms of the achievement of programmatic goals are superseded by high expectations related to personal goal attainment. A crisis intervention mentality is replaced by a proactive crisis prevention perspective that identifies formal and informal resources, develops multiple backup strategies, and is based on the premise that support is not a program that ends, but a long-term commitment.

In 1990, the Family Support and Empowerment Project at Cornell University asked workers involved with traditionally oppressed people, as they struggled to gain control over their own destiny, to define what it meant to provide support. It is striking how the themes that emerged from their efforts parallel those that run throughout the studies related to people with disabilities in this book. One of the larger ideas that emerges is the need for professional roles to be transformed along lines such as the following, described by (Cochran, 1990b):

1. Ability and commitment to identifying strengths in people and groups:

   • Genuine respect for diverse perspectives and lifestyles
   • A capacity to listen and reflect

2. An ability to subordinate one's own ego (to put one's self aside in the interest of the group):

   • Skill and creativity in helping people become more aware and confident of their own abilities
   • Appreciation of when to step back and the ability to help the individual or group assume decision making and action
   • Ability to analyze power relationships and help others to do so
   • Knowledge about how to gain access to information

3. Ability to reflect on and criticize ongoing processes, including one's own role in those processes (p. 25)

Subsequent efforts to explore the meaning of these skills specifically targeted implications for research and evaluation enterprises (Barr and Cochran, 1992; Cochran, 1991). Racino adds more to the base of information on this important topic. All of the studies presented in Part IV bring us face to face with this aspect of change. A consistent theme presented in this book is an acknowledgment of the unique perspective of each individual who engages us in the process of understanding—those people who in another time we would call our "subjects." Here, Racino confronts us with the fundamental realization that if we truly have experienced a basic change in the field of services and research related to people with disabilities, we must acknowledge the movement from seeing people as passive objects of our inquiry to seeing them as active partners.

Read and reflect. The challenge is significant.

Chapter 12

The Role of Family Case Study Research in Family Policy: Local Agency Delivery Systems

Julie Ann Racino

FATHER AND SON:
A BRIEF CASE STUDY OF RESIDENTIAL
SCHOOL PLACEMENT IN NEW YORK

When we met in March of 1989, Bill Jamison lived in a midsize city in central New York with his biracial, ten-year-old son, Jerry. By all accounts, Bill, who is divorced, wanted Jerry to continue living at home and was reluctant to even consider temporary residential school placement. However, when the family name was crossed off the list of potential family support participants, I learned that Jerry had been placed in a residential school (i.e., a large children's institution) located in southern New York (about five hours away) in January 1989.

The Research

The study included two visits and interviews with Bill in his family home (one prior to his first visit to see Jerry at the residential school), an interview with a family friend and family support worker at her office, an interview with one of Jerry's longtime baby-sitters in her home in the neighborhood, a participant observation visit during Jerry's first visit

---

This research case study is excerpted from Racino, J. (1989). *Father and Son: A Brief Story of Residential School Placement.* Syracuse, NY: Syracuse University, Center on Human Policy, unpublished research field memo.

home after placement (including with his half sister who lives nearby with Jerry's mother), a review of official records kept by one agency, and numerous telephone and related conversations.

Jerry

People who know and care about Jerry describe him as affectionate, really sweet, a precious little kid, and very loving. On the day we met, he wore a big, warm smile, was constantly on the move, and, at one point, took my hand, sat me down on the floor, and leaned on my shoulder. His father, upon inquiry, said Jerry loves going places in the car, going to the playground, and digging mud holes. Jerry demonstrated his love of music and dancing in front of the television, watching himself in the mirror. He also demonstrated the family fun routines of ball rolling across the room to each other and balloon breaking (two activities Jerry seems to enjoy). By all accounts, Jerry and Bill have a close relationship.

At the same time, everyone agrees Jerry is spoiled rotten, can be a little pill sometimes, can be outrageous, and will run roughshod if a person does not know how to handle him. Though described by his baby-sitter as a smart kid, he was labeled as multiply handicapped, moderately retarded, autisticlike, and as having mild cerebral palsy and epilepsy. His father says he must have been assigned twenty labels by twenty different people. Other than a report of a single word, his father says he uses forty personal signs, including a sign for ice cream, one of his favorites.

Bill

Bill is a soft-spoken, gentle man who values individuality and common sense, and who tries not to blame other people even when he believes they are in the wrong. Probably considered a liberal in his view on lifestyles (interracial marriages, homosexuality), he is a university basketball fan, frequents a book warehouse, and enjoys classical music and watching baseball.

Though a pacifist who believes "war is a bunch of old men sending out young boys to be killed," he joined the Navy for adventure and served in Vietnam and Japan. A graduate of a well-known university, he works as a clerk in a local grocery store (part of a larger chain); he appreciates the flexibility of the job, but could not take opportunities to advance in the company due to child care. A "confirmed atheist," who has been married twice, he "believes in the Chinese philosophy that it is better that people change their wants."

EMERGING RESEARCH THEMES

These excerpts from the confidential field memo include emerging themes from the coded data on the interviews and visits. It was written in 1989 and edited in 1998, after being placed on a public database without permission of the researcher.*

Life at Home: Doing Everything Together

Jerry and Bill literally do everything together when they are at home. They eat together, play together, shower together, and even slept together for eight years. Other than work, Bill seldom was able to get out of the house alone, even for a walk, more than twice a month. Life is structured heavily around Jerry; for example, Bill sleeping with his arm around Jerry, since otherwise he gets up and cries.

The Life of the Father: When "Abnormal" Becomes "Normal"

Probably the most important aspect of life at home was summed up by Bill. He said when Jerry was three, what Bill considered abnormal became normal and vice versa. It became "normal" not to leave the house and to do everything with Jerry, only a few feet away at most.

On Friends and Family: Growing Up

Bill has two sisters, both out-of-state, who keep in touch, with cards and an occasional visit. Bill's mother sends birthday cards, but did not approve of his interracial marriage or Jerry's birth. Other relatives live out-of-state, except for an aunt in another central New York city. Jerry grew up playing with the neighborhood children, but this practice tapered off as he grew older. In public school, Jerry, who started in kindergarten in "early childhood development," does not have much opportunity to be with other children.

On Coming to the Out-of-Home Placement Decision

One of the most important parts of the study was the process of how a father, friends, the school, and agencies came to the decision that the

---

*The field memo is "contained in" the research study Racino, J. (1988). "Innovations in Family Support: What Are We Learning?" *Journal of Child & Family Studies,* 7(4), 433-449.

"best" place for his son was a residential school. As Bill related, the process started with his first program of early childhood development (see, for example, Able-Boone, H., Sandall, S. and Loughry, A., 1989) and came to include:

1. the daily routine and constant fight (the father always needing to "be on," and fighting systems meant to "help");
2. the end of the line of good options ("everything works good for awhile");
3. the residential school as just another program, with the father now asking, Is it home-like? Are the staff good? Is the parent welcomed and has input? Will they treat my child well?
4. professionals know what is best for your child, with, in this case, "the last resort" being posed after other options were exhausted;
5. the child must change as the "last hope";
6. from temporary placement to possible lifetime, custodial care;
7. the child's future: emphasizing the positives (he has children to play with, even if he is covered with bruises from them);
8. the parent deserves a life, too, with the passage of one's own life's goals as one becomes older;
9. critical incidents (the rationale or excuse), in this case, as the rationale for placement, with a dispute regarding the reported accidental hitting of another child in the nose in school; and
10. placements as a way for bureaucracies to ease themselves of hassles.

On the Complexity and Interconnectedness of Relationships

Jerry's relationships, as one suspects of most children, were heavily dependent upon family relationships and his interactions in school and the neighborhood. Jerry's social network was expanded by his baby-sitter who was described as a "goer," a "doer," and a "family connector." Jerry himself initiates relationships and exerts control in his relationships. He is the raison d'être for other relationships; he has given meaning and purpose to the lives of different people. All the relationships in the study intertwine, including Jerry's relationship with his mother (and her extent of contact with him), with diverse contributions and demands as these relationships, including new ones, affect one another.

On Services and Service Systems

The first themes that began to emerge were:

- *schools and families* and their "unified" role in supporting children in their families, homes, and communities with state-funded "family support" provided by community agencies;
- *control and decision making* and efforts at maintaining control of one's child, self, and family, while seeking services, with the cost of the social workers not always worth the price paid;
- *learning the system*, as survival and caring for the child, knowing the available programs and the people who are willing to go to bat for you;
- *the role of agencies and services*, including the expensive resources for out-of-home care versus the minimal in-home supports, and their roles in blessing relationships that already exist or are doing the "dirty work" of placement; and
- *the relationship of informal and formal supports*, including the meanings and implications when viewed from different individual perspectives and from closer or distant relationships.

*   *   *

INTRODUCTION

With national interest in examining issues through a support and empowerment paradigm that emerged in the late 1980s and early 1990s (American Association on Mental Retardation, 1992; Smull and Bellamy, 1991), the importance of hearing the voices of all family members for program and policy development comes to the forefront. This theme and imperative raises the value of qualitative methodologies (Taylor and Bogdan, 1994) that seek to understand the diverse perspectives of families in societies around the world.

This chapter briefly describes three primary areas of research, policy, and practice affecting the lives of the case study family. These are the literatures on school exclusion and inclusion, the status of family support programs, and family support policy. The body of the chapter then describes the use of family case study research and selected research methodological concerns. The chapter concludes with an example of the use of family case studies in evaluation research and the contrast between agency evaluations using traditional methods and those using participant observation and interviewing over an extended time frame.

School Exclusion and Inclusion

The case study introducing this chapter began as a study of family support, with service demonstration funding awarded to the private, nonprofit agency led by parents of children and adults with disabilities (Racino, 1998). However, the school system, not the community agency, was considered responsible for decision making regarding the nature of the primary day services for the young boy, and secondarily his father. The father's position predates one of the main findings in an article published in 1993 comparing two case studies on when, how, and why educational placement decisions are made (Hallenbeck, Kauffman, and Lloyd, 1993). As described in the field notes, the elimination of options on a placement continuum may have had the effect of forcing more restrictive environments. Students with "emotional and behavioral" disorders represent an increasing percentage of students served in separate facilities of all types, and these youngsters (like Jerry) are disproportionately those of color (Stephens et al., 1990). The literature describes a movement toward excluding acting out, aggressive students from the special education system (Cline, 1990), including through the legal system, adding to previous exclusionary rationales (Wolfensberger, nd).

The exclusionary practices used in transferring Jerry from public school to an institution (residential school) contrast with the movement toward integration, inclusion, and inclusive schooling of children with disabilities (Biklen, 1985; Knoll and Meyer, 1987). Inclusion has been defined as moving toward community, with classrooms of diversity, offering natural support and accommodation, flexibility, empowerment, and the promotion of understanding of individual differences (Stainback and Stainback, 1990). Such inclusion, say its strongest adherents, means schooling in regular classrooms within the academic arena (e.g., O'Brien et al., 1989). Principles and best practices for regular school settings continue to evolve (Taylor, 1982; Stainback, Stainback, and Ayres, 1996), together with analyses of the factors supporting integrated placements (Hunt et al., 1993).

Yet, residential schools and centers (Sunshine et al., 1991), with from 20 to 200 children, often away from their home communities, continue as a primary alternative to public schooling for children in trouble (see, for example, a comparison of children in residential centers and school settings in Silver et al., 1992; history of residential schools in Kauffmann and Smucker, 1995; and standards for residential treatment centers). Special education placements and relationships with segregated options vary markedly by state (Danielson and Bellamy, 1989), as do local capacities in specialty areas of mental health and behavioral supports in schools (Lovett, 1996).

Status of Family Programs

In the 1980s, family support programs were highlighted (Kagan et al., 1987; Taylor et al., 1986), with implications for family policy. These analyses drew upon local programs in neighborhoods, early intervention and early childhood efforts by the federal government, and parent training and support. These were followed by disability family support books based on programs in the United States and internationally (Gartner, Lipsky, and Turnbull, 1991; Mittler and Mittler, 1995), emphasizing parent-to-parent support (Ziegler, 1988) and emerging empowerment, community, and organizing themes.

Social support continued as a focus of investigators (Cochran, 1990a; Newton et al., 1994; Vaux, 1988), including studies on the effect of support on the family. Social support was studied in the context of service systems (Racino, O'Connor, Walker, and Taylor, 1991), contrasting perspectives of service users and workers on the meaning of support (Racino and O'Connor, 1994). The popular and theoretical versions of formal and informal support (Bulmer, 1987) formed the basis for research in diverse community settings, homes, and employment sites.

Vaux described support as having buffering effects on stressors (the stress-support theory) and proposed specific support mechanisms, such as protective direct actions. As Vaux described (1988, p. 292), support programs, however, are "rarely located conceptually within the full context of support." Several common errors occur in their development: (1) the potential to disrupt or supplant existing support can be overlooked; (2) various targets of change may not be explicitly recognized; (3) an understanding that all strategies from group creation to community seed funding have inherent strengths and limitations may not exist; and (4) tactics within programs have advantages and disadvantages (with false assumptions that what works in one situation would work in another).

Support programs may not acknowledge adult needs in the context of families and parenting, may miss the component of parental involvement and collective decision making, and may be targeted to low-income people versus all people in a neighborhood (Zigler and Weiss, 1985). Most important, congruent with the position of McKnight (1989b) of Northwestern University (1988, p. 142), Vaux states that "inept supportive behavior may harm," and Riley and Eckenrode (1986) note that the mobilization of support, in the absence of resources, may result in what has been termed *negative support.* Flynn (1989b) summarizes her review of the research describing social support as moderating the damaging effects of stressful life events and being related to good health.

Neighborhoods as the "inevitable" focal point of service, in ecological models (Garbarino and Sherman, 1980), did not appear in the disability literature until the 1990s (Friedman, 1994; Racino and O'Connor, 1994; Walker, 1995), with the former neighborhood-based systems concurrent with the urban child mental health initiative of the Annie E. Casey Foundation. Studies of the ecology of neighborhoods have investigated, for example, variations in playmates, child supervision, fear of exploitation arising from neighboring, and relationships with professionals in high- and low-risk neighborhoods (Garbarino and Sherman, 1980). The neighborhood-based initiatives, as part of mental health service system reform, became tied to prevention and family support and an increase in flexibility in funding and modifications of fiscal incentives (Friedman, 1994). Yet, no discussion appears of Bronfenbrenner's (1974) thesis of the larger events in society that will determine with whom and how a child will spend his or her time in the context of the neighborhood approaches.

Status of Family Support Policy

Family support policy continues to be divorced from education policy (Taylor et al., 1989), with the United States criticized for lack of coherent family policy for all its people (e.g., health care, housing, employment, leisure, community, and economic development). Family support, which has developed as part of the process of community agencies working with families, has been reflected in state laws (Turnbull, Garlow, and Barber, 1991) and has been a major form of national organizing. In the 1980s, family-centered services became a central theme (Nelkin, 1987) in family support, entering the mental health field from the fields of assistive technology and mental retardation.

The medicalizing of family support (Knoll, 1992; Krauss, 1993), with the advent of Medicaid, has remained a critical issue, with the states having more control to demedicalize and shift financing than they generally exercise. While a state's commitment to family support may be seen in its use of Medicaid funds (Knoll et al., 1992b), little differentiation has been made between the use of Medicaid funds for people with medical and physical needs and those which may be of a different nature, and more likely to be supported through the use of state funds.

Income support, reimbursement schemes, vouchers, cash assistance, and individual payment schemes for families (Bertsch, 1992; Bradley, Knoll and Agosta, 1992) emerged in prominence as state family support budgets increased. However, concerns about differential allocations and impacts on families, conflicting policy goals (adults' rights and those of their parents), and unintended consequences of these efforts were minimized as programs were solidified, and both grassroots and legislative support was gained.

Respite (Cohen and Warren, 1985; Edinger, Schultz, and Morse, 1984; New York State Office of Mental Retardation and Developmental Disabilities [NYSOMRDD], 1985) continues to be a central family support service, with the focus of research on the central concepts of burden and stress (Grant and McGrath, 1990). In contrast, a strand of work in recreation involving the use of generic services by choice of the adolescents ("recreational respite") attempts to reverse the concept of burden (Heumann and Racino, 1988; Racino, 1985a). As of 1990, recreation was a fundable support service for families in over thirteen states (Bradley, Knoll, and Agosta, 1992), with expansion in mental health and in generic day care (Yuan Baker-McCue, and Witkin, 1996). However, the concept was often still defined by parental (not youth) needs.

Major themes arising in family support were greater movement toward diversity, particularly ethnic, cultural, and racial variations (Dilworth-Andersen, Burton, and Turner, 1993; Kaylanpur and Rao, 1991); involvement of fathers (Davis and May, 1991) and gender concerns with support arrangements (Traustadottir, 1988); and the changing nature of the family, including the movement toward single parenting (Shank and Turnbull, 1993). Beginning with a medical and clinical emphasis, the fields of brain injury and mental health moved forward to nonclinical family support approaches. In disability, on the research level, family-home-school relationships or the home-family-school interface often becomes the subject of research and change efforts (Sieber, 1981), to date, more from the education perspective (Sailor et al., 1996) than the family-home perspective.

FAMILY CASE STUDY RESEARCH

Sharing some of the characteristics of miniethnographies or life histories (Bogdan and Biklen, 1982) and the observational techniques of natural environments (Adler and Adler, 1994), family case study research contributes to the understanding of the diversity and complexity of families and their relationships with society. On the basis of social policy and service practices and interventions, family case study research offers concrete examples for policymakers and planners, families, researchers, administrators, and potential and current service users.

Depending upon research designs, case studies offer effective ways to analyze data in a comparative fashion. Such analyses may occur across similar or diverse programs, and people and families of diverse demographic backgrounds, geographic and political locations, departments and disciplines, agencies and systems, neighborhoods and communities, etiological and clinical backgrounds, and affiliations by organizations and associations. The literature on multisite evaluations (Mowbray and Herman, 1991) and multicase study design, (Yin, 1989) is relevant to these designs. Yin (1989, p. 113) states, "case studies are the preferred strategy when 'how' or 'why' questions are being posed, when the investigator has little control, and when the focus is a contemporary phenomenon within some real life context."

Research Principles

In the late 1980s, principles guiding family research described research as a collaborative endeavor (e.g., Turnbull, Turnbull, and Senior Staff, 1989) that could lead to action and change. While qualitative research is nearer to collaborative designs than most quantitative studies, by their nature, they, too, vary in the degree to which families and potential audiences are involved in all aspects of the research. Movement toward participatory action strategies, popular in the late 1980s and early 1990s, began to create other options for research design, building on the empowerment aspects of action research (Foster, 1976; Reason, 1994).

The Holistic Nature of Family Research

Family research involves all aspects of family members lives when approached from an ethnographic perspective (see Lewis, 1959). These aspects may be considered private by one family member (e.g., employment of the father, or relationship with his son), and not held or known the same way, if at all, by another family member, such as a spouse. This situation may be particularly true for cases involving divorce, remarriage, and changes in custody of children. Entry into homes opens another private domain, with extended observations and interviews often revealing beliefs, prejudices, and practices. These beliefs may reflect attitudes toward, or about, leisure, education, religion, employment, and politics, as well as about family members, friends, professionals, and community members.

Basic Methods of Family Case Study Research

In qualitative research designs, three primary methods contribute to the collection of data, data analysis, and the form of the research studies. These are in-depth interviewing, participant observation, and document review, described as follows:

1. *Participant observation* can be described as "research which involves the researcher and informants in the milieu of the latter,

during which data are systematically and unobtrusively collected" (Bruyn, 1966). Taylor and Bogdan (1984, pp. 15-75), in their basic text on qualitative research methods, describe the process of entering and leaving the field, role negotiation, establishing rapport with informants, selection of key informants, observer comments (i.e., researcher notes and self-reflection), and difficult aspects of field relations. Levels of field involvement are compared by Stainback and Stainback (1989), following descriptions of the participant-observer or observer-participant roles in classic ethnographic texts.

2. *In-depth interviewing* can be defined as "repeated face to face encounters between the researcher and informants directed toward understanding the informants' perspectives on their lives, experiences and situations as expressed in their own words" (Taylor and Bogdan, 1984, p. 77). In-depth interviewing that is open-ended and involves reflection, as in Carl Roger's approaches, is helpful in these contexts.

3. *Document reviews* (Taylor and Bogdan, 1984) contained in this book include newspaper and media articles, first-person accounts, private and public letters, legislation and regulations, historical documents, court papers, agency-prepared materials and program descriptions, photographs, personal commentaries, and books and publicly prepared drafts and final articles.

RESEARCH METHODOLOGY

This section describes several design and field concerns in family case study research: literature reviews, interviews with people with disabilities, access and entry into families, selection of methodologies, basic content and types of case studies, multicase studies, triangulation with organizational studies, and common concerns and misconceptions in family studies.

Literature Reviews

As indicated by Chelimsky (1995), literature reviews can increase credibility and decision making on new policies and programs. Compared to the design of quantitative studies, qualitative researchers often review the relevant literatures upon completion of the research data collection and analyses. This process is, in part, due to the inductive nature of the research study design, data collection, analyses, and theoretical developments. This methodology for reviews allows for informants to raise concerns (e.g., outpatient commitment to personal assistance services) not anticipated by the researcher, with subsequent review of the relevant literatures in relationship to these findings.

Interviews with People with Disabilities

A series of research articles and papers in the late 1970s and early 1980s (Sigelman et al., 1981) concentrated on methodological concerns with interviewing people with mental retardation. An excellent example of in-depth interviewing is contained in the rereleased version of *Inside Out* (Bogdan and Taylor, 1982), describing the lives of two primary informants with mental retardation. In addition to on-site interviews in the homes of people with mild or moderate mental retardation (Halpern et al., 1986), this was followed in the late 1980s by an article from Syracuse University on participant observation and interviewing with people with mental retardation (Biklen and Moseley, 1988). The article which cited a selection of public case studies from a major study of national organizations (Racino, 1991c; Taylor, Bogdan, and Racino, 1991).

Interviews in Chapters 2, 5, and 12 through 15 also involved people with mental retardation, in person and onsite. Interviews in Chapter 9 were by telephone, with people who have not been met in person. The same field guides were used with the informants, with and without disabilities, in all studies. This is, in part, because unlike other published analyses involving yes-no and either-or responses, the interviews were semistructured, open-ended, and based on the person's experiences. The major exception in these studies was the use of a facilitator by one informant from California, with the facilitator interviewed separately for the study of personal assistance services.

In the family case study research, which involved home visits, not all people with disabilities had a visible way of communicating directly with strangers, either through language, nonverbal response to an entering stranger, or communication technology. This finding was similar to the results in national technical assistance visits involving people with disabilities who may have had broken communication boards or ones that were stored away and not used (or, in other cases, not available) in the home setting. No cases of facilitated communication (Heckler, 1994) arose in this set of studies, though training was taking place in states and the local community.

Access

Access to research informants, especially through organizations, is viewed as problematic and a perennial concern, often described as entry through "gatekeepers" (Taylor and Bogdan, 1984). This difficulty of access is in part due to the nature of the relationships between universities and community and governmental organizations and of the centrality of research and evaluation concerns to both types of organizational entities (e.g., media, profit making). Yet, organizations often serve as training and placement sites for universities, with confidentiality a perennial concern to the sites, and with universities viewing this position by agencies as a protection of the agencies, not of their clientele. Today, community agencies and government, both often with their own research staff, may compete with research organizations and the educational sector for the same research funding.

Entry into the Lives of Families

Agency ownership of families remains a prevalent public position, with the agency claiming control over future research with the families. This position is an outgrowth of a standard service position on the relationship between agencies and their clients, whereby the agency relegates the person and/or family to a form of clienthood for life. Entry can take place through informal networks of professionals and parents, through formal proposals to family support and disability action groups, and through studies that secondarily identify families which may use service agencies, be part of community associations, or be involved in a set of recreation events or activities. Family privacy, of different family members, and the complexity involved, presents a challenge to all researchers.

Selection of Case Study Methodologies

Case study methodologies can be selected to examine critical national and local concerns and applied issues being faced by families, agencies, communities, and government. These include: persistent concerns with family support and out-of-home placements, community, relationships and empowerment, agency versus consumer-operated and -directed services, program management and quality in foster care, and agency change in new program adoption (e.g., Birnebaum and Cohen, 1993; Racino, 1998) (see Table 12.1 for sample areas of inquiry). Case studies can focus on an individual within an environmental context or program, or at that of life histories, for example, highlighting the experiences of a person coming out as a lesbian (Shoultz, 1995) or in conflict with his or her family (Shaw, 1929). Ecological approaches, involving diverse environments and neighborhood life (Brooks-Gunn et al., 1993), can be studied through interlocking, multicase study designs (Yin, 1989).

TABLE 12.1. Sample Areas of Inquiry

Parenting styles and behaviors
Beliefs, values, and philosophy of living
Relationships and their formation, nature, and development
Support interventions in diverse settings
Disability and community networks
Family life and its nature
Empowerment and leadership
Intergenerational and/or age-specific dynamics
Divorce and remarriage
Process of family reunification
Unemployment and its effect on the family life cycle
Experiences of families with courts and legal systems
Family unit analyses
Homes and their meaning
Ethnicity, culture, gender, disability: multiculturalism
Assistive technology and its use across environments
Effect of the Fair Housing Act on families
Process of socialization into disability
School-community relations
School inclusion/exclusion with children with emotional needs and/or
  behavioral problems
Communication processes in families and with agencies
Relationship between foster and birth/natural families
Parent-professional leadership
Hospitalization of adolescents and process of institutionalization
Return of children with brain injury to local communities
Disparities among low-, middle-, and high-income families in service usage

Common Concerns and Misconceptions in Family Studies

Early tendencies in family research case studies of limited duration appear to include the following: (1) a tendency to attribute to disability processes, circumstances, or outcomes, which may be caused or mediated by other factors; (2) a framing of studies on the basis of existing forms of services, practices, and disability assumptions; (3) prejudices or perspectives of researchers based on lack of knowledge or experiences with people of diverse social classes, ethnicities, cultures, and values; (4) confusion among gender-, class-, or ethnicity-based frameworks of analysis, with a broader multicultural framework; (5) level of research involvement, including in relationships as a participant observer; (6) degree of intimacy and access based on organizational affiliation interpreted as personal access; (7) lack of comparative knowledge of the phenomenon under study, with unwarranted generalizations; and (8) breaches of privacy and confidentiality. These affect understanding and the validity and reliability of the studies (see Chapter 16).

Basic Content of Case Studies

Family case study methodologies differ from family interview studies (Copeland and White, 1991), which have been conducted at the family support agency and county levels, with agencies as the major service delivery mechanism in the United States. Case studies of families often involve a description of the family and its members in details of appearance, personality, interaction, interests, values and beliefs, reaction to the researcher, own perceptions and reflections and other reports (e.g., see Table 12.2a, a description of a low incidence disorder [Table 12.2b]). Other common background areas of description are: friends and relationships, relatives, community activities and participation, employment, work and schooling, leisure and recreation, religious and spiritual practices, services, neighborhoods, and housing (for a critique of exemplary case studies, see Yin, 1989, pp. 146-151). Relationships with the researcher, and the researcher's reactions, prejudices, and previous knowledge base, may be part of an entry field memo or described in observers' comments, and may or may not be included in public case studies. Case studies may be constructed based upon one or more of the themes that arise from data collection as one reporting design. An initial report by a mother of the onset of disability in her daughter is presented in Table 12.3.

Multicase Studies

Multicase studies (Yin, 1989), as described in Chapter 15, are ideal for multisites, multifamily comparisons (see sample comparison of four families in Table 12.4), with one case often being sufficient to challenge existing assumptions. One method of selection in small agency or regional studies is similar to the selection of informants in statewide change projects involving person-centered planning and regulatory, legislative, financing, and programmatic changes. The agency studies may involve a selection of a range of high-risk families with diverse family or household

TABLE 12.2a. A Brief Family Sketch and Introduction to Rett's Syndrome

Mr. and Mrs. Jeffries, together with their only daughter Michelle, live in one of the surburban towns located west of Syracuse. They have resided there for ten years, having previously lived in other parts of the country while Mr. Jeffries was in the military. Until their son Chauncey entered military school in Vermont, he also lived at home and is the recipient of a Congressional Merit Award. He continues in college with lacrosse and skiing, both downhill and cross-country.

Michelle is fourteen years old and is one of about 1,000 girls in this country who have been diagnosed as having Rett's Syndrome. She was one of the first to be diagnosed as such, and is higher functioning than many Rett's girls. Mrs. Jeffries (Wendy) is actively involved in the international/national Rett's Association and maintains contact with families across the country. Mrs. Jeffries also is active in other ways in disability concerns, including serving as a "parent rep" on school committees for the handicapped and raising money for award banquets. She enjoys handicrafts, and likes to be on the go, skiing, jogging, refinishing tables, going to rummage and garage sales, and walking outdoors.

Mr. Jeffries is co-owner and manager of a well-known corporation and continues to travel extensively as part of his work. Described by his wife as a private man, he is medically retired from the military, after also serving in Vietnam six weeks following their honeymoon. Chauncey has traveled to Europe with his father, who has a boat near their home with water rights (to the nearby lake). Mr. Jeffries keeps in touch with his mother regularly.

Michelle, whom I spent time with in her home and at the pool, attended a segregated school for one year before her mother "fought and got her back into school," where she has a one-to-one aide. Michelle is transported by van to a YMCA about a half hour from the school for a special water therapy program. At home, Michelle watches videotapes on television in the den, especially Mickey Mouse, which seems to be one of her favorites. She also spends time with her mother in and near their inground backyard swimming pool and on outings when the weather is nice. Her bedroom is decorated classically all girl in pastels and frills.

Source: Racino, J. (1990b, October). *A Case Study of the Jeffries Family.* Syracuse, NY: Syracuse University Center on Human Policy.

TABLE 12.2b. Background on Rett's Syndrome

1. It is a neurological disorder (with research centering on abnormalities in the x chromosome).
2. It happens only in girls, though one researcher predicts it will be found in boys.
3. It strikes girls from sixteen to eighteen months of age.
4. It causes loss of functional hand use and includes abnormal movements.
5. It leads to severe mental retardation and physical handicaps.
6. Epileptic seizures are common.
7. There is no known cause, treatment, or cure.

Herald Journal, 1990

Primary Source: LaRue, A. (1990). Rare Rett's syndrome afflicts only girls. *Syracuse Herald American. New Studies:* Burd, L., Randall, T., Martsolf, J. T., and Kerbeshian, J. (1991). Rett's syndrome symptomology of institutionalized adults with mental retardation: Comparison of males and females. *American Journal of Mental Retardation*, 95(5), 596-601.Padgett, W. and Raymer, R. (1989). Diagnosis and treatment of Rett's syndrome. *Psychiatric Aspects of Mental Retardation Reviews,* 8(9), 59-62. Perry, A. (1991). Rett's syndrome: A comprehensive review of the literature. *American Journal of Mental Retardation,* 96(3), 275-290. Wilcox, D. (1991, March). Heather's story: The long road for a family in search of a diagnosis. *Exceptional Parent,* 21(2), 92-94.

characteristics (e.g., income, ethnicity, household composition, levels and types of disability, neighborhoods), expected diversity in support needs, and desire for out-of-home placement of their children (Racino, O'Connor, Walker, et al., 1991). The statewide projects may involve the selection of children, adolescents, and adults in a variety of settings, including the family home, the person's own home, foster care, residential centers, and group homes (Racino, 1985-1992).

Use of Case Studies

Family case studies can explore the phenomena of family life, communities, and societies with research involving all family members. It can be pursued from the perspectives of service systems, highlighting similarities and discrepancies between consumer agencies' and service users' perspectives. Such studies can offer new data for the development of new interpretive frames, and they can be used to introduce controversial and under-

TABLE 12.3. Brief Case Study Memo: Byron Family

This brief case study memo is based on several telephone calls and two visits in 1990 to the home of Mr. and Mrs. Byron and their two children, Mike, a senior in high school, and Becky, who is a disabled teenager. It includes visits with all four family members.

As described in the preliminary information, Mr. Byron works the graveyard shift at a local manufacturing company, enjoys the outdoors, and is active in the Hillite Lodge and a range of other activities. Mrs. Byron is working part-time (soon to be full-time) in a secretarial position for a small company, enjoys camping, and is actively involved as a sponsor/organizer of a foreign student exchange program. Mike is graduating this year, currently plays lacrosse, and will be attending a college in New York State starting this fall. Becky was in a segregated class where her mother says she is the highest functioning, has been on waiting lists for residential placement for seven years, and has continued to reside at home since awakening from a coma caused by meningitis at the age of four months.

Early History/Experiences with Becky

Becky became sick when she was four months old. Her mother Johanna explained:

> She was fine until she was four months. She had meningitis. Don't know how she got it. Was in a coma for four days.* I call the doctor with fevers. Some people don't, but I do. If I hadn't called, she wouldn't have lived the night. The doctor said "take her home; we don't know what she can do." She's been like this ever since. You just do what you can (Set #1, 14).

> Becky has been in physical therapy since she was very small. She didn't sit until the age of 2½, or walk until 9. They needed to work with her on these things. At 9½ her medications changed, and she became awake to the world around her.

In 1977, they moved to [this city], and became hooked up with a private, non-profit agency for therapy and also the state agency. Becky has remained primarily in segregated programs, first one at the local institution, at BOCES since 1986. . . . When she was small, the county also recommended home care to teach feeding techniques and positioning.

To the extent possible, the family has tried to maintain "as normal a family life as can be" (Set #1, 9). However, much of the responsibility for this has been placed on Mrs. Byron. As she explains:

> I'm the one who is usually home. It's a sore subject. He [her husband] says just go. Get a sitter. Sitters cost money. Going places costs money. And who am I going to go with? You can't have people come here all the time. Nothing gets done if Mom doesn't do it. (Set #1, 9).

*Five days instead of four days in a coma (Review by mother, 1998, March).

Source: Racino, J. (1990a, June). *Brief Case Study Memo: Byron Family.* Syracuse, NY: Syracuse University, Center on Human Policy.

TABLE 12.4. An Excerpt from a Case Study of Four Families

The Meaning of Labels

In some families, for example, disability does not present a major problem, but rather becomes part of who they are as a family. This is true in many cultures. In these families, the child is not viewed as disabled or as a major trouble. Disability becomes a public issue only within the structures of the system that define it. In the Henry family, Chas was seen as a member of the family. His actions, typically described by people in the system as autistic behaviors, were described by his family as moods, phases, and habits that he was going through. When discussing how much their son liked things to be the same, otherwise known as ritualistic behaviors, typical to how autism is defined, his mother said, "He likes things to be the same—you know, kind of a habit."

The Loss of Cultural Identity

Many people with disabilities receiving services are viewed in terms of their disability labels. This often determines the treatment or intervention. Workers and professionals do not look beyond the label to see the ethnic, racial, or gender identities of either people with disabilities or their families. Thomas, a young Arab-American man, was very fond of Arab music. While talking to a staff member at the group home in which he lived, I asked if he listened to Arab music there. With a puzzled look on her face, the staff person said, "Oh, is he Arab?"

Source: O'Connor, S. (1992). *Supporting Families: What They Want versus What They Get.* Syracuse, NY: Syracuse University, Center on Human Policy.

represented views (e.g., sexuality and abortion, psychiatric survivors' position on case management) or new service models.

Use of Case Studies for Financial Analyses

Case studies can be used to compare aspects of service design, such as local financial models for family support services and use of direct financial assistance (Knoll et al., 1992b; Langer-Ellison et al., 1992). These can involve the diversity of families, states, and agencies in multicase study designs. Primary financial concerns have included the priority need in families for financial assistance compared to services (Arnold and Case, 1993), the skewing in the use and allocation of resources (Turnbull and Turnbull, 1987), the use of cash subsidies going directly to families (Caro and McKaig, 1987), the use of state versus Medicaid funding (Knoll et al.,

1992b; Racino, 1985-1992), leveraging of funds and cost shifting and intergenerational transfers of wealth (Bergman and Singer, 1996), and agency policies and regulations on use and distribution of funds (Bersani, 1987; Racino, 1988c, 1998).

Practice and Policy Implications and Case Studies

Case studies can directly connect with aspects of family policy often neglected in this type of research. These include a reexamination of the approach to family support innovations in the United States, national policy (on labor, health care, education, transportation, welfare, family, and economic policy), and international developments (e.g., societies of acceptance).

Triangulation with Organizational Studies

Family research case studies can be triangulated with other qualitative research studies (Greene and McClintock, 1985), and national findings can be examined locally, including in the service sector demonstrations. However, this process involves a form of deductive reasoning, which varies from the inductive process involved in participant observation research and the emergence of case study themes (see Taylor and Bogdan, 1984, for comparison of deductive and inductive reasoning). As an example of deductive reasoning, basic findings in organizational studies, on the importance of families being able to select their own workers (Racino, 1988c, pp. 24-25, for example, through contracts; Racino, 1991c) continue to be supplanted by agency reliance on the families' workers to supplement their own staff.

THE ROLE OF FAMILY CASE STUDIES
IN EVALUATION RESEARCH

Case studies are important in presenting divergent perspectives, particularly those which vary from official positions of truth (Rose and Black, 1985). For example, it is often taken for granted that workers and the agency have the right facts to support the real or true story behind events that occur and, subsequently, the right solutions, inclusive of major decisions such as out-of-home placements of children (Racino, O'Connor, Walker, and Taylor, 1991). In other words, positions of the families that vary may be discounted.

Evaluation Research Designs

Evaluation research designs are often described in comparative terms as either formative or summative (Weiss, 1972, pp. 16-17) or process-, impact-, descriptive-, and/or outcome-based evaluations. Qualitative designs, by their nature, tend to be formative (i.e., part of an ongoing change process). Often termed descriptive (as opposed to empirical, which is equated with scientific, not statistical data) by quantitative researchers, qualitative studies, by their nature, result in the collection of data on processes (Rist, 1984), interactive effects, and mediating variables and can, by design, examine impacts and outcomes.

Cornell University researchers Jennifer Greene and Charles McClintock (1985) attempted to describe some of the problems that occur in combining quantitative (deductive by nature) and qualitative (inductive by nature) evaluation research conducted by separate teams, explaining the inherent divergence in the underlying frameworks. Yet, most major studies in the policy domain tend to be designed for statistical analyses on large samples, with qualitative interviews or multisites in ethnographic studies contributing to an explication of the quantitative models.

In ethnographic studies, Gitlin, Siegel, and Boru (1989) note that the basic problem influencing schools has been the inability of ethnographers to arrive at a shared understanding of the situation with the people participating in the studies. Instead, understanding has been separated from application with the researcher/participant observer using his or her privileged position to say what things mean as opposed to describing events, experiences, and interpretations from the viewpoints of the informants or participants (Bogdan and Biklen, 1982).

An Agency Evaluation Research Example

This section describes an excerpt from a local family support evaluation that incorporated the use of case studies of families based on extended participant observation and interviewing over a period of seven months, with over 1,000 pages of field data (see Racino, 1998).

The *Family Support Agency* has over a decade of experience in providing supports and advocacy for families with children with disabilities, operates all family support services (e.g., respite), has a board and staff of whom the majority are parents or relatives of children with disabilities, and a community reputation of responsiveness to families. The agency was one of two local family support agencies competing for county selection for the project, both with long histories of participation in research and service demonstrations in family support.

The *Family Support Project* was one of four voucher (i.e., reimburse-ment) programs funded in a large northeastern state (New York) as part of its fiscal year (FY) 1989-1990 family support initiatives. Located in a midsize city of 100,000, the nonprofit agency was selected to demonstrate a family-directed approach to family support. The proposal for the project had three basic design components:

1. The availability of an average of $2,500 for each family, which was part of the agency's project budget and could be individualized and flexibly used based on the needs and preferences of the family
2. Availability of a family support worker (i.e., family guide) who could work with the family to develop an individualized family support and spending plan, and whose role could be flexible depend-ing on the needs and preferences of the families
3. Development of a family support project advisory group that would serve in an ongoing role throughout the project to maximize coor-dination among agencies, maximize resources, and provide recom-mendations for systemic change

Family Perspectives: Research Findings

The purposeful sample of six case studies of families resulted in find-ings on when agencies and families come together (socialization into services, nature of daily life, who the family is as defined by the workers, disability as a part of family life, and the meaning of family support); roles of workers and services (role flexibility of workers, implicit and explicit roles of workers, good families and family meetings, being with families, and how families view the system); and cash assistance and its implica-tions (learning what the agency thinks is good, what cash assistance means financially, and agency accountability and cash assistance). These findings are reported elsewhere (Racino, 1998).

Agency-Based Evaluation Research Findings

The program was found to vary at inception, at the time of funding, and in implementation (Weiss, 1970). Another set of findings was based on interviews with agency personnel, telephone interviews with all of the other participating families, review of agency records, meetings, and facil-itated sessions with an advisory group. These data resulted in findings on the families' use of family support funds (reported usage by service cate-gories and goods, clusters of usage, and by family) and five implementation issues of concern to policymakers: the role of the agency in informal supports, role of the family guide, flexibility and guidelines, agency accountability and decision making, and the relationship of family support programs with existing agency services (for the report reference, see Racino, O'Connor, Walker, and Taylor, 1991).

Families' use of the family support funds. The project, as originally proposed, had no formal, externally imposed limitations upon how the funding could be used and was presented by the agency as family-determined. In other words, families had the option of deciding which goods or services the funding would be spent on, depending upon what they believed would best meet the needs of their families. This differed from what actually occurred in submission, funding, and project implementation.

Goods and services. In practice, all goods and services identified by the families could be classified in one or more of eight major categories: child care/respite; medical, therapy, or personal care; recreation; transportation; basic household/personal items; household appliances; household bills; and regulatory requirements. For example, transportation included payment for costs of trips for specific activities (e.g., to camp or work), car repair, and an auto insurance payment; household items included mattresses and clothing; household bills were telephone/utility, mortgage/ taxes, lawyer fees, and moving expenses.

Family patterns of usage. Each family had a unique pattern of use for the family support funds, such as the types of items purchased and the frequency and timing of purchases. Use across categories indicated several clusters of items: (1) household appliances, household bills, basic household/personal items; (2) transportation and respite; (3) respite and medical/personal therapy; and (4) respite and recreation. Respite, transportation and recreation could be obtained through the current family support system, whereas items in cluster one (i.e., household appliances, bills, and household items) were typically excluded as reimbursable items. Most expenditures during this period were one-time expenses for a family (a practice implemented by the agency), although repeated patterns were most common in the areas of recreation, respite, and purchase of incontinence garments.[1]

---

1. The categories of usage have become one of the most common data collected at the state level survey evaluation of family support programs (see, for example, Knoll et al. 1992b, p. 81, for taxonomy; Yuan, Baker-McCue, and Witkin, 1996, p. 371, for aggregate use of flexible funding in Vermont). Family patterns do not appear to be analyzed and reported on these levels, though data by family are available. See also options such as gift certificates to families and subsidized housing (Caro and McKaig, 1987).

Cash subsidy process. In response to semistructured interviews on the telephone, respondents (mainly women identified as the primary contact) described the cash subsidy process as purchasing goods and services and then being reimbursed. This is consistent with the state's subsequent report on model reimbursement programs (NYSOMRDD, 1990). The exceptions were instances in which agency vouchers were used for large purchases (e.g., appliances). All respondents reported in the telephone interviews that the cash assistance was important and that they determined how the money would be spent with input from the family guide.

Role of Agency in Informal Supports

The agency developed a community-oriented assessment guide,[2] modeled after one used at an excellent support agency in the Midwest (Brost and Johnson, 1982; Wisconsin Department of Health and Social Services, 1985). The family guide attempted to learn more about the informal supports and relationships. He concluded that the use of a questionnaire, even as a guide, was not a helpful way to talk with families about their lives: "Most people do not think in terms of words like supports. I am learning to get away from the language, just sort of get away from the interviewing so much and just try to be there and be conversational." One area the family guide explored in the early stages of the project was how to "build on the family's support network."

Role of Family Guide

The family guide described his role as more flexible than those of many other professionals, which he defined as people who are paid to help other people. He contrasted his role with other workers who were there primarily to work on specific activities (e.g., teaching) with specific family members (e.g., mother, child with a disability) and said he was thus in a better position to obtain a fuller picture of the family. The roles and tasks of the family guide were originally proposed as determined by the needs and preferences of each family. The worker's role was to find other ways to meet needs through seeking or identifying other funding sources, creating new services, identifying community opportunities, and so forth. One

---

2. General public policy position in the United States is to first use informal supports before accessing formal supports; options of payments to parents and friends are available in some areas (for discussion, see Bulmer (1987) on informal and formal support relationships).

family support worker reported spending time on the following nine tasks: communication with other agencies about the needs of families that were not being met; setting up and accompanying people to appointments; processing vouchers, managing funds, and documenting work; providing transportation; getting to know and understand families; coordinating interagency meetings; referring people to other services; and supporting families and setting up new services.[3]

Flexibility and Guidelines or Procedures

The project, as proposed, was designed to be flexible and to respond to the individual families.[4] In practice, although families could suggest services and goods, the agency wanted internal procedures that indicated to the state that the agency acted responsibly in approving these purchases. For example, the family guide was responsible for reviewing "out of the ordinary" requests with his supervisor; medical documentation was sought when the agency saw this as appropriate; and the way in which respite would be handled was developed based on existing respite services *operated by the agency.* The agency tended to act conservatively, siding with perceived accountability over family flexibility. The family guide, responsibly, started to let families know about these agency-imposed limitations in the project.

Agency Accountability and Family Decision Making

In this project, two additional factors influenced the agency's concerns about accountability. First, funding for the project had been delayed by the state office, actually resulting in the termination of the initial family guide and letters to families notifying them of the end of the project. Second, the agency was conscious of its role as a demonstration project and therefore tended to be conservative in approaching the project.

*Role of the Family Support Agency
and Relationship with Existing Services*

The agency considered this to be a short-term project and not an opportunity to examine the structure and functioning of the agency as a whole. It

---

3. The major trend in the United States is toward the use of parents as case managers or service coordinators, with most analyses considering the service coordinator role to be an essential service. Parents and people with disabilities have expressed concern regarding required case managers to receive services or subsidies.

4. Cash subsidy versus agency forms of assistance was one area of important study; see, for example, recommendations in Pennsylvania on no vouchers or accountability mechanisms in cash assistance schemes (Langer-Ellison et al., 1992).

viewed the project primarily as a way to expand the kinds of services and goods offered to families and as an opportunity to prove to people outside the agency that a voucher (cash subsidy/reimbursement) system could be expanded to better meet the needs of families. The tendency of the agency was to try to fit the project into the agency as opposed to examining how the project might actually impact on the nature of all agency services and supports.[5]

Systems Issues: Professional Perspectives

The advisory board identified the following barriers and issues as negatively affecting families and children with disabilities: case management roles (training, time commitment, and relationships); lack of family directiveness (of own services); funding incentives for out-of-home placements (e.g., institutions and residential schools); rigid and inadequate funding for family supports; unavailability of child care (particularly in rural areas); lack of willingness for strong state family policy; schools as a source of trauma for some families; lack of national family policy; and disruptions in home care funding, together with inordinate administrative expenses.[6]

Agency Implementation Issues

The agency identified the following as occurring over the course of the project (i.e., agency implementation issues). Family credits were not exempted from income reporting for public assistance, Medicaid, and food stamps, and initially with Social Security (though the latter was resolved by the agency for SSI recipients). The project was hampered by the lack of child care and respite, particularly in suburbs and for teenagers after school, and lack of available transportation to move goods purchased with the family credits. The program coordinator's role (supervisor of the family guide; respected parent in local community) with families with issues beyond disability (chronic unemployment, drug or alcohol dependency, and/or physical abuse in family) was another major concern. The agency identified the need for dialogue with the families about requests (agency

---

5. Similar to supported employment, many family support programs are treated as agency add-ons and need to fit in with the existing agency structure, regulations, and procedures versus serving as a mechanism for creating change in how agencies work with families and service users.

6. These barriers and issues reflected a relatively sophisticated approach to boundary issues and concerns, and to the relationships among community, governmental subsidy and services, and specialized disability services.

reports 99 percent of requests met); resources would be used to first help some working families meet survival needs (e.g., shelter, clothing, and utilities), then for an emergency fund, for long-term family support with decrease in advocacy by the family guide, and for a one-time purchase allocation.

CONCLUSION

Family case study research (D. Ferguson, P. Ferguson, and S. Taylor, 1992; McWilliams and Bailey, 1993; O'Connor, 1995; Taylor, 1991a, c, d; Wickham-Searl, 1992) remains a critical component of qualitative research and evaluation strategies. Considered to be relatively new in the field of family research (see Copeland and White, 1991), the methods have the strength to develop new ideas and to inform existing family theory (e.g., family systems theory, popular in the field of psychology and social work) through "analytic generalization" (Yin, 1989, p. 38). In the field of disability, the methods hold promise in addressing intransigent, long-term approaches to working with families, in contributing to the development of family policy, and in the necessary reform of the U.S. agency-vendor system of community services.

Chapter 13

State Policy in Housing and Support: Evaluation and Policy Analysis of State Systems

Julie Ann Racino

In line with the national shift toward the support and empowerment paradigm (see Chapter 1), this chapter describes the policy analysis findings of a proposed statewide change from traditional residential services for adults with developmental disabilities to a housing and support approach, known as person centered or individualized (Racino et al., 1989). Primary service characteristics of these approaches (identified through field research in states, e.g., Racino, 1995a, in Wisconsin, Minnesota, California, North Dakota, and New Hampshire) include the following: the separation of housing and support services; the promotion of home ownership and integrated housing; individualized and flexible services and supports; individual assessment, planning, and funding; and consumer-directedness in housing and services.

EVALUATION RESEARCH: EFFORTS AT STATEWIDE CHANGE

Major analyses through the support and empowerment paradigm were: the use of the continuum concept for analysis of the system (Taylor, 1988; Taylor et al., 1986); analyses of changing residential program models to nonfacility-based services (see also Taylor, Racino, and Rothenberg, 1988);

This evaluation research case study is modified from Racino, J., O'Connor, S., Shoultz, B., Taylor, S. J., and Walker, P. (1989). *Moving into the 1990s: A Policy Analysis of Community Living for Adults with Developmental Disabilities in South Dakota.* Syracuse, NY: Syracuse University, Center on Human Policy, Research and Training Center on Community Integration.

multiple analyses of the vendor system (the primary delivery mechanism in the United States) in the state; thematic identification of concerns and issues from qualitative research field data collection (Taylor and Bogdan, 1984); and analyses based on the emerging major service characteristics of a housing and support approach.

The Continuum Concept: Toward Support Approaches

As in all states, the design of residential services in South Dakota is based on the principle of the least restrictive environment (LRE), with its status in federal education law and implementation as a continuum. Analysis on the basis of the flaws with the continuum concept for service design (Taylor, 1988; Taylor et al., 1987b) had not previously been conducted as part of statewide evaluations. This is, in part, because these ideas were not reflected in the design of many research studies, such as those on movement in residential settings, which were designed to study movement from institutional care to the community (the major theme of the last generation, with the community majority now reached; Lakin, 1991) and to monitor quality outcomes. Specifically, the following reflect South Dakota's status on one critique of LRE (Taylor et al., 1986):

- *People with the most severe disabilities get relegated to the most restrictive end of the continuum.* In South Dakota, this included the assumption that people must move from one institution to another before community placement.
- *The most restrictive placements, such as institutions, are not necessary.* The state had a particularly strong institutional bias, with legislation stating that one institution shall be maintained and community services may be established.
- *The continuum implies people need to leave their homes every time they acquire new skills.* Physical movement from site to site was generally viewed as a sign of positive growth in this state, with movement sometimes based on minor changes in staffing, space, or integration, with less concern over personal relationships and community connections.
- *The most restrictive placements do not prepare people for the least restrictive placements.* The readiness model in South Dakota was seen as one of the system's strengths; teachers were not "pushing" the adult services system to reflect new approaches in supporting people with severe disabilities with information introduced in the state through statewide technical assistance in 1986.
- *The continuum concept confuses people's rights with the intensity of their service needs.* People still needed to "earn" the right to live in a

typical home, though there could be "exceptions" to the rule. Choosing between a home or appropriate supports was an unfair and unnecessary choice, and intensive supports should not be equated with the abridgement of rights.

- *The continuum directs attention to physical settings rather than to the supports and services people need to be integrated in the community.* For example, in 1989 in housing, a supervised apartment building for people with developmental disabilities was financed to "fill a hole" in the system, instead of examining the system of housing and supports in the locality.

From Residential Program Models to Non-Facility-Based Services

The primary structures on the local levels for the delivery of community services for adults with developmental disabilities were the (seventeen) adjustment training centers (ATCs). Each operated as a private, nonprofit organization, providing a range of different residential and day services, generally in a geographical area of the state, except for specialty centers. Evaluation of the private vendor system in the state included multiple analyses by residential program models and distributions, thematic analyses of ATC characteristics, the state relationship to the regions (ATCs), community residential service types, and the major characteristics of facility-based services.

Residential Program Models and Distribution

These models included, as described by the "state office" in 1989, ten major types: state-operated institutional services, private institutions for children, private nursing homes, intermediate care facilities, community residential facilities, supervised apartments, monitored apartments, adult foster care, family homes, and "independent apartments." As of 1992, community services options of six or fewer people were termed monitored apartments, supervised apartments, and individualized supported living (Braddock et al., 1995).

Thematic Analysis of the Characteristics of the Adjustment and Training Centers

Regional agencies' (ATCs) themes identified through qualitative analyses were: the size, nature of the local community, characteristics of the people served, and the progressive nature of all ATCs. There were two larger and expanding ATCs, with 35 percent of the ATC population, and a mean number of sixty people at each ATC in the state. At least three ATCs worked with Native Americans; specialized ATCs were developing in the state (e.g., people with challenging behaviors); and being in the forefront was viewed as important.

The State Relationship with the ATCs

A description of the state political stakeholders and community services structures can be found in Smith's and Gettings' 1988 assessment report on South Dakota from the National Association of State Mental Retardation Program Directors.

Community Residential Services Types

Four major types of community residential services existed in this state, with only one of the four—the intermediate care facilities (ICFs)—tied by definition to facility type: community living training, follow along/outreach, home and community-based services, and community intermediate care facilities.

The Major Characteristics of Facility-Based Services

Identified through previous research, major characteristics of facilities were agency-owned or rented facilities, licensed or certified facilities, agency staffed, staffing ratios based on groups not individuals, linkage of housing and support services, core funding tied to facility, weak relationship between funding and individual planning, and facility classification based on supervision needs (see Taylor, Racino, and Rothenberg, 1988).

Relationship to Person-Centered Approaches

These analyses, based upon the continuum, the residential program models, the thematic analysis of the ATCs, the community residential service types, and the major characteristics of facility-based services, varied from person-centered technical assistance approaches, which started from the selection of a range of people who resided in diverse settings (e.g., Pocatello, Idaho). The major purpose of this analysis was to increase flexibility in the systems and identify major (systemic) impediments to

person-centered approaches (Mount, 1994). Initially, this practice was introduced as part of state and regional planning processes for funding allocations
(1986), and later (1988) as an effort in states to explicitly change funding and
residential categories. Carl Rogers described person-centered approaches in
difficult situations such as terrorism (Rogers, 1980), with the community
change efforts in the 1990s oriented more toward better quality of lives
through local group processes.

Strengthening the Current System

South Dakota was considered to be at a critical juncture in its development of services for people with severe disabilities (Scheinost, 1988), with
the creation of a shared vision of the future with parents and people with
disabilities. Strengthening the current system centered around seven major
issues, which were common to state systems: community integration,
planning, waiting lists for community services, community supports, toward community funding, personnel, and quality.

Community Integration

Community integration (Racino et al., 1989, pp. 56-59) in this state
analysis included physical integration in recreation, work, and neighborhoods; size, concentration, and appearance of homes and facilities; location near community resources; transportation and the use of vans; community participation, including in churches, community groups, and in
culturally diverse ways; relationships of people with disabilities and community members; tension between home and program; and continued
emphasis on readiness and transition (i.e., physical movement as a sign of
independence). Wolfensberger's frameworks on normalization (1972),
particularly model coherency (i.e., how it all fits together), and social role
valorization (Wolfensberger, 1983), are particularly relevant.

Planning

No regional authority existed with mandated responsibility for planning
supports and services for or with people from the region (e.g., responsibility for the people who were in the institutions) (Wolfensberger, 1977).
Four major concerns with planning and communication were the communication between the regional structures (ATCs) and the state office (Division of Developmental Disabilities); the reported lack of support by parents of community integration (with parents on the boards and committees

of most ATCs); emerging self-advocacy (with several people on ATC committees); and communication with other organizations (i.e., major relationships were with the special education cooperatives in the region [see Graney, 1988; Racino and Merrill, 1988], regional offices of the Department of Vocational Rehabilitation, Department of Health for monitoring, Department of Social Services for foster care, and the county boards of mental retardation and institutions).

Waiting Lists for Community Services

As documented nationally (Hayden and DePaepe, 1994), the ATCs in South Dakota had waiting lists for services. In addition, people from institutions and other out-of-home placements were not always included on the lists; sometimes the same name would appear on multiple lists; some people would be included on lists although not accepted for services; and more places were available for people with mild disabilities than were needed. Although institutional closure was an emerging issue (see New Hampshire's closing of its only public institution in Chapters 3 and 4), South Dakota was still discussing the future of its institutions, with a new generation of children still being institutionalized out-of-step with national trends.

Community Supports

Extending services to people previously excluded from community options was a priority. These included people who needed assistance with toileting, injections, or tube feeding (see nursing practices acts, e.g., Flanagan and Green, 1997) or who were assessed as needing a high staffing ratio (e.g., due to challenging behaviors or criminal justice system involvement). Some ATCs may specialize in a particular area that requires a person to move to another area of the state. Also, interest was emerging in providing supports for parents with mental retardation, elders in the state institution, people with medical needs, and youth transitioning from the school systems.

Toward Community Funding

South Dakota was one of the early states to use the Medicaid Home and Community-Based Services waiver program for community services for people with mental retardation and related conditions (see Smith and Gettings, 1988). Increasing its Medicaid waiver services rate, which remained lower than the rate for institutional facilities (e.g., intermediate care facilities), was a major concern (see Lakin, Hill, and Bruininks, 1985). The state reported increasing per diems and pending expenditures of major capital costs in at least one of its state institutions. Financing cutbacks in the Medicaid Home and Community-Based Services waiver program at the time resulted in optical (e.g, eyeglasses) and dental costs being eliminated. Other funding options by the state mental retardation and developmental disabilities department were being explored. Broadening the funding base from Medicaid was recommended, together with expansion of local ATC and community efforts to address problems in the localities (e.g., day care for children).

Personnel

Staff training, including in normalization/social role valorization, with movement away from medical/behavioral emphases to participation in home and community life, was recommended. Some ATCs were still in conflict over custodial care (taking care of people) versus staff running the programs (staff as trainer), with a new approach to personal and community lives needed. Therapists had not yet moved to more consultant roles. Dissemination of information on assistive technology, nonaversives with people with challenging behaviors, and support approaches with children and adults with medical needs were other state issues, similar to concerns at a number of other state technical sites (Center on Human Policy, 1985-1992). Staff salaries in direct care and staff turnover were emerging national issues (Mitchell and Braddock, 1994), and parents in South Dakota ranked low staff salaries as a major issue for their service system.

Quality

Quality of services included existing citizen advocacy, a family advisory board, self-advocacy, and guardianship programs, with recommendations for a new conceptual framework that would differentiate between facility-based and community-based support services (Taylor, 1989, in Racino et al., 1989). Self-advocacy was gaining in national importance, with citizen advocacy (Hildebrand, 1992) still emerging in some states (see Wolfensberger and Zauha, 1973). Provider concerns with quality primarily revolved around the national accreditation standards (with debate about use of Accreditation Council on Services for People with Developmental Disabilities [ACDD], Gardner and Parsons, 1990; or Commission on the Accreditation of Rehabilitation Facilities [CARF] standards, 1985) in contrast to quality-of-life standards at the agency level (e.g., Options in Community Living, 1987).

Conclusion

This evaluation was designed as an example of one action research and change approach. The purposes were to lead the developmental disabilities system into housing and community development (Kelly and Van Vlaendern, 1995), to promote approaches to funding and support that could be used across state departments, and to allow for major reorganization in the state, including local agency and person-centered change. The evaluation differs from approaches through the Americans with Disabilities Act, with the primary clients being the state offices and service systems, yet with a focus on actual and potential service users and local communities. It varies from person-centered evaluations, which require equal work and access across all systems (e.g., employment, transportation, recreation, education) for systemic change. An excerpt from the second half of the evaluation, based on the evolving support and empowerment paradigm, is contained in Table 13.1.

Concurrently, the state entered into an agreement offering a joint statewide conference on community integration. A keynote address was presented by a leading self-advocate (M. Kennedy, 1993) who lived in a New York institution most of his life and also a panel of South Dakotans with disabilities. The evaluation, as a study of the conceptualization of the nonrestrictive environment, constitutes a major breakthrough in the field of disability, which differs from the use of the concept of the least restrictive environment with children in schools. The evaluation was linked with national developments in housing and support, which aimed to differentiate local, state, and national points of responsibility and to move from a national crisis within the now established community systems (Smull, 1989) to the next generation of participation in community life.

*   *   *

INTRODUCTION

Housing evaluations and research for people with disabilities tend to be problematic for two major reasons: first, due to the separation of specialized (for a particular group) and generic community housing development (Marcuse, 1989), and, second, because housing systems are not closed and initiatives by one group influence other groups seeking housing (Abt, 1979). Indeed, Bronfenbrenner (1974) of Cornell University explained that an ecological orientation, for example, to the policies of housing organizations points to the relationships between systems as being critical to a child's development. This chapter highlights affordable and accessible

TABLE 13.1. A Housing and Support (Person-Centered) Approach to Community Living

The basic principle with adults with disabilities is that all people can live in typical homes in the community, with support services. This approach has been pioneered by agencies such as Options in Community Living in Wisconsin, together with the Madison Mutual Housing Association and Cooperative, with aspects of an individualized approach found in Colorado, Ohio, Minnesota, North Dakota, and Michigan. It is described in the book, *Housing, Support, and Community: Choices and Strategies for Adults with Disabilities* (Racino et al., 1993) and highlighted in national distribution.

Individualized and Flexible Supports

An individualized approach focuses on support options (secondarily, of course, to the person and his or her relationships and life), as opposed to supervision (Taylor and Racino, 1989), and a reliance on paid, shift staff. Major areas reviewed were: the types of services and supports available and fundable; barriers to providing in-home support services; individualization of supports; flexibility of supports; the role of service coordination; the role of service agencies; and monitoring of supports.

De facto limitations existed for in-home services, in part due to the state Nursing Practices Act. These state acts were also problematic in states such as Idaho, with a waiver on training as one option to allow for people with medical needs to live in their own homes. Although open to these options, no examples of an attendant hired by a person with a developmental disability (Litvak, Zukas, and Heumann, 1987), paid roommates or companions, or hiring of staff matched to work with a particular individual (Racino, et al., 1993), were identified. Legitimate concerns were expressed about stipends with neighbors and potential effects on relationships. State limitations and access by people with developmental disabilities to the Social Services Department program on attendant care, designed for people with physical disabilities, was cited by informants as barriers.

Individualization was occurring within the context of residential settings (sometimes known as community living arrangements). This was consistent with the emerging studies of community support within facilities, such as small ICF/MRs, with apartments of four persons each in New York—the most creative use nationally of this restrictive facility category. Emerging approaches offered support in people's own homes. Flexibility in the state included the capacity to respond in an emergency across settings (i.e., sharing of resources). No capacity existed in practice to combine funding sources. A temporary services or exceptions payment mechanism, such as in Connecticut or Michigan (see also Taylor, Racino, and Rothenberg, 1988) was recommended. As in New York, case management was occurring within the agencies, with difficulty in moving to service brokerage roles with advocacy, supports planning, and evaluation (Salisbury, Dickey, and Crawford, 1987).

Source: Modified excerpt from Racino, J., O'Connor, S., Shoultz, B., Taylor, S. J., and Walker, P. (1989). *Moving into the 1990s: A Policy Analysis of Community Living Arrangements for Adults with Developmental Disabilities in South Dakota*. Syracuse, NY: Syracuse University, Center on Human Policy, Research and Training Center on Community Integration.

housing, communities and neighborhoods, particularly the efforts at reform of the disability community living systems, and the debates on housing construction and allowances.

Housing and Community Planning

Housing policy has traditionally been driven in the United States by the
housing building industries, which include major banking institutions,
homebuilders associations, and, secondarily, real estate boards and cham-
bers of commerce (Heidenheimer, Heclo, and Adams, 1990). In housing
terms, major impacts of housing initiatives are described as transfers among
three major participants: federal government, local programs, and the home-
steaders (Abt, 1979); instead of shelter programs, housing programs have
become a form of income redistribution (Heidenheimer, Heclo, and Adams,
1990).

Local community housing plans (CHAS, Comprehensive Housing Affordability Strategy) are one governmental method for community planning, with each state having its own housing development programs
(Brandon and Economu, 1973). Yet, initially, planning for community
housing excluded people who were in institutions, similar to the "comprehensive needs studies" of the 1970s (The Urban Institute, 1975). Governmental planning either assumed that people in institutions had homes or
that another process outside of regular community planning would occur,
often as segregated and congregate housing developments, such as large
"community" intermediate care facilities (ICFs).

Housing Allowances and Construction for Housing

One of the major policy decisions regarding housing is the allocation of
financing between housing allowances and/or subsidies and housing
construction, with resistance to diversion of funds from construction to
cash allowances (Heidenheimer, Heclo, and Adams, 1990). Housing allowances are payments made directly to eligible households to help them
pay the costs of living in housing of their choice (Allen, Fitts, and Glatt,
1981); they are used internationally as a government policy instrument
(Granberg, 1989). Some countries have experimented with a mechanism
for housing assistance for people of all income levels (e.g., Sweden, Great
Britain) (Heidenheimer, Heclo, and Adams, 1990). In the United States,
subsidies have started to be directed to the white suburbs (Orfield, Eaton,
and the Harvard Project on School Desegregation, 1996).

Section 202 loans were created by the Housing Act of 1937 for "nonprofit sponsors to help them create new housing for the elderly and dis-

abled with low incomes" (Millman, 1992, p.7). As reported by David Braddock (1987), in the Housing and Community Development Act of 1974 (PL 93-383), coordination was required between Section 202 loan applications and Section 8 rental assistance payment programs. The section 8 certificate program was the nation's main housing assistance strategy for helping the poor afford a decent place to live (Newman, 1994). Although "mobile Section 8" was described as staying with the person if he or she moved to decent housing, some rental assistance programs are tied to the dwelling instead of the person (O'Connor and Racino, 1993; Transitional Living Services of Onondaga County [TLS], 1979).

As reported by Racino (1989), in the developmental disability service provider and governmental sectors in the United States, almost universal support existed for the "mobile" Section 8 program. A two-year waiting list, however, was virtually consistent across states. Interim or bridge subsidies were created by state departments for people with disabilities to move into regular housing until the generic housing subsidy became available (O'Connor and Racino, 1993; Taylor, Racino, and Rothenberg, 1988). Subsidies of home start-up costs, such as mental health in New York, were initiated in some places as early as the 1970s (see TLS, 1979), with subsequent studies of independent housing, Section 8 certificates, and individuals with chronic mental illness (Newman, 1994).

A number of studies in the 1970s and 1980s compared housing allowances to housing construction and the options of cash assistance or income transfers (Bradbury and Downs, 1981; Friedman and Weinberg, 1982). In a 1982 study, Friedman and Weinberg explained that "comparative analysis unequivocally showed that housing allowances can provide decent housing at a fraction of the cost of construction oriented programs and are capable of serving two to three times as many households per dollar of subsidy" (1982, p. 142). The Abt study (Abt, 1979; see also Van Willigen, 1986, pp. 182-184) found that "the poor could effectively operate in the open housing market in terms of their own choice;" however, the study was not successful in breaking down housing segregation.

The federal debate between construction and housing assistance led to efforts to create set-asides for people with disabilities in new housing (Consortium of Citizens with Disabilities, 1992). This reform created competition among equally deserving groups and led to the development of new supportive facilities. The concerns of elders who were sharing housing projects with families and persons with mental illness reached the national policy level. In the 1980s, regulations were adjusted so that foster care payments and income of a live-in aide were included as income in determining rental subsidies (Millman, 1992), with adjustments made for child care and handicapped assistance expenses.

Housing Laws and Rights

Major U.S. legislation that affected people with disabilities during this period included the Fair Housing Amendments Act of 1988, the national Affordable Housing Act (1990), the Stewart B. McKinney Homeless Assistance Act (1987), the Housing and Community Development Act of 1974, the Architectural Barriers Act of 1968, Section 504 of the Rehabilitation Act of 1973, and the Americans with Disabilities Act (1990) (Kregel, 1993). Dissemination of information on rights under state and federal housing laws remains a primary function of advocacy and rights agencies. State laws continue to prohibit housing discrimination based on disability (e.g., in New York), and federal tenancy rights now include the right to refuse accommodation, aid, service, opportunity, or benefit, if the person chooses not to accept (Milstein and Hitov, 1993).

Barriers to Integrated Community Housing

Based upon development of congregate facilities financed through Housing and Urban Development (HUD) funds and the Farmers Home Administration, several other barriers existed in states regarding movement to regular community housing. These barriers included the creation of housing, which stood out from the local neighborhoods, against the basic principles of normalization and designed as facilities with medicalized funding and long-term mortgages (Racino, 1989; see Newman, 1995, for twenty-, thirty-, and forty-year commitments of federal revenues). Second, financing for accessibility was tied to the facilities, and not always available for home rehabilitation and modification in people's own homes.

Affordable and Accessible Housing

Accessible, affordable housing can be considered to be a right of all people of all ages and abilities and a matter of social justice, inclusive of all people and families-at-risk. Affordable housing (Mulroy and Ewalt, 1996; U.S. Department of Housing and Urban Development, 1991) was reflected as a basic principle of housing leadership, including organizations and associations such as the United States Catholic Conference (1981). Fair housing without discrimination was embodied in federal and state laws, as one of the most important bodies of federal law affecting people with disabilities (Arranda-Coddou, 1992).

American National Standards Institute (ANSI) standards, available for accessibility of housing in the 1970s, incorporated universal design principles in housing for local communities (DeJong and Lifchez, 1983). Most recently, accessibility has been described as part of architectural home design features in descriptions, illustrations, and photographs of beautiful homes (Rhule, 1998). Requirements through the Americans with Disabilities Act (ADA) for accessibility in existing housing are reportedly more stringent than the Fair Housing Amendments of 1993, with program accessibility tied to integration (Milstein and Hitov, 1993).

Housing Quality

All communities in the country did not have housing standards in place (see Newman, 1995, on minimum housing standards nationwide). As described earlier, the function of the housing allowances has been, in part, to upgrade the stock of community housing and to encourage people to live in better-quality housing (Abt, 1979). Housing standards internationally have often been described in such terms as space allocation per person (Mayo, 1995), external features, and other physical characteristics such as heating, lighting, and plumbing (Newman, 1994). Housing quality continues to be affected at the tenant level by disputes between tenants and landlords about disrepair and upkeep, from plumbing to painting, appliance replacements, window repair, and pest control (Rosenbaum, 1996), and who is to cover the costs of repair (and accessibility costs, if any). While standards have been developed by disability agencies (Options in Community Living, 1987), people with disabilities continue to live in boarding and care homes and other congregate or substandard housing (U.S. Congressional Committee on Government Operations, 1988).

Housing, Mental Health, and Positive Life Outcomes

In the public media, concern about housing quality was dwarfed by homelessness, with new funding being diverted to these causes (Cress, 1997). As Howie the Harp (1993, p. 413), a leading consumer activist, explained, "homelessness is a symptom of a society that refuses to provide what it is that people really need." A general consensus exists that poverty, housing, and employment are key factors in child development (Bath and Haapala, 1994) and in positive outcomes for people with severe mental illness (Newman, 1995); poor housing has been associated with the "emergence of child maltreatment problems that lead to the need for child welfare services" (Bath and Haapala, 1994, p. 395). Housing has been the focus of studies of mental health and family life, space, neighboring and child supervision, socialization of children, employment, and leisure and recreation use (e.g., Bartlett, 1997; Wilner et al., 1962).

RESIDENTIAL REFORM
AND DEINSTITUTIONALIZATION

During the period of the mid-1980s to the mid-1990s, major efforts were initiated in the developmental disabilities services systems to reform the state of residential services, which were often congregate and facility based in nature (Center on Human Policy, 1989b; Racino, O'Connor, Shoultz, et al., 1991). In Great Britain, as in the United States, six-to-eight-person staffed residences were developed for people with severe handicaps (Felce, 1989), with U.S. facility size for group homes exceeding twelve or more persons. These group homes, apartments, or complexes and duplexes were developed, in part, as an alternative to institutions that had been the subject of exposés for their conditions and violations of constitutional rights (see Chapter 3).

Developmental Disabilities: Group Housing
to Supported Living and "Own Homes"

Most typically, residential services in developmental disabilities have come to be viewed as housing and related services provided to people in out-of-home placements (Lakin, Bruininks, and Larson, 1992, p. 198). This conceptualization, however, does not differentiate between adults and families, or agency and parent, or housing owned or rented by adults with disabilities. People with disabilities moved to smaller homes from institutions, with efforts to reduce placements of twelve to twenty people per home to six or fewer (Lakin, Braddock, and Smith, 1994). Greater choice of places, roommates, and support services occurred, which was nationwide in scope (Racino, O'Connor, Shoultz, et al., 1991). In some states, moving to people living in their own homes involved administrative, technical, political, technological, attitudinal, and managerial changes (sometimes as an interim step to federal change) (Center on Human Policy, 1989b); these changes continued to occur through the 1990s.

Supported Housing and Mental Health

In the field of mental health, the Center on Community Change through Housing and Support in Vermont (Carling et al., 1988; Center for Community Change through Housing and Support, 1990) worked nationwide with state housing coordinators to move toward housing reflecting principles of stability, consumer preferences, and more regular, integrated, and valued housing (e.g., Tanzman, 1993). Continuing through the 1990s, supported housing in mental health moved into state practices (Livingston and Srebnik, 1991), together with efforts at moving back to homes that people select (e.g., Michigan's supported independence program in mental health and developmental disabilities).

However, the term supported housing was applied to situations such as single-room occupancy (SROs), as well as apartment and other home options. The separation of housing from participation in treatment is considered to be a cornerstone of the mental health system (Milstein and Hitov, 1993). Yet, in mental health and addictions, "self-run houses," followed work a decade earlier on consumer-controlled housing (Chamberlin, 1978) and on Fairweather Lodges, also operated by people with psychiatric disabilities.

International Reform: Great Britain and Israel

Reform initiatives were occurring in Great Britain (e.g., Towell, 1988) in its National Health Service. Housing reform offered an opportunity for attention to feminist concerns (Austerberry and Watson, 1985) and reform based on similar principles to those embodied in normalization and consumer involvement. Yet, in Israel, one community housed adults with mental retardation, embodying some principles of normalization (kibbutz living, a minority housing style in Israel), without integration in housing shared with nondisabled people (Aharoni, 1991). This Israeli community may bear some resemblance to intentional communities (Lutfiyya, 1991c) that are found worldwide, often with a spiritual relationship, the best known being L'Arche, (Vanier, 1982) which is international, and to those in the United States which are funded through residential funding schemes.

HOUSING AND SUPPORT SERVICES

Housing and support services were an effort to return to the roots of housing in the community, with a movement toward community supports for all people (Taylor, Bogdan, and Racino, 1991). The movement is tied to basic principles of normalization, with people having choices in their lives and homes being considered to be homes (Shoultz, 1992a; Wolfensberger, 1977). To achieve consensus and offer guidance, principles were developed regarding people with disabilities owning or renting their own homes (see also Table 13.2) and on housing and support services (Research and Training Center on Accessible Housing, 1993).

Facility-Based Systems in the United States

The design of residential services in disability are generally driven by facilities, which are bundled together, with the majority of funding for support services in congregate settings (Taylor, 1988). This design results in reform approaches emphasizing decreases in facility size or living arrangements (Lakin, Braddock, and Smith, 1994), program individualization, and zero exclusion to accommodate people with significant disabilities in existing options (Singer, 1987). This differs from approaches that seek to change the nature of community living arrangements, with new assumptions about residential services reform (Taylor, Racino, and Rothenberg, 1988).

New Program Options in Housing

In the late 1980s and early 1990s, program modifications (support services in apartment buildings and homes, sometimes funded by foster care) were at times promoted as best practices in community living (M. Kennedy, 1993). As described in Chapter 7 on supported living, new options, modeled in part after organizations such as Options in Community Living in Wisconsin (Johnson, 1985) that could support people with severe disabilities were developed nationwide. These options were termed residential supports, housing and support, or supportive/supported living (Horner et al., 1996; Klein, 1992; O'Brien and Lyle-O'Brien, 1994; Racino and Taylor, 1993). Yet, these developments presented confusion in some places where supported apartments, semi-independent living, or supported living were only for people considered to be more capable (Halpern et al., 1986).

Housing and personal assistance services were combined in the fields of developmental disabilities (Flanagan and Green, 1997; National Council on the Handicapped, 1988) to include people with significant disabilities. Mental health explored this option (Carling, 1995), with emerging interest in brain injury (Racino and Williams, 1994). Table 13.3 represents a traditional approach to reform in disability housing and support, in this case, as part of an effort to return people with brain injuries from out-of-state placements to the state of New York. The study of housing cooperatives that do indeed

TABLE 13.2. Advantages of Consumer-Controlled Housing

Ten Reasons Why People Should Rent or Own Their Own Homes

All across the United States more and more people with developmental disabilities rent or purchase their own homes. The common threat in this "consumer-controlled housing" is that the people have the homes they want with the services and other supports they need brought to them, not them being forced to live in the "homes" of their services. Thus, they are able to live life more on their own terms. They can become the "kings and queens of their own castles," no longer just guests in places that are owned by or rented and controlled by the agencies that provide needed services. There are at least ten very significant advantages to people who live in consumer-controlled housing:

1. *Permanency:* The risk is reduced that other people will decide one must move from one's own home. People who live in their own homes are free to choose new service providers or even to reject service providers without also losing their homes.
2. *Community inclusion:* People who control their own housing have greater choice in living near people and places that support their participation in the community.
3. *Freedom:* People who live in homes they control make their own rules. The basic right to privacy desired by all human beings is more easily met in one's own home. The place where one can "be oneself" is more easily achieved in one's own home.
4. *Respect:* A home of one's own is a typical and important achievement of American adults. It gives the owner or leaseholder a valued social role. Both owners and renters contribute to the local economy.
5. *Responsibility:* A home of one's own makes an individual responsible for a number of economic and domestic activities. Responding to these responsibilities helps people to grow in social competence, both in actual terms and as they are seen by others in their community.
6. *Economic gain:* People who buy their own homes have found that careful purchase and long-term residence can yield an equity build-up that increases an owner's financial resources. Those who rent often can choose housing and housing arrangements at costs that free funds for other economic decisions.
7. *Location:* People who choose their own homes can live where it is most convenient to their jobs, families, friends, stores, transportation, and so forth. They can live close to places they enjoy and thus be able to participate more frequently and with less dependence on others.
8. *Choice:* To most people, the prospect of spending their whole lives with strangers whom they have had no voice in selecting is dismal at best. Yet this is the typical experience of persons with developmental disabilities. Controlling one's home includes controlling not only where one lives, but with whom.
9. *Self-Determination:* People should have a right to control as much of their lives as possible. Few areas are more basic and unambiguous in self-determination than selecting the housing one wants within one's resource limits.
10. *Independence:* People who live in their own homes can exercise independence in seeking a new service provider. In contrast, people who live in buildings owned by a service-provider agency must weigh the loss of home, neighborhood, and proximity to friends against seeking services from another individual or agency.

Source: Reprinted with permission from Fields, T., Lakin, K. C., Seltzer, B., and Wobschall, R. (1995, September). *A Guidebook on Consumer Controlled Housing for Minnesotans with Developmental Disabilities.* Minneapolis, MN: ARC Minnesota and the Research and Training Center on Residential Services and Community Living, College of Education and Human Development, University of Minnesota, pp. 1-2.

TABLE 13.3. Residential Systems Reform: An Example in New York

New York, as with all states, was facing challenging economic conditions that made it extremely difficult to find the fiscal resources necessary for the development of a new system of housing and community support services. Yet an expected cost savings of $27.3 million was documented by the repatriation of people with traumatic brain injuries from out-of-state facilities (NYSDOH, 1992), with a decision to pursue a targeted home and community-based Medicaid waiver.

Support Resources

Probably the most challenging concern in financing support services from the consumer perspective is to ensure that adequate funding is available, including for people with the most significant needs on a long-term basis, to have flexible mechanisms in place that respond to the changing needs of individual people, and to have more consumer control of the financing.

Development and Infrastructure Costs

Supporting people in personalized ways involves both initial and ongoing development costs. Unlike a situation in which an agency facility is established, supporting people in their own places means that financial capacity must exist to assist people to move to different sites and to locate to other places, to change supports, to facilitate local capacities, and so forth. Technical assistance capacity, including leadership development, must remain as a central budget item, and funding should be available to assist local efforts.

Financing Housing

Financing housing must be considered on a long- and short-term basis, since the long-term integration of people with traumatic brain injury into community housing may require an increase in the available housing stock and modifications in federal policies. The major long-term strategy is to have housing of different kinds, from apartments to duplexes to cooperatives to small houses, available in local communities so people who have sustained traumatic brain injuries can choose where to live.

Personnel

Five major areas related to personnel should be considered, including the development of the professional specialist base, a cadre of paraprofessional support staff, the provider system, the regional-state infrastructure, and cross-departmental collaborations. In particular, initial efforts should be targeted at identifying existing resource people, expanding the quantity and quality of staff knowledgeable about people with traumatic brain injuries and their families, and retraining existing personnel from a medical to a community support service orientation.

TABLE 13.3 *(continued)*

Policies

It is well accepted that making housing and services in New York work for people with traumatic brain injury will require multiple cooperative systems relationships. The development of new community housing should remain the responsibility of the state housing agency, not the Department of Health (DOH), yet with a contribution of resources by the latter. On the local level, a strong case can be made to develop independent living centers as the locus of coordination for housing and support services, though this may vary from region to region. In New York, the closest service parallels are in the field of developmental disabilities, and the DOH needs to build on this growing state and local expertise in the development of individual and family support services.

Regulations

New York is considered to be one of the most heavily regulated states in the country. Its systems also are very provider driven, including in areas ranging from residential and vocational facilities to personal assistance and support services. In creating new programs and infrastructure, one of the keys will be to minimize centralized regulatory control and avoid creation of duplicate administrative structures.

Source: Adapted from Racino, J. (1993c). *Living in the Community: Toward Supportive Policies in Housing and Community Services.* Syracuse, NY: Community and Policy Studies.

have tenants with severe disabilities (Racino, 1993b) moved again outside the United States, to places without U.S. funding structures and the state-federal relationship (Kappel and Wetherow, 1986; Walker and O'Connor, 1997).

Creative Financing for Housing

Leading the reform movement in the proverbial order of financing and technology first (Racino, 1991c), were creative approaches to housing financing (Randolph, Laux, and Carling, 1987). In the latter case, in New York, these approaches involved the goal of maximizing the use of funding for housing by mixing diverse financing sources through forms of leveraging. These financial approaches could be used for supporting person-centered options and for adults with disabilities to live in places of their own versus in agency facilities (see O'Connor and Racino, 1993). However, many of the initial options for creating regular housing involved elaborate interagency collaboration (see Table 13.4) for the development of options ranging from clustered apartments to independent living services offered in apartment sites (Taylor, 1987a; and for critique of clus-

TABLE 13.4. Supported Housing Demonstration Project, Allegheny County, Pittsburgh, Pennsylvania: Interagency Collaboration

United Cerebral Palsy of Pittsburgh
Three Rivers Center for Independent Living
Long-Term Care Assessment and Management Program (LAMP), Allegheny County Office of Long-Term Care Coordination
Office of Policy, Planning and Evaluation, Department of Public Welfare (DPW)
Pennsylvania Developmental Disabilities Council
Kane Regional Centers, Allegheny County Board of Commissioners
ACCESS, Pittsburgh Port Authority
Allegheny County Adult Service, Area Agency
Department of Aging
Office of Vocational Rehabilitation, Department of Labor and Industry
Improvement Program of Allegheny County (IMPAC)
Forbes Fund of the Pittsburgh Foundation
Handicapped Challenge Foundation
Westinghouse Foundation
Department of Public Welfare
University of Pittsburgh
Allegheny County Board of Commissioners

Source: Taylor, S. J. (1987a, July). *A Policy Analysis of the Supported Housing Demonstration Project: Pittsburgh, PA* (pp. 22-25). Syracuse, NY: Syracuse University, Center on Human Policy, Research and Training Center on Community Integration.

tered sites, see Taylor and Racino, 1987b). By 1995, these options involved new collaborative agreements with housing departments, including for homeownership (Smith, 1995).

Support Services Financing

The major concern expressed by funders and providers in reform was the lack of funding for support services with housing (Racino et al., 1993), which Newman (1995, p. 412) identified as one of the two primary features of the "threshold of a new phase of housing policy." Efforts nationwide in the field of developmental disabilities resulted in modifications in support services financing structures that were orchestrated with regular housing options, with variations by state (G. Smith, 1990). This reform was followed by a call in children's mental health for more flexibility in financing for children and families (Meyers, 1994), with continued questions concerning the place of adults with mental illness in long term-care. Support services represented separate funding streams with particular restrictions on twenty-four-hour support services in regular homes (ARISE Independent Living Center, 1988; Racino et al., 1993).

Coordination of Housing and Support Services

Coordination of housing and support services has taken diverse forms around the world (e.g., Housing and Intellectual Disability Project, 1988, in Australia). Recent efforts in the 1990s were to "debundle" these two aspects of community financing. In the United States, public policy equated housing and health coordination on the federal level with the coordination between two state systems and local public housing authorities (Newman, 1995), instead of coordination among systems that comprise community living for people with disabilities (e.g., three to four state departments, each with separate local service networks).

Person-centered forms of planning (Chapter 15) were used as part of the process of reexamining coordination structures and the necessity of mix-and-match approaches to support services wherever the person might choose to live (see Table 13.5). Forms of the Canadian service brokerage approach were well received in the United States, consistent with service coordination, advocacy, individualized financing, and the movement toward community (Snow and Racino, 1991). Yet, in federal planning, linkages with home-based care often referred to more medical based services. One "model" of housing and support services coordination is HUD 202 buildings, which has a service coordination position onsite.

Homeownership and Consumer-Controlled Housing

In the late 1980s through the 1990s, homeownership (Achtenberg, 1989; American Association on Mental Retardation, nd, a), building on developments of cooperative ownership, was a focus of efforts in the disability sector. The first strategy was parent-owned housing, followed later by consumer-controlled housing (Skarnulis and Lakin, 1990) and other options for adults with disabilities, such as condominiums. Homeownership options, such as home equity conversions, life estates, sales/leasebacks, and deferral arrangements for payments were explored (Millman, 1992), together with the removal of legal impediments (American Bar Association, 1995). Life (investments and futures) planning for parents who were becoming older encouraged the exploration of more options for housing and support services, with a tendency toward parent-owned homes.

TABLE 13.5. Services and Funding Sources, State of Minnesota

Adult foster care
Assistive technology
Caregiver training and education
Chore services
Environmental modifications
Homemaker
Home health care
Housing access coordination
Housing service
In-home family support
Money management
Personal care attendant
Personal support
Semi-independent living services
Specialist services
Supportive living services
Twenty-four-hour emergency assistance

Funding sources may include home and community-based services, medical assistance, accessibility housing loans, state semi-independent living services grant program, Community Social Services Act (includes services a county may fund), and Community Health Services Program.

Source: Fields, T., Lakin, K. C., Seltzer, B., and Wobschall, R. (1995, September). *A Guidebook on Consumer-Controlled Housing for Minnesotans with Developmental Disabilities* (p. 37). Minneapolis, MN: ARC of Minnesota and the Research and Training Center on Residential Services and Community Living, College of Education and Human Development, University of Minnesota.

HOUSING, NEIGHBORHOODS, AND COMMUNITIES

Housing, as a community process linked to community development, tends to involve key stakeholders, user or consumer groups, and community participatory processes. Aspects of generic community housing, which have been marginally addressed in a primarily specialized disability housing system, are efforts at resident management of housing (Ryzin, 1996) and intergenerational and multigenerational housing (Rosenthal, 1986), with families and people of diversity, and of all abilities and income levels (Furman, 1987). Yet another type of mixed housing that holds promise is cohousing, which, by design, has a cross-section of old and young, families and singles (McCamant and Durrett, 1991).

Neighborhoods

Neighborhoods are often the focus of service efforts (Hagedorn, 1995), the location of people's homes, and sources of support (Warren, 1980), identity, permanence, and relationship (Racino and O'Connor, 1994). Good relations with neighbors in localities are considered important in the United States and United Kingdom (Flynn, 1989a), such as the 1980s theme of the New York Office on Mental Retardation and Developmental Disabilities (i.e., people with mental retardation make good neighbors). Neighborhoods may reflect the culture and racial composition of the area, and be determined to be areas of "high risk" for infant mortality, drug abuse, and teenage pregnancy. Neighborhoods have been the sites of outreach efforts, for example, family support programs to increase participation of low-income black families. Such efforts may include suppers open to all, child care and transportation (Wojdyla, 1990). Neighborhoods designated or perceived to be high in poverty or low in safety, remain as a target of study of interventions and change, with studies in high-rises and apartment complexes of particular interest in the 1970s (e.g., Zito, 1974).

Community

As a major area of sociological study (e.g., Reiss, 1959) and public policy, community has diverse meanings derived from research, including the "specific institutions that constitute the community" (church, parochial school, and social, civic, and political organizations) (Gans, 1962, pp. 104-119). The loss of communities in Western society has been a dominant theme, including in the disability field. Efforts to rebuild and regenerate community (McKnight, 1987) are often associated with particular ideologies, such as communitarianism (Etzioni, 1993), and the central theme of social justice (Weil, 1996). As described by people with disabilities, community may be the antithesis of institutions; community access involves changes in physical and attitudinal access. Community and neighborhoods are associated with "place," which has been studied in relationship to housing selection (Lindstrom, 1997), neighborhood associations, and community (and citizen) control (Hagedorn, 1995). Bronfenbrenner (1986, p. 731) cites outstanding studies of families and community that indicated community factors may be more important than intrafamilial factors and that "adverse effects of city environments on children may be indirect, resulting from disruption of the families in which they live."

Community Development

> Community development is a process of social action in which the people of a community organize themselves for planning and action. (International Cooperation Administration, 1955, in Van Willigen, 1986, p. 94)

According to anthropological concepts, community development is most frequently associated with self-help group action through community participation and voluntary cooperation, with the primary goals of self-determination, democracy, self-reliance, or local self-government and a deemphasis on material goods (e.g., better living standards, improved housing, diet and health). The concept of "felt needs" of the community is considered central, together with an optimistic spirit of human potential (Van Willigen, 1986). This philosophy bears similarities with what has been termed the "self-determination of peoples" (Moynihan, 1993). It differs from, yet is congruent with, community development geared toward "upgrading the physical characteristics of neighborhoods to make them more attractive as residential and commercial locations" (Struyk, Tuccillo, and Zais, 1982).

Linkages to regular community development efforts have been minimal, in relationship to contributions to stabilize, revitalize, and regenerate neighborhoods and communities (Lehman, 1988). However, beginning in the 1970s, with the development of residential programs in the United States, connections were made with neighborhood housing associations and tenant organizations (TLS, 1979), similar to the situation in the United Kingdom. Yet, in the 1980s and 1990s, community integration began to move toward community building.

The roots of urban development corporations in many cities are found in activist groups (Vidal, 1992), which are similar in some ways to homelessness activist groups (Cress, 1997) that formally incorporated as nonprofit organizations. As the province of community development, urban studies, public policy, and administration, housing and community support services for all people continued to be relegated to specialized roles and facilities.

Community and Social Acceptance

Traditionally, in the fields of disability, community presence revolved around an expectation of social life and community participation (Taylor,

Biklen, and Knoll, 1987). Evolving away from approaches that are devaluing and stigmatizing (e.g., large congregate settings), community acceptance has often been the rationale for community endeavors that could overcome social deviancy (e.g., Becker, 1963) and instead reflect social acceptance (see Bogdan and Taylor, 1987, for the sociology of acceptance).

Community acceptance refers to more local acceptance, including in associations, clubs, civic organizations, public places, and public events, with access to transportation, banking, parks, and arts centers. Strategies for community acceptance (O'Brien, nd) often involve people with disabilities and their supporters in community projects and in the life of the community (e.g., city, town, borough, suburban or urban neighborhood, building, and/or rural farmland). In Great Britain and some parts of the United States, community acceptance is considered an integral part of the movement toward community integration of people with severe handicaps (Felce, 1988).

Housing and Anthropological Research

Anthropological and sociological methods of studying regular housing in relationship to disability appear to be relatively new (Van Willigen, 1986). Potential methodological contributions can include the practice of intervention anthropology (action, research and development, community development, advocacy anthropology, cultural brokerage), policy research (social impact assessment, evaluation research, technology development research, cultural resource assessment, and social soundness analysis) (Van Willigen, 1986, xviii), and multisite, qualitative evaluation research case studies (Yin, 1989).

CONCLUSION

Tremendous work continues to need to be done to foster the integration and inclusion of people with disabilities in regular housing, together with the opportunities enjoyed by many Americans for homeownership and hopes for more cooperation in the community. As society begins to recognize the need for societal supports for all citizens at the same level of pubic policy as housing, movement can occur toward universal family, employment, education, and housing policy. Qualitative evaluation research holds promise, especially in making available to everyday people and policymakers the choices and options that can be accessible for better futures for people of all ethnicities, cultures, income classes, and abilities.

Chapter 14

A Policy Analysis of Foster Care: Children, Adolescents, and Adults

Julie Ann Racino

ADULT FAMILY HOME PROGRAM IN MILWAUKEE COUNTY, WISCONSIN

As in many states, Wisconsin, one of leading states in human services innovations, established a foster or family care program for adults with developmental disabilities (Taylor et al., 1987). This brief evaluation excerpt (Racino, 1988a) examines the adult family home program in Milwaukee County, a large urban area located in southeastern Wisconsin, which has been known more recently in the news media for its efforts at the education of African-American youths in separate schools (Hudley, 1995).

Background

Milwaukee County and Deinstitutionalization

As of April 1, 1985, Milwaukee County had 500 people still living in the state's three major institutions for people with mental retardation. According to the 1984 Department of Health nursing home census, Milwaukee county had a total of 746 people with developmental disabilities in nursing homes ranging in size from 16 to 350 beds (Biklen and Knoll, 1987b). As of April 1986, only one person had returned to the county under the state's Medicaid services waiver Community Integration Program (Racino, 1988b; Wisconsin Department of Health and Social Ser-

This evaluation research case study was modified from Racino, J. (1988a). *An Evaluation of the Adult Family Home Program: Milwaukee, Wisconsin.* Syracuse, NY: Syracuse University, Center on Human Policy, Community Integration Project.

vices, 1983), with extensive waiting lists for residential services in the county (Doherty et al., 1984).

Milwaukee County System of Foster Care

Since January 1983, the adult family home program for people with developmental disabilities in Milwaukee County has been operated by Community Services for Milwaukee, Incorporated, a private, nonprofit provider. Under contract with the Milwaukee Combined Community Services Board, which once operated these services directly, Community Services for Milwaukee provided support and case management for up to seventy individuals living in adult foster homes. In the county, foster care services for children were administered by the Milwaukee County Department of Social Services (DSS), which also contracted with the agency for juvenile foster homes. The Wisconsin Department of Health and Social Services (DHSS) was the state department responsible for the licensing homes housing three or four unrelated adults.

Milwaukee County Combined Community Services Boards (CCSB)

Wisconsin had a strong county-based system of services (see Taylor, 1991b), with the Combined Community Services Boards created under state statutes 51.42 and 51.437, to plan and coordinate a comprehensive system of services in alcohol and other drug abuse, mental health, and developmental disabilities. In Milwaukee County, the CCSB coordinated services and allocated funds to over forty-five public and private agencies. CCSB funding came primarily through the state, with secondary funding from county tax levies, private contributions, federal Title XIX, program fees, and insurance.

Strengths of the Adult Family Home Program

> The children are most important in our lives. We are not a business. We are a home. An institution is a place where there are doctors, nurses, and all of this, while we are a home. We help to build these kids on a home atmosphere, on a family life atmosphere. I have two boys of my own, and we try to make it a family.
>
> Foster parent, Milwaukee, WI, 1988

The key strengths of the adult family home program in Milwaukee County were described as follows:

Foster Families' Commitment to the People Living in the Homes

Many of the people living in the homes were placed there by the Department of Social Services when they were children and moved to a new administering agency as adults. In a few situations, the caring appears to be so deep and significant that it can be characterized by the word love, something that no service system can provide.

The Opportunity to Live in Homes in the Community
"As Opposed to Institutional Living"

The homes were typical homes, in typical communities, yet fundable through the state Medicaid services waiver for people returning to the county from state centers (which were large institutions, all located outside the county). The funding could be potentially beneficial to people already living in the county who may not have been institutionalized through shared living situations.

An Opportunity for Family Life,
and for a Family of Their Own

The family homes offered the opportunity to know neighbors and relatives; to be part of family outings, celebrations, and tragedies; an opportunity for people to feel good about themselves and their families; and to share meals, household chores, and family routines.

An Effective Transition Process
Between Children and Adult Services

Planning meetings included a representative of the Department of Social Services, the county case manager, the foster care agency, and the foster family. The major concern in planning was the difference in rates paid by the county for children and for adults in foster care.

Committed Staff

The staff included a clinical psychologist who made in-home visits, generally every other week, for which he was not always reimbursed, and access to support or administrative staff "any time day or night."

Issues and Recommendations

Following data collection at agency, county, and family homes, the site using field guides (Racino, 1986), the next section briefly describes eleven areas common to adult foster care programs, for which recommendations were offered. These areas were: the definition of the adult family program, community living options for adults, respite and other support services, training, case management, recruitment, certification and monitoring, quality of lives, rate and reimbursement structures, regulatory and legal concerns, and future program expansion.

Definition of the Adult Family Program

> We believe there is dignity to be found in all people and, as such, all people will be treated with respect.
>
>   Foster parent, Milwaukee, WI, 1988

The adult family program was designed as a parental model of foster care, a model generally suited more to the needs of children than adults (see Taylor and Racino, 1987a). Community Services of Milwaukee needed to enhance its role in supporting the integrity and decisions of the foster family, while supporting the adulthood of the child and assisting the adult to make more substantial life decisions.

Yet, although some adults had grown up in these homes since childhood, in other situations, new homes and matches would be located for adults. In the former, support for transition to adulthood from adolescence, as with natural families, was a focus, including opportunities for employment, housing, and adult recreation. As with birth families, the foster families who raised children from when they were young had varying expectations for the children's futures as adults. Some expected them to stay forever, and others expected them to move, maybe to a group home. New approaches, such as roommate options for adults, distinct from a parental model, could be developed as new matches (Racino, 1988a). These could emphasize roommate matching, shared decision making, companionship, joint responsibility for household tasks, and shared ownership or leasing (as opposed to moving into the home of another).

Community Living Options for Adults

> Group homes and nursing homes do not take people like Jane. This is her only chance to live in the community.
>
>   Foster parent, Milwaukee, WI, 1988

One major theme was the people who lived in foster homes were being excluded from adult living options, such as group homes, because of difficult behaviors, with adult family homes being the backup option. The debate was centering on how disabled a person could be and still live in a family (see Taylor et al., 1986, for children around the country living in families, no matter how severe their disability, including in Wisconsin).

The balance between home and program was in debate, with the dominant view being that homes needed to take precedence. The measure of effectiveness was the movement to independent living (including group homes), with foster homes on a continuum of services as a less restrictive option having fewer resources (see Taylor et al., 1986). Learning to do things for oneself versus getting a job, wanting a change, moving closer to friends, or marrying, was seen as the reason for a person to move from a foster home to independent living.

Respite and Other Support Services

> We cannot get assistance . . . no respite. In an emergency, the family takes over. One of us needs to stay home always, even for things like funerals. We can't do things as a family. We need to do things in shifts.

> Foster parent (provider), Milwaukee, WI, 1988

One of the major reported weaknesses was the lack of a support system for providers, with the perception that the adult family home providers were not a priority for respite. Only one informant stated that the supports were currently adequate. In Milwaukee County, respite services were provided through another private, nonprofit provider in southeastern Wisconsin. Expansion of other respite options, such as families fostering for one another, were proposed to fill the need for emergency respite (Warren and Cohen, 1985).

Twelve people in the adult family home programs received Community Options Program (COP) funding, including for day services, attendant or homemaker care, medical day treatment, and clothing and household damage. At the time, restrictions existed for use of Title XIX funds for respite, for psychologists/behavior management specialists, and for payments to improve physical access to buildings, such as the construction of ramps and removal of physical barriers.

Support services plans, described as minimal, could be funded through the Community Integration Program (CIP) Medicaid waiver (Wisconsin Department of Health and Social Services, 1983). The program was not currently being used in the county, partially out of concern that the program costs would later be shifted from the state to the county. Similar to Wisconsin's family support program, services through the Community Integration Program could be individualized and flexible for each family home and could include, but not be limited to, the following: in-home respite, out-of-home respite, sitter or companion services, homemaker services, home health aides, social and recreational programs, family or provider training, home modifications, special equipment, clothing or appliances not covered by other sources, transportation, and other goods and services that would support the family.

Training

Individual training was viewed as the responsibility of the case managers by the agency administrator, but not by the case managers. Individual training, for example, in positioning, may be needed for an individual, or family members may need to know what to do if a person is self-abusive. Five in-service training courses were offered on such topics as parent-guardian interaction, group home management, and behavior modification, but there was a lack of funds to pay for training, and, often, attendance was low. As one provider explained:

> For me it is obsolete; it is not necessary for me. For people who have been parents, it is more or less a waste of time.

Adult family home providers named only medication training as a needed area of instruction. Most key informants (e.g., county and agency personnel) considered values-based training as a high need. Yet, as one case manager explained, "No one wants to be told how to do things in their own home or how to be a good parent."

An orientation for new adult home providers could include the following topics: philosophy of homes (including age-appropriate expectations for adults); role of the provider; teaching within the home, including partial participation (Baumgart et al., 1982); orientation to supported work and work services; accessing resources in the community (e.g., medical, recreation); and relationships with natural families and guardians. People with disabilities and families could be involved in the training sessions.

Case Management

Historically, the case management system had shifted from the county to the agency. Although the case manager was considered the key person in the system by several informants, differing views were held about the roles of case managers by the agency, the county, and the state. However, as one family home provider stated, "I would like to know what the case managers are supposed to do." Or, in contrast, another family, explaining its relationship with their case manager, said "Changing case workers amounts to losing a friend."

Emerging concerns included the assumption of case management functions by contract agencies from the county, without expressed payment or agreement; distinctions between family homes and group homes; monitoring, coordination, and hands-on support roles of case managers for the individual and the family, including in advocacy and times of crisis; and authority for coordination functions (e.g., records access). The recommendations included training and supervision of case managers and regular visits to the homes, with the ratio of families to case managers appearing adequate. As one mother stated:

> I would think they would call every couple of months just to see if things are going all right. Come in every three or four months just to see the kids; some could be abused or not taken care of. In my case, they say, "We know you are taking care of the kids; that's why we don't bother you."

Recruitment

Recruitment was viewed as a major barrier to the expansion of the adult family home program, though an active program was not occurring at the time of the evaluation. The most effective approach identified for recruitment of foster families was word of mouth, common for these programs, with resources and a recruitment plan needed at the agency (see Taylor et al., 1986; particularly in Michigan, Macomb-Oakland, Regional Center, nd). Recommendations included use of nontraditional providers, such as roommates, and adult living options, such as those offered by Options in Community Living in Madison, Wisconsin (Johnson, 1985), and a wider range of recruitment techniques.

Certification and Monitoring

Yearly recertification of homes and certification of new homes remained the responsibility of the county. Major concerns were: licensing and certification (with a recommendation that they remain unlicensed with minimal certification standards); the lack of a state statute on adult family homes (leading to a perception of bias, especially against poor families, and arbitrariness); rules and standards that apply to the homes (with recommended guidelines to restrict homes to no more than two adults, with a regional waiver for those who grew up in the same homes); the respective roles of the county and agency in oversight (discontinue monthly home narratives to the county);

and quality (with a yearly evaluation of agency services, inclusive of consumer satisfaction).

Quality of Lives

Major areas discussed were the need for more leisure options for the adults apart from the family, addressing continued segregation in schools and at work (with limited supported employment options), more opportunities to gain competence and to participate fully in household routines, and individual services plans that would enhance participation in home and community life.

Rate and Reimbursement Structures

The funding for the program appeared to be inadequate, as expressed by the informants, with the county, however, stating that the funding was sufficient, unless the aim was for a "cadillac program." As one family provider described:

> The rates are low; the bills are high. Under certain circumstances, things like diapers are not covered, or stool medication. Things just do not last that long. I have to keep replacing things. Foster parents need to pay annual dental bills and, a lot of [the] time, transportation costs.

The rate for children was substantially higher than for the adult program, with cutbacks of up to $250 per month upon reaching adulthood. The providers experienced increased demands ("As adults, they are harder to handle. They are bigger and harder to bathe."), and sometimes, medical and dental expenses. Addressing this inequity was one of the recommendations, together with support service funds.

Regulatory/Legal Concerns

> We have been contacted by foster families who were concerned about funding, the tax situation, and about resources they felt should be available and were not.
>
> Milwaukee County Administrator, 1988

New and extensive records were being required, including receipts, depreciation of homes and cars, and so forth, with efforts to address this situation (e.g., county meetings) exacerbating the providers' concerns.

The county and case managers needed to play an active role in clarifying requirements and in assisting providers with the requirements stemming from federal and state changes.

Future Expansion

Competition for community services dollars in Milwaukee County resulted in providers being pitted against one another, as is the situation in other areas of the country. Priority for expansion of the adult foster care program, as compared to other community options, was considered the primary focus. Increasing the "community services pie" by shifting institutional resources to the community (e.g., through the Community Integration Medicaid waiver) was recommended. However, many expressed concern about the regional waiting lists and the political problems associated with these Medicaid waiver funds, for example, when parents know their child's place on the waiting lists, and their child, who may have lived at home, is "bumped" by someone in the institution for the next day program option.

INTRODUCTION

Evaluations of generic foster and family care programs, and those specialized programs exclusively developed for people with a categorical disability, such as mental retardation or a psychiatric disability, have a long history in the United States (Borthwick-Duffy et al., 1992). Foster care has been considered to be integral to the deinstitutionalization movement in the United States (Browder, Ellis, and Neal, 1974; Intagliata, Crosby, and Neider, 1981), and its forms and future have been debated (Linn et al., 1977) and compared with those developed in Europe (Pollock, 1936).

Foster care remains a key linchpin in family services in child welfare, offering an affordable model compared to institutional treatment that is consistent with American family values. In mental health, foster care in its noninstitutional forms remains one of the residential service components in the development of local care systems (Stroul and Goldman, 1996), with specialized foster care systems developing in juvenile justice for seriously delinquent youth (P. Chamberlin, 1990).

PHILOSOPHIES OF FOSTER CARE

Adoption Assistance and the Child Welfare Act of 1980 (PL 96-272)

As part of the long-term effort to reform child welfare in the United States, this act addressed the antifamily bias that pervaded the system, along with the following three major problems: (1) more children in foster care and out-of-home placements than deemed necessary; (2) too many children without hope of returning to their natural families; and (3) children in foster care and other out-of-home placements being bounced from setting to setting (Taylor, Lakin, and Hill, 1989). This act required the use of case plans and review; however, such plans may mirror plans made prior to neglect charges and not have a direct relationship to reunification of the family (Racino, 1997a; Ratterman, 1987).

Three primary philosophies are embedded in federal law and affect public policy regarding foster care: permanency planning, family preservation and independent living.

Permanency Planning

Permanency planning (Petr et al., 1990; Taylor et al., 1992), part of family preservation approaches, is based on a number of philosophical and policy assumptions including the following: (1) first priority is to return the child to the birth parents; (2) if the child is in an out-of-home placement, the priority is to use resources to facilitate reunification with the family (Pine, Warsh, and Maluccio, 1993); (3) if reunification is not possible and there is no active parental involvement, then adoption planning should be pursued (e.g., see Lindsay, 1987, for open adoption); and (4) for some children, strengthening the ties with the birth family while the child is in foster care may be appropriate.

In mental health, in contrast to the field of mental retardation, supportive and preventive services are seen as beyond permanency planning, as opposed to integral to it (e.g., Pelton, 1991), and, in some cases, are tied to efforts to move toward unconditional care (Lourie, Katz-Leavy, and Stroul, 1996). Independent living with late adolescents may be seen as the goal, for example, when reunification with the family is not possible (Child Welfare League of America, 1993).

Family Preservation

Child welfare systems are often characterized by their focus on child protective activities, with a priority on crisis intervention. Family preservation, as described in the Family Preservation and Support Services Act (PL 103-66), emphasizes short-term intensive services, lower caseloads, a separate funding stream, and twenty-four-hour worker accessibility (Danzy and Jackson, 1997; Wells and Biegel, 1991). However, family preservation, unlike family support, is not tied directly to the long-term support services of the specialized service systems.

Independent Living Program

Title IV of the Social Security Act was designed to provide all states with funds to assist youth in out-of-home care to prepare for self-sufficiency and independence as adults (Child Welfare League of America [CWLA], 1989a). Youth independence was an area overlooked by the landmark Child Welfare and Adoption Assistance Act of 1980, receiving permanent authorization by Congress and President Clinton in 1993. The Stark-Moynihan bill (PL 99-273) was designed to "enable states to implement or expand programs to assist youth in making the transition from out-of-home care to self-sufficiency" (CWLA, 1993, p. 29). All states and the District of Columbia were providing independent living services to youth in foster care (CWLA, 1993).

SPECIALIZED AND GENERIC FOSTER CARE SYSTEMS

Specialized and Generic Systems

Foster care in child welfare has been studied from the perspectives of the specialized support fields of mental retardation (Hill et al., 1987) and mental health (Miller and Yelton, 1991), through the perspectives of people who come in contact with this system (Taylor, 1991a), and through child welfare and generic evaluation researchers (English, 1993). Enough abuses in foster care have been documented in the media to "warn against an overreliance on this approach" (Roeher, 1975).

Generic Foster Care

The generic child welfare service systems, which operate under separate state departments, are not generally designed to be long-term in nature. Unlike their disability counterparts, they remain crisis, short-term oriented approaches (Miller and Yelton, 1991; Taylor and Racino, 1987a). This category of crisis intervention is a highly valued form of family preservation services (Bath and Haapala, 1994), with characteristics of these services defined by the Child Welfare League of America (CWLA, 1989b). Out-of-state placements in foster care have needed to be reformed through court orders in some states. Yet child welfare agencies have proposed a role for themselves as brokers of services with businesses, business associations, juvenile justice, and churches (CWLA, 1989b).

Specialized Foster Care Systems in the United States

In addition to foster care through child welfare (Stone, 1969), states operate specialized foster or family care programs for people with mental retardation and developmental disabilities (Morrissey, 1966; Hill et al., 1989; Taylor and Racino, 1987a; see Table 14.1), in mental health (Friedman, 1988), and for juvenile delinquency (P. Chamberlin, 1990). These systems have diverse names in the field of developmental disabilities, for instance, community training homes, family care, specialized foster or family care, shared homes, host homes, professionalized foster homes, adult foster care, and personal care (e.g., Bogdan, 1986; Walker, 1989; Walker, Salon, and Shoultz, 1987; Taylor, Lutfiyya, et al., 1986). Specialized foster care differs from generic foster care in its mission, funding, program, and regulatory schemes. Delivery systems occur through county, regional, and private, for-profit, and non-profit agencies, and vendor arrangements at the local levels.

COMMON CONCERNS IN FOSTER CARE

One of the problems that occurs when people with mental retardation, mental health, or other disabilities become involved with the child welfare systems is that these state systems are unfamiliar with their needs and with the practices in the related fields. The relationship between these social service and specialized disability systems is seldom characterized by shared responsibility, and both systems function largely autonomously, with little coordination between them (Miller and Yelton, 1991; Taylor and Racino, 1987a).

Foster or family care has been viewed as an ideal option for children who cannot live with their birth or natural families, next to permanent adoption. Specialized foster care has been used to prevent institutionalizations of children (West Virginia Medley Project, 1988), for placements from institutions, nursing homes, and hospitals, for return and diversion of children from out-of-state placements to residential treatment, and for situations when the birth family can no longer care for the children. These new or expanded programs are part of reform efforts and a developing consciousness in states toward their children which followed major calls for reform, especially in children's mental health (Knitzer, 1982).

In the late 1980s and 1990s (Taylor and Racino, 1987a), these programs shared several common problems. They tended not to differentiate between children and adults in combined programs (see Table 14.2 for selection with adults), were often ill-equipped in situations that overlap with generic, crisis-oriented foster care programs (i.e., child abuse and neglect), and tended not to be characterized by an overriding philosophy, policy, and practice framework (i.e., permanency planning and family preservation). Notable exceptions of leaders were in the state of Michigan and its Macomb-Oakland Regional

TABLE 14.1. National Studies of Organizations Supporting People with Severe Disabilities

As part of the specialized family care program (SFC), STEP offers different foster care options, including full-time foster care and shared foster care. Currently, of the sixteen children in the SFC program, three are in full-time foster placements and six have "shared foster care arrangements." One staff member commented that "shared foster care is becoming the most popular option." She said this option usually involves the child spending from two to five days per week out of the natural home and in a foster family home. (pp. 9-10)

Source: Walker, P. (1989). *Family Supports in Montana: Region III—Special Training for Exceptional People (STEP).* Syracuse, NY: Syracuse University, Center on Human Policy, RTC on Community Integration.

* * *

The "professional foster homes program," also referred to as the "professional parents program" or "professional developmental homes," serves forty clients who live with families in the community. The clients have severe disabilities and range in age from six to sixty-three with a mean age of sixteen. Fifteen of the forty are adults. There are three support staff, a coordinator with a special education degree, a three-quarter time psychologist who provides consultant services to the parents, and a case manager. Respite is available, and the professional parents have a network to help one another. All services are provided in the home or by generic local agencies. (p. 7)

Source: Bogdan, R. (1986). *It's a Nice Place to Live: Professional Foster Homes and Supervised Apartments in Washington County, Vermont.* Syracuse, NY: Syracuse University, Center on Human Policy, RTC on Community Integration.

* * *

Seven Counties Services, Inc., supports families, both natural families and "foster" families. As stated by the MR/DD (mental retardation/developmental disabilities) director, "children belong in a family not a group home." . . . Children who do not have or can no longer live with their natural family are "matched" with a family selected for them through Community Living or Community Connections. The hallmarks of this approach that distinguish it from traditional foster care are (1) the degree of emphasis placed on a "match" between the child and family; (2) the ability to match "medically fragile" and "behaviorally challenging" children with families; (3) the empowerment of the "foster" family in decision making regarding the child's life and; (4) the availability of accessible supports for the family. (pp. 6-7)

Source: Racino, J. (1985b). *Site Visit Report: Seven Counties Services, Louisville, Kentucky.* Syracuse, NY: Syracuse University, Center on Human Policy, Community Integration Project.

TABLE 14.2. Common Issues in Family Care

Policies on Placement of Adults in Foster Care

Policies should provide guidance for the placement of adults in individual family homes. As a general rule, adults should have the opportunity to live in their own homes, and placement with an individual or family in an existing community home should be made only when this can be justified on the basis of individual needs and preferences. Placement guidelines should address the situations in which the placement of adults in families and community homes is appropriate:

- The individual expresses a clear choice to live with a family (see also Roecker, 1971).
- The individual has a preexisting relationship with an individual or family and expresses a desire to live in that home.
- The individual needs companionship and a close personal relationship beyond that which is ordinarily provided by friends and acquaintances.
- The individual has experienced long-term separation from the community and family members and is not likely to form relationships with community members otherwise.

In instances in which an adult is served in foster care, it is critical that families are supported in viewing the person with a disability as an adult. Training and supports should be tailored to promoting the choices, participation, and competencies reflective of an adult.

Source: Taylor, S. and Racino, J. (1987a). Common Issues in Foster Care. *TASH Newsletter, 13*(2), 1-4.

Center, which integrated its family support framework with other systems of family placement (see Taylor, Bogdan, and Racino, 1991).

Foster Care and Community Participation

Foster care has been compared to other options such as group homes (Hill et al., 1989; Willer and Intagliata, 1982). As reflected in the evaluation excerpt, foster care studies and evaluations may examine the participation of residents in foster homes in the activities of the home, community, and neighborhood; development of daily living skills and domestic participation; employment and schooling; transportation; and family relationships and social connections (inclusion through families and their networks) (Hill et al., 1989; Lakin et al., 1993; Willer and Intagliata, 1984). This is particularly the case where integration or inclusion in schools, employment, and recreation is still in progress and with adults with significant disabilities.

Children and Adults with Medical Needs

Earlier myths regarding children with disabilities, including those with multiple disabilities being served in families, were dispelled throughout the 1980s and 1990s (Taylor, Bogdan, and Racino, 1991). In other words, all children, no matter how severe their disabilities, can be supported to live in families (Center on Human Policy, 1987). Yet, adults with disabilities such as seizures, which were not controlled by medications, were still in institutions in some of the more progressive states in the late 1980s (Shoultz and Racino, 1988).

Adolescents and Adults with Challenging Behaviors

During the 1980s and 1990s, major concerns were the return of youth from out-of-state placements, including from residential schools, and the use of nonaversive technology instead of punishment approaches (Berkman and Meyer, 1988). Adults with challenging behaviors, and sometimes involved in criminal behavior, were being supported in apartments in the community with intensive staffing in many states and the use of positive interventions for increased life quality (e.g., New Hampshire) (Knoll and Racino, 1988). The mental health system appeared to support the use of foster families with adolescents, especially those who had been hospitalized, removed from the home, or in residential treatment centers (Pinderhughes, 1996).

FOSTER CARE MODELS IN THE UNITED STATES

Foster care has been a "model" that included four to six residents (Hill et al., 1989) in "families." Two or three people with disabilities living together with the foster family was common in the 1980s in New York (Willer and Intagliata, 1984). At times, foster care has been compared to the unstructured room and board homes and facilities, which often do not need to meet standards, are larger, even institutional in size, and have been the subject of exposés from California to the East Coast. Foster care, generally the generic crisis service, has continued to be publicly criticized for the instability of its placements (Kahkonen, 1997). This section describes selected foster care models for children, adolescents, and adults, as well as enhanced foster care models such as therapeutic and professional foster care.

Foster Care Models for Children

The philosophy and planning framework for permanency planning and family preservation provides for the option for shared foster care options between the birth and foster families (see also Table 14.1), and for adoption when family reunification is not possible. The preferred option, if out-of-home placement is to occur, is for children to live with families, as opposed to in group facilities, residential centers, treatment facilities, or even small groups (Center on Human Policy, 1987). A similar position was reflected in Swedish legislation where Council "must in the first instance offer children a home with another family, i.e., a foster home" which was considered to be permanent, "unlike a backup family" (Tanner, nd). The position is congruent with Bronfenbrenner's (1979, p. 159) call for "the enduring, irrational involvement of one or more adults in care and joint activity with the child" as essential for human well-being.

However, parents often oppose the option of their child living with another family, for example, reporting that physicians recommended institutionalization or foster care when their child was very young (Racino, O'Connor, Walker, and Taylor, 1991). Nancy Roseneau and Jerry Provencal at Macomb-Oakland have found ways in the field of mental retardation to explore foster care options with birth families, instead of admissions of children to nursing homes, state institutions, and private institutions (Roseneau and Provencal, 1981). Stoneman and Crapps (1990) reported on the relationships between foster families and families of origins across the life span, with family involvement with placement the strongest predictor of future contact.

Foster Care Models for Adolescents

One of the concerns of the 1980s, as reflected in the "generic" child welfare literature, was the preparation of adolescents for independent living (Child Welfare League of America, 1993). As described in the Westat study (1988) of 1,650 youth leaving out-of-home care, all youth need assistance as they become adults. Yet, youth in foster care may have histories of abuse, neglect, and exploitation; they may lack independent financial stability, have low education and training, and need employment and a place to live. Goals of adolescents were viewed as the movement toward self-sufficiency, goal of permanence, with the role of the family as the primary resource of teaching independent living skills for children (CWLA, 1989a). Reflecting the movement toward diversity, youth programs have been developed in conjunction with foster care to promote ethnic identity and values in order to promote adolescent identity related to occupation, ideology, and interpersonal relationships (Gavazzi, Alford, and McHenry, 1996).

Adult Foster Care

In community living and disability, distinctions are not always made between children and adults (Racino, Walker and Lutfiyya, 1987), for example, with foster care described as "most normalized for people with mental retardation" (Hill et al., 1989, p. 9). In some places (e.g., Region V, Nebraska; Rucker, 1986), separately funded adult foster care programs have been available since the 1970s, although paralleling children's models, with the first foster homes in mental retardation designated for adults (Borthwick-Duffy et al., 1992). However, agency contracts for foster care in places such as Milwaukee "went to large, white-led, traditional providers, not based in central city" (Hagedorn, 1995, p. 65).

Throughout the United States, adult foster care has traditionally meant moving into the home of the family care provider, who may be licensed or certified. However, in the mid- to late 1980s, states began to explore options that allowed adults to select and live in their own homes (Hill et al., 1989; Racino, 1985-1992). As described next, such options had been possible under states' legislation and regulation, not by planning, but apparently by coincidence through the phrasing of the laws, which assumed that the home would be that of the family care provider.

Foster Care As a Funding Option

During this period, technical assistance efforts supported movement from facility-based approaches to greater choice in where and with whom people would live (see Chapter 13). Programmatic modifications of foster care were relatively easy to accomplish in most states—to, in effect, reverse the selection process with adults to more roommate approaches and mutual selection of homes, apartments, flats, duplexes, and condominiums. This partially addressed one of the primary concerns of the Canadian National Institute on Mental Retardation (Roeher, 1975) regarding entering the host home (foster home) without the same rights or status as the other household members. With the "add-on" of Medicaid supplements (Lakin, 1995) or personal care (see Willer and Intagliata, 1984, in New York), foster care with more intensive services became an affordable option in some states for people with more significant disabilities. However, these supplements were not tied typically to changes to other adult program models, but to training and other provider requirements.

Enhanced Foster Care Models

As institutions began to move toward closure in some states (see Chapters 3 and 4), new forms of enhanced foster care models that utilized state employees from institutions began to develop on a small scale in states from Idaho to New York (Christian and Whitmer, 1988). The stated intent was to match employees who already had a good relationship with institutional residents, thereby moving both or a group out together into the community, usually into the home of a staff member. As in Idaho (see also Tables 14.3 and 14.4), these models were combined with efforts to reexamine foster care for children, young people, and adults, to ensure that

TABLE 14.3. Idaho Personal Care Services "Home" Program

The 1980 legislature authorized personal care services (PCS) for people with severe disabilities. However, not until 1983 did the Idaho Department of Health and Welfare enact a program to provide these services under provisions of the Medicaid waiver authorized by the federal Omnibus Reconciliation Act of 1981. Originally designed for people with severe physical disabilities who choose to live in their own homes in the community rather than in skilled nursing facilities, the PCS program and regulations have a strong medical orientation. . . . During the waiver modification process, the definition of personal care services was changed to allow more intensive training requirements for the developmentally disabled services provider (Final Task Force Report, 1987).

A model project that moved sixteen people out of the institution and into community placements in regions throughout the state was designed by the Community Integration Task Force (Mulkey, personal communication, 1987). The model contains settings which strongly resemble what has been traditionally known as adult foster care. However, individuals placed have a wide range of disabilities and often have physical disabilities, medical needs, behavioral program needs, or some, or all of these, and have tended to be persons the ICF/MR system has tended to overlook.

The providers maintain the homes in which they and the resident(s) live, and coordinate with various day programs to provide around-the-clock training and personal care services to the individuals in their homes. The number of people who are developmentally disabled in any one PCS home is limited to two. Providers are often former staff of the Idaho State School and Hospital, and most of the PCS placements are in the Nampa-Caldwell-Boise area (Mulkey, McCowan, personal communication, 1987). The funding sources of state supplemental payments and Medicaid waiver options have been utilized to develop the residential. Case management and other services are coordinated in the region by the provider and Department personnel.

Source: Christian, G. and Whitmer, J. (1988, July). *Foster Care in Idaho and Twelve Other States.* Boise, Idaho: Idaho State Council on Developmental Disabilities, pp. 9-10.

TABLE 14.4. Case Study: From a Staff-Client to a Family Relationship, the Idaho Personal Care Home Program

Sheila and Bob Keith live, together with their young children and two people labeled disabled, in a ranch-style house on the outskirts of Nampa, Idaho. Sheila and Bob, a young couple in their thirties, are participants in a "personal care home program" funded under the state's Medicaid waiver. Through this program, two adults, Don and Sara, were able to move into their home from the Idaho State School and Hospital (ISSH), the state (public) institution for people labeled mentally retarded in 1985.

Sara: How the System Viewed Her

Sara is a thirty-year-old woman who has been labeled by both the mental health and mental retardation systems, a "dual diagnosis" person. At Idaho State School and Hospital, she was on a locked behavioral unit and was described as violent. She has been in a lot of placements, including State Hospital South in Oakland, a mental health facility. Everyone said the personal care home wouldn't work out for her.

Sara: How Bob and Sheila View Her

Sheila and Bob see Sara and her situation in a very different way. To them, Sara is a victim of the system. Bob said, "The problem is that people act as if they are dealing with charges instead of with people and don't use common sense." Sheila explained that in some of her placements, Sara "saw stuff that no one should see." Both felt living on the locked unit was bad for Sara; it taught her to do things to defend herself and to get the things that she needed.

Sheila and Bob staunchly state that Sara is not a violent person. They said people who think that way about Sara did not know her. There have been no major problems since she moved into this home. As Sheila said, "She's learned self-discipline. She didn't know how to work things out alone. She needed help." Sara concurred, saying, " I showed them. I made it for a year. Someday I will live on my own."

Sheila and Bob's Description of Their Relationship

Sheila and Bob have known Sara for a long time. Sheila met Sara at State Hospital South and then again at the State School where she worked. Bob met Sara when he worked as an employee of the Idaho State School and Hospital. Bob and Sheila consider Sara to be family. Even though Sheila, Bob, and Sara knew one another for years before she moved into their home, it "never dawned on [us] that there would be so many first-time experiences."

Source: Racino, J. (1987). *Memorandum, Case Study: From a Staff-Client to a Family Relationship.* Syracuse, NY: Syracuse University, Center on Human Policy, Community Integration Project.

funding was available for benefits and/or support services. Use of state employees was a preferred model, on a small scale in some states, where employment for state workers in the community was considered one of the major barriers to institutional downsizing or closure. In other states, such as New York, one of the prototypes was a model of foster care developed in Michigan that removed mothers from the public assistance roles and matched them with developmentally disabled children (Judson Center, in Michigan, 1990).

Therapeutic Foster Care

In mental health and juvenile delinquency, treatment or therapeutic models of foster care were developed. More explicit expectations for the foster care parents were to "apply systematic interventions" and to act in roles such as "therapist trainees" (Chamberlin and Reid, 1991). As recommended earlier by Carling (1984), in the field of mental health, differential development of foster care for different subpopulations has been supported, however, at times, with the assumption of the capacity to identify and match model components and types of children.

Therapeutic foster care has been identified as a key component of residential options in mental health (Stroul and Friedman, 1986), including crisis options considered integral to a comprehensive mental health system (Kutash and Rivera, 1996). Although not supporting a single model of therapeutic foster care, Friedman (1988) identified a number of common features of successful programs: intensive work with the child and family, individualized programming for the youngsters, training and other support for the parents, small caseloads for the program staff, and the capacity to respond immediately in a crisis (p. 13). He explains that these features are similar to the Homebuilders' model, described as an archetypal family preservation model (Bath and Haapala, 1994).

PROFESSIONALIZATION OF FOSTER CARE

During the 1980s and 1990s, efforts increased the professionalization of foster care providers nationwide (e.g., Bogdan, 1986; Willer and Intagliata, 1984) by upgrading training and other requirements, some imposed by standards related to Medicaid or other funds, which were used to supplement foster care state payments in some states (Racino, 1985-1992).

Training and Attitude Change

A review of the foster care literature indicates that such efforts at training and attitude change have occurred throughout earlier periods in foster care programs (Intagliata and Willer, 1981; Mamula, 1970), with foster care continuing to attract people with similar characteristics and motivations (Beatty and Seeley, 1980; Wolins, 1963; see, for example, Table 14.5). These included the desire for additional family income, the desire to help others, and the desire for companionship (Roecker, 1971). Foster parents have been screened for meeting morality standards and for being reputable in character (Wolins, 1963), similar to other governmental approaches to selection.

As expressed by people with disabilities, individual approaches to training work best. Community preservice for foster parents or providers is almost universally recommended, with training of foster care field staff critical during periods of major change or field demonstration (Roecker, 1971). As with other types of group training, the sessions are opportunities for foster families to meet one another, to get an overview of the program

TABLE 14.5. Connecticut Community Training Homes: Excerpts from Foster Families

---

Preface

"We treat the kids like kings and queens. But that's the only way. Children should always get the best."

"DMR's expectation is to offer all kinds of services for the basic room and board rate."

"Someday I will need help, someone to care for me. . . . If I do a good job now, maybe somebody else will do the same for me."

"To see her happy and smiling is like money in my pocket."

"I have continued despite the system. No one else is doing this because the system is so crappy and wide open for abuse because of lack of support, funding, and training."

"The Lord calls you to do things."

"We couldn't have children of our own. This gives us our family."

"It is fulfillment for me, a way of doing some good."

Source: Taylor, S., Lutfiyya, Z. M., Racino, J., Walker, P., and Knoll J. (1986). *An Evaluation of Connecticut's Community Training Home Program.* Syracuse, NY: Syracuse University, Center on Human Policy, Community Integration Project.

and its rules, and an introduction to basics of philosophy, disability, and their roles. Presentations may be given by experienced foster families (with no record of training by people who live in foster care in this review). Some early programs incorporated visits to institutions, where people may have lived, and other foster homes (Mamula, 1970).

The Child Welfare League (1989b) standards include a section on training for family programs, and a greater emphasis on family preservation. However, training programs often overconcentrate on potentially problematic areas (e.g., behavior), which may not apply to the specific person, or may incorporate training similar to that of community residences, such as emergencies, medications, first aid (offered by the American Red Cross) and nutrition (Carling, 1984, p. 14). The most recent addition in this category is a HIV/AIDS education program (Scott et al., 1996) designed for foster care providers.

Training for youth in out-of-home care have been in hygiene and general health, accessing medical care and insurance, legal assistance in reading housing documents, legal rights and responsibilities, food preparation and nutrition, locating and renting apartments and tenant/landlord rights, and addressing the "triple threat to youth" of sexual activity, chemical dependency, and infection (Child Welfare League of America, 1993). Recommendations for adults with disabilities have included opportunities to participate in family and household routines, community activities and social networks, companionship and relationships, age-appropriate activities and routines, and choices and decision making (Taylor, Lutfiyya, et al., 1986).

Foster Care and Adoption Recruitment

Early leaders in the field of mental retardation and developmental disabilities, were in the Macomb-Oakland Region of Michigan. These leaders included longtime regional director Jerry Provencal and state leadership of Sheri Falvey, Paul Newman, and the late Ben Censoni (Taylor, 1985). Renewed efforts at the diversification of foster care and adoption recruitment in both the generic and foster care fields occurred in the 1980s. These strategies were the recruitment of single parents, people of different ethnic backgrounds, and a greater diversity of family and household compositions (Smith and Guthiel, 1988; see Roecker, 1971, for interracial placements). Some foster care regulations were revised to allow for greater opportunities for foster parents to work outside the home, though some evaluators recommended the importance of an independent income in selection of families (Taylor, Lutfiyya, et al., 1986).

SUPPORT SERVICES

Major debate areas with support services in foster care include adult protective services and adult rights, parents with disabilities, inequities between birth and foster families, family support services, court-mandated services, and the use of treatment and behavioral plans in homes. This section briefly highlights adult protective services and adult rights and parenting.

Adult Protective Services and the Rights of Adults

The rights of adults include the assumption of competency, the right to refuse services that may be offered (Boyajian, 1990), and the right to marry and have children (Hayman, 1990; Marafino, 1990). Yet, adults with disabilities still may be denied legal access to maintain their constitutional rights (e.g., sterilization by parents/guardians without the person's knowledge).

Agencies that provide support services to adults may have assumed the right to "draw the line between parental interaction, or parental restrictions, and the desire or right of a person with severe disabilities to adult activities and interpersonal relationships such as dating, sexual activity, or even community integration" (Virginia Community Services Board, in Racino et al., 1993, p. 128). These rights of adults vary from the distribution of rights of children in foster care, including the rights of the foster parents, the natural parents, and the agency. In some communities, services are accessible for the children of parents with disabilities, although the parents themselves still face barriers to obtaining family services as parents and as a family (e.g., specialized service systems that do not offer services to babies of parents with disabilities).

Personal Finances

The handling of one's own money is a primary concern of people who are self-advocates (Whittico, 1994). The traditional foster care program in the United States is designed for payments to be made to the foster parents, with foster "adults allowed to keep part of their income for personal needs, such as clothing, personal articles, and spending money." In "keeping with the philosophy of encouraging self-reliance in each adult commensurate with each foster adult's ability, all foster adults should be encouraged to manage their own money to the extent they are able to" (Luecking, 1986, pp. iv-1). As Wolfensberger (see also Roeher 1975) had argued earlier in his career in regard to payments to families, the introduction of payment into human relationships creates a serious conflict of interest, which does not negate the importance of family subsidies.

Options that provide funding to the adult directly, changes the program/funding category in most places and affects the income status of the person who may be receiving disability benefits. However, pooled household funds, and forms of shared decision making on use of funds, can occur without such program changes in situations that are more akin to roommates and a shared living situation. Support services can be purchased through arrangements such as personal care or supportive home care (e.g., New York, Wisconsin) or through other approaches such as housing and support, whereby individualized funding may be pursued (Racino et al., 1993).

Parents with Disabilities: Foster Care and In-Home Supports

"Parenting is a complex endeavor requiring the acquisition of knowledge and skills in child development and management," including responding to household emergencies, decision making, and skills in dealing with a child's problematic behavior (Tymchuck, 1992, p. 53). Parents with disabilities are at high risk of having their children removed from their homes, which reportedly occurs if the mother has a "problem in addition to mental retardation" or if she was "unwilling to attend and actively participate in a training program designed to improve her parenting abilities," and/or did not have someone to "provide support" (Tymchuck and Andron, 1990, p. 321).

Parenting with support can include support from paid neighbors, intercoms, shared living with a boarder, in-home support (Racino and Taylor, 1993), personal response systems (Chambler, Beverly, and Beck, 1997), and family foster care (for the entire birth family,) as well as shared foster care. Parents advocating for their own rights (Peter, 1991) and emerging efforts to foster generic community approaches for parents in parenting, child care, and recreation (Pennsylvania Developmental Disabilities Planning Council, 1997; Racino, 1997a) hold promise.

Some approaches to supported parenting parallel approaches to adolescent pregnancy and parenting (Warren, 1990; Levy et al., 1992), including Section 8 housing, church support, crisis pregnancy and community maternity, family mediators, peer support, transportation, home responsibilities, parent programs, sex education, employment and school, home visiting programs, respite care, homemaker services, child and family advocacy, health care and nutrition, psychological support and counseling, and information delivery (Wasik and Roberts, 1994).

QUALITY OF HOMES AND THE SAFETY OF CHILDREN

Quality of homes for people living in, or funded by, foster care remains a perennial concern, with certification (or licensing) of homes standard practice in most places in the specialized field of mental retardation. However, concern about housing standards (or lack of such standards) in some communities disproportionately affects people in mental health. Citizen monitoring has been implemented as an option, together with increased efforts to differentiate between approaches to quality in homes versus in facilities (see Bersani, 1990).

Individual service plans for people living in foster homes have a long history (Mamula, 1971) and vary from family-centered plans. Person-centered planning (O'Brien, 1987) has been used in foster care situations with adults to identify system impediments to change (e.g., Idaho) to improve life quality (Racino and Lutfiyya, 1988).

As has been publicized, abuse and neglect can occur in foster homes (Rosenthal et al., 1991) with children and youth who may have been removed from their birth families for these very same reasons (i.e, neglect and abuse). Different standards are applied to the natural or birth family than to the foster family, with particular societal concerns when more resources are devoted to the latter. Significant circumstances have included children and adolescents who move from foster care to state institutions, in part due to disputes over who is responsible for payment in community settings.

CRITIQUES OF FOSTER CARE EVALUATIONS

The major critiques of foster care systems evaluations are the continued separation of evaluations by categorical group, the lack of match between public policy goals of preventing out-of-home placement and actual practices, the continued incoherency between possible and actual practices in states and localities, the diversion of funding to segregated facilities (e.g., institutional foster care, residential treatment centers) instead of local schools and communities, and the lack of transfer of positive practices between the child welfare and disability fields.

Valued Outcomes

Valued outcomes of foster care reflect a movement toward quality of life (Borthwick-Duffy et al., 1992). Possible outcome measures can be, and have been, drawn from the diverse schema in independent living, standards for family preservation programs (Jones, 1991), out-of-home placement measures, treatment outcomes, quality-of-life measures in homes, families, and community life, and their antitheses (e.g., records of arrests, recidivism to institutional settings). As defined by the Children's Defense Fund (1992), outcomes for children would include good health care, education, housing, family income, and family access to child care, among others.

CONCLUSION

Foster care, as family living, will continue to offer opportunities for children and youth who have no possibility of living with their birth family and for adults who choose a family option. However, a more coherent and just system for children with specialized needs and a reaffirmation of supporting birth families, including those headed by parents with disabilities, are critical for the future of all our children and societies.

Chapter 15

Organizational Case Studies: Creating Change in Housing, Employment, Families, and Community Support

Julie Ann Racino

A CASE STUDY OF A FOR-PROFIT AGENCY IN MINNESOTA

Nonprofits are run by a Board of Directors and by people all with their set agenda who are charged with guiding the agency administration. . . . [This company] is built on my philosophy and other people I believe in. Ownership is based on the beliefs, the values I choose. . . . We manage better because we provide the best services available in our product—services for people with mental retardation.

Company Owner, 1988

The Minnesota Context

Minnesota had one of the highest out-of-home placement rates in the nation in intermediate care facilities for people with mental retardation (ICF/MRs) (Minnesota Department of Human Services, 1987b. Based on a report from its state Office of the Legislative Auditor (1987), the Minnesota legislature called for a moratorium on the development of ICF/MRs and directed the Department of Human Services to apply for a Medicaid

This organizational research case study was excerpted from Racino, J. (1988c). *Individualized Family Support and Community Living for Adults: A Case Study of a For-Profit Agency in Minnesota.* Syracuse, NY: Syracuse University, Center on Human Policy, Research and Training Center on Community Integration.

Home and Community-Based Services waiver (Minnesota Department of Human Services, 1987a).

As of July 1984, Minnesota had obtained a Title XIX Medicaid waiver to support people to remain in or return to their homes or, if necessary, to live in "out-of-home, normalized, community settings" (Minnesota Department of Human Services, 1987b). As defined by the state department, services offered under this waiver included case management, respite care, homemaker, residential habilitation (i.e., in-home family support services, supportive living services for children and adults), day habilitation (including supported employment), and adaptive aids (see Fields et al., 1995, for updates in Minnesota).

The waiver was administered on the state level by the Mental Retardation Division, Long-Term Care Management Division, and Health Care Program Division within the Department of Human Services. On the local level, eighty-seven counties were responsible for determining income and service eligibility for clients, assuring program development and monitoring, providing case management, and contracting for services with private for-profit or nonprofit companies.

Minnesota's major deinstitutionalization lawsuit, *Welsch v. Gardebring* (see Chapter 3 for a similar lawsuit in New Hampshire), continued to have a major impact in the state. The agency utilized a semi-independent living state and county grant program and a family subsidy program.

The Company and Its Services

Community Living Services (a pseudonym), incorporated in 1985, partially in response to the Medicaid Home and Community-Based Services waiver program. As of August 1987, the agency supported twenty-five families in their in-home program and thirty-five people in supportive and independent living. The company had about 125 employees, mainly part-time workers, many of whom were hired on temporary contracts for individuals or families. The owners operated ten intermediate care facilities for seventy-two people through a company they started in 1977, together with seven other businesses (furniture and household furnishings, property management, and electrical services).

Family Support Services

Keeping the family together is one of the best things you can do.

Family support worker, 1988

For the in-home program, the agency negotiated a contract with the county for each individual family, with guidelines allowing an average of $64 per day per family. Additional funds were available for minor physical adaptations of about $3,400 for the year. Individual service plans could include an array of services (e.g., consultation on day services, communication, respite, psychological evaluation, assistance in daily living).

The program was designed for flexible changes in support staff, based on changes in families; family control of how and when service hours were used; and family selection of service types. One family support worker described support services for a teenager:

> Kathy, who returned from two years in residential treatment, had a support person for every morning routine, and for getting to learn the bus to school, the grocery store, her grandparents' house, and sometimes help with homework. Her psychologist helped her make a relaxation tape.

Direct arrangements in this agency could be made between the families and the support workers. For example, one father who had custody of a nine-year-old son with profound mental retardation, had two workers he could call directly. An emerging issue at the time was intrusiveness of support staff in the lives of families, especially regarding parent decision making on behavioral programming in homes. As another worker explained, "The parents stopped doing it . . . it is so intrusive to families. . . . Families can be very creative in saying no." In this agency, the cost of support services varied from family-to-family (from $6,000 to $25,000 per year), indicative of individual planning with each family.

Supportive Living Services for Youth and Adults

> We help people decide in what neighborhood they will live and look for a place that seems right to the people.
>
> Supportive living services worker, 1988

According to regulations and policies, supportive living (Smith, 1990) services could be provided to adults in their own homes, in adult foster homes, and in group living situations of six or fewer people; in this agency, serving adolescents was a new experience, especially through supportive living services. Hennepin County, where Minneapolis is located, allowed people to own or lease their own places, though this practice was newer in the state.

The array of individually tailored services could include involvement in communities and neighborhoods, consultations on difficult behaviors or situations, recreation and leisure at home and in the community, individual counseling, public transportation use, and budgeting and personal finances, as well as related services (e.g., nursing, occupation and physical therapy). Another worker at one of the sites described the supportive living services:

> We are more one to one than group homes. We are more able to go out in smaller groups to do activities. Three handicapped adults are the most we have in one facility. Some handicapped adults prefer to live alone.

However, though enabling people to live wherever they choose, supportive living services here did mean smaller, agency-rented group homes housing people who have little in common with one another (other than similar needs, such as challenging behaviors and speech difficulties). It meant, for one young man with many complex life conditions, living alone with staff instead of with the support of families and a peer group. Even though allowing for individual budgets, agencies could, and did, combine budgets for groups of people and pay for staff based on facility needs versus for the person. Small homes could continue to be viewed by localities and agencies primarily as congregate, agency homes, with the people living there viewed as clients.

Semi-Independent Living Services

Semi-independent living services, from a few to twenty hours per week of support services, is offered to a small number of people through state-county funding. It was a new program, only two years old. The person receiving services could remain in the same home they lived in with the same staff instead of being required to move when funding shifts from the county to the Medicaid waiver; this was an option for people served by this agency. The agency found that people who resent staff intrusion or are aggressive in group homes sometimes do better living in their own place.

Key Practices: Beyond Services

> I like Jane. She's a super, super lady. I give her a hard time. She takes it, takes it, then gives it right back to me. That's what I like. I stayed with this agency because of Jane. I could get waivered services elsewhere. We couldn't replace Jane.
>
> Family support services user, 1988

The organization's two key strengths were the emphasis placed upon relationships between employees and families and individuals with disabilities and staff support provided by the agency.

Relationships and Commitment

> Bev is so new at it, she doesn't have bad habits. Her philosophy of life fits right in . . . a firm, soft-hearted person. She works at those relationships.

> Company manager, 1988

As one of the middle managers explained, the agency often looks for people who already have good rapport with the family or individual with a disability to be workers, since the technical skills can always be taught. Staff were hired to work with specific people, even though they have a contract with the company. Respect was valued, and the major focus was on the relationships of the clients with the staff, versus nonpaid relationships with others in the community.

Staff Support

> Support is simple. Pay more to hire a high-caliber person. You train them and give them adequate support and supervision. . . . It is critical that there are people who can provide support to staff. They need on-site support . . . a person they can call [who] will come.

> Company manager, 1988

Staff support, particularly at scattered sites, was a high management priority. Behavior analysts work in the homes, and staff can propose additional on-site support. Commitment, understanding the value of what people were doing, and pride in this work were important organizational themes. The agency heightened its own profile of being a client advocate and of being committed to quality and excellence.

* * *

INTRODUCTION

The excerpt beginning this chapter is from a case study of a for-profit agency selected as one of the best examples of community living for children and adults with developmental disabilities in Minnesota (Racino, 1988c). The site was part of a nationwide organizational study of leading agencies (Racino, 1991c; Taylor, Bogdan, and Racino, 1991).

The tradition of organizational studies in disability is to highlight emerging best practices in the community, whether in the private, for-profit, nonprofit, or governmental sectors. However, research studies in disability based upon strict sampling, on-site visits with taped and recorded notes, participant observations, and research analyses (e.g., Glaser and Strauss, 1967) may be identified by competing groups as anecdotal accounts.

Case studies may be written as personal accounts from the perspectives of one or more participants in an agency, especially directors and staff members (Fratangelo, 1994; Klein, 1992). These may follow, or be followed by, public evaluations of their programs (O'Brien and Lyle-O'Brien, 1991b), and be used by organizational change consultants (e.g., Kiracofe, 1994). Some case studies resemble descriptive accounts of services by authors native to an area or a country (Tate and Chadderdon, 1982). Others are based upon collaboration between universities and management and co-authored and may highlight provider and state concerns in a historical context (Hogan, Johnson, and Jones, 1989).

This chapter briefly describes research methodology in multisite case studies at the organizational level and the use of case studies in teaching, research, and field work. It concludes with hope for the future in the agency-based vendor system characteristic of social and human services in the United States.

RESEARCH METHODOLOGY

Excellent theoretical and methodological texts (Denzin and Lincoln, 1994) include chapters on case study methods (Stake, 1994), which can be used to study a range of phenomena. These phenomena may range from studies of public service localization in Great Britain (Barker, Hambleton, and Hoggett, 1987) to Chicago school reform (Hess, Flinspach, and Ryan, 1993) to agency development in Connecticut (Hogan, Johnson, and Jones, 1989).

Places can be units of case study, such as cities (Price, 1972), schools (Salisbury, Palombaro, and Hollowood, 1993), hometowns (Lamb, 1952), classrooms (Rose, 1995), state departments (Wolf, 1990), and agencies (Rothman and Rothman, 1984). Case studies often reflect disciplinary approaches, for example, in early intervention, social work, public administration, and therapeutic recreation (Keller and Wilhite, 1995; Gilgun, 1994; McWilliams and Bailey, 1993).

Multicase studies (Yin, 1989) in major evaluation research projects are one multimethod approach to understanding the processes and outcomes at multiple local sites, within or across states, counties or regions, cities, neighborhoods, and countries. For example, Bogdan and Taylor (1990) describe one design using national nominations, purposeful sampling, two-to-four-day on-site visits, detailed field notes, diverse forms of analyses, document review, and public case studies of twenty-five to thirty-five pages in length per site as a form of policy evaluation.

Research Questions, Field Guides, and Triangulation

Qualitative studies of organizations, which involve team approaches, may be structured through the use of field guides (see Bogdan and Biklen, 1982, p. 71). Each field guide can include the research questions (generally two or three) for the study, which may have emerged from previous studies, literature reviews, and fieldwork. Research questions may be formulated across multistudies in which raw data and research products (e.g., case studies) can be compared and triangulated (Greene and McClintock, 1985) for better understanding.

Theoretical and Purposeful Sampling

Theoretical and purposeful sampling (see Bogdan and Biklen, 1982, p. 67; Glaser and Strauss, 1967) are ways of studying phenomena through samples selected to inform the evolving or developing theory(ies). Snowballing techniques, as one method of sampling in qualitative studies, have proven to be effective in major studies (e.g., Racino, 1991c; Taylor, Bogdan, and Racino, 1991). However, snowballing techniques (see Bogdan and Biklen, 1982, p. 66), in the hands of a novice, can result in the identification of an informant base whose characteristics, situations, and circumstances in relationship to the theory are unclear. A perception of replication based on an understanding of quantitative sampling methods alone differs markedly from theoretical sampling, leading to different debates on applicability of the findings.

Theory Building

The concept of theory being grounded in, or generated from, the research data appears to be best understood (and is indeed developed) over time and through the use of diverse methodological designs (Strauss and Corbin, 1994). In particular, the concept of the role of negative cases (see Bogdan and Biklen, 1982, pp. 66-67) and deviant cases (see Whyte, 1991, p. 10) in discounting theories is crucial. Many study designs neither begin with theory testing, nor do they intend to contribute systematically to theory building. A recent example in the disability field is the research on supports related to employment that ignored prior research on supports in homes and community living.

Interviewing

Interviewing, universal in the social sciences (Hayman, 1954), is central to qualitative research in organizations, especially multisite studies. Participant observation opportunities may be controlled to some extent by the agency, if access was gained by this method. Basic interviewing and related interview design skills include choosing to interview, selecting and approaching informants, descriptive questioning and soliciting narratives, log or diary interviews, interview guides, probing, cross-checks, recording, journals, and relations with informants (see Taylor and Bogdan, 1984, pp. 76-105). Yet, interviewing skills alone may require substantial field time and analysis to develop proficiency (e.g., recorded and critiqued interviews and interview series) (Macklin, 1974). Analyses are necessary to compare anthropological, sociological, and ethnographic studies, with psychiatric, psychoanalytic, personnel, counseling, social work, human and industrial relations, and other forms of common professional, disciplinary interview training.

Research Methods Within Methods

Case study research visits or observations can incorporate diverse methodologies, including group interviews (Denzin and Lincoln, 1994; Taylor and Bogdan, 1984, pp. 111-112), individual interviews (semi-structured, formal and informal, open-ended), and participant observation. Group interviews can resemble focus groups (see Chapter 1), exploring how and why phenomena occur; may be guided by separate field guides; can be used to explore group phenomena and interactions; and may be structured by the participants and/or by the participant observers/researchers. Participant observation in formal organizational studies can include, for example, informal exchanges and observations at the airport upon meeting, while riding in a car, during lunch or dinner in a restaurant, and at agency and funding offices, program sites, homes of friends and family, and community, recreational, cultural, and employment sites.

Coding and Analytic Methods

For those trained in a constant coding and recording process during the course of analysis (see Bogdan and Biklen, 1982; Taylor and Bogdan, 1984; see also, analytic induction, Robinson, 1951), for computer programs, such as Ethnograph, impose additional restrictions. Multiple codes by hand may be used on the same data sets by the same researcher depending upon the focus of analyses. Similar to writing, which is intimately tied to thought and perspective, investigators and researchers seldom use the same codes or coding methods, unless codes have been predetermined at some point in the analyses.

Validity (Understanding) and Reliability

The debate on validity and reliability in qualitative research has centered either on the misapplication of quantitative (positivistic) concepts of validity to qualitative ethnographic research, or on the nature of validity in qualitative research (see Kirk and Miller, 1986; Maxwell, 1992). The latter typically involves the creation and explication of new concepts (authenticity, understanding) that are considered more fundamental. Social validity is one of the most important forms of validity in disability research (see educational or ecological validity, Voeltz and Evans, 1983) and in qualitative methods ascertaining "the trustworthiness of observations, interpretations, and generalizations" (Maxwell, 1992, p. 280). Maxwell's schema has five categories of descriptive validity, interpretative validity, theoretical validity, generalizability, and evaluative validity.

Reliability as a concept of replication (LeCompte and Goetz, 1982) is a foreign and inapplicable concept, in its traditional sense, in ethnographic research. Yet, reliability in its broadest sense applies to efforts involving team research (e.g., observer reliability), the use of any form of instrument, including field guides, and the conditions, processes, and informants who are part of the research process. Kirk and Miller (1986) suggest field notes as a form of reliability check and explain that reliability and validity are meaningful only in reference to some theory.

Analytical Frameworks

Qualitative research has a rich history of conceptual leaders in methodology who have drawn upon their interdisciplinary experiences in anthropology, sociology, and psychology, at times combined with political science and public policy. Yin (1989) describes three major modes of analysis in multicase study designs: pattern matching, explanation building, and time analyses. Bogdan and Biklen (1982) identify their major analytic techniques as analytic induction and the constant comparative method of Glaser and Strauss (1967). Taylor and Bogdan (1984) particularly stress the role of inductive reasoning (Rist, 1977) (in contrast to deductive reasoning) and the inseperability of methodology and theoretical perspectives. Schwartzman (1993), in analyses of organizations, relies on a method of context analysis (pp. 53-54), more similar to organizational development approaches, evaluation research, and policy analyses.

ORGANIZATIONAL STUDIES

Organizational studies in business and management, and sociological studies of organizations have contributed to an understanding of the nature and definitions of organizations (Etzioni, 1961). These include the key elements of leadership, participation, and ongoing, concerned commitment to the field of disability (Becker, 1960; Kofman and Senge, 1993; Mills, Turk, and Marguiles, 1987).

A review of the rich history of organizational studies highlights all of the major concerns of traditional disability organizations, including feminist concerns (Martin, 1990; Cunningham with Schumer, 1984). These include: organizational structures and their relationships to outcomes (Foster, 1976), quality management (Jablonski, 1991), organizations and their roles (Aiken and Hage, 1971), organizational behavior (Argyris, 1978), culture (Austin, Ahearn, and English, 1997), socialization (Manning, 1970), and organizational change (Hasenfeld, 1980). Organizational development and consultancy approaches (Albin, 1992; Schein, 1969) remain essential in the change processes in moving to a new generation of community services.

Types of Case Studies

Robert Bogdan and Sari Biklen (1982), in their typology of case studies, differentiate the following: historical organizational studies, observational case studies, life history, community studies, situational analyses, microethnographies, and comparative and multicase studies. Yin's pilot case study (1989) is similar to Bogdan and Biklen's description of the first multisite case study (see Bogdan and Biklen, 1982, p. 65).

Agency Case Studies

Common components to case study reports on agencies, which may range in size from a few people to thousands or more (Racino, 1991c), include descriptive material on the locations or sites (neighborhoods, city, county, and countryside), reason for visit, researcher's entry, history, services, size and structure of the organization, organizational purpose, goals and/or mission, funding and organizational relationships with communities and constituency groups, clientele, staffing and personnel practices, and themes arising from the research visit. Many reports include the perspectives of service users, staff members and management, executives, board members, family members, neighbors, friends, and, in highly visible, positively selected samples, organizational supporters (e.g., legislators, national spokespersons, community leaders).

CASE STUDIES: TEACHING, RESEARCH, AND FIELD USE

This section briefly highlights several uses of case studies (e.g., see Ruckdeschel, Earnshaw, and Firrek, 1994). These include the study of change; comparative studies of organizations; programs and funding at local, state, and federal levels; as multicultural analyses; as evaluation research; the study of support; as a source of empowerment; in communications research; as illustrations; as a form of organizational development; as a form of policy development; as a means of disseminating new ideas; as a matter of their public and private nature; in teaching, and in field development.

Use of Case Studies in the Study of Change

Case studies can be used in diverse forms of time series designs to compare changes in organizations and the influence and reflection of field changes in organizations, organizational life, and the community-organization-individual interfaces. Case studies can be explicitly designed to study the crucial events of change, the nature of change, the impediments and barriers to change, the ways that change occurs and why, and the intended and unintended outcomes, impacts, and consequences.

Case studies can report on the experiences of people in an initiated change process, for example, the conversion from sheltered work to supported, integrated, and competitive employment (Beare, Severson, and Lynch, 1992; Murphy and Rogan, 1995) or the transition from group homes and facilities to homes with support services (e.g., Walker, 1993); they can report on new innovative agencies in employment (Racino, 1985c; see Table 15.3). Aspects of change can be discovered as themes in organizational studies, for example, changes in agency contracting processes to support integration (Rogan, 1992), and as the ways in which organizations view their roles in social change (e.g., Bogdan, 1991; Walker, 1991).

Use of Comparative Case Study Designs

Case studies can compare organizational types, such as disability and nondisability (Racino, 1991a, 1991b); service types (see Tables 15.1, 15.2, and 15.3, on family support, small group homes, and employment); organizations of diverse sizes; sponsorship (private, nonprofit, and for-profit); and geographical location or state (Taylor, Bogdan, and Racino, 1991). Common themes from case studies of good organizations, such as leadership and commitment, can lead to extensive bodies of research in organizational studies, commonly not taught in the fields of disability, and to popular management books (e.g., *In Search of Excellence: Lessons from America's Best Run Companies* by Peters and Waterman, 1982).

Use of Case Studies: Programs and Funding at the Local, State, and Federal Levels

As described elsewhere (see Chapter 2), qualitative policy research studies have often focused on programs generally operated by a particular state department or by primary funding sources (Kennedy and Litvak, 1991). These studies are often designed to be descriptive in nature and sometimes to compare programs to theoretical models (Mowbray and Herman, 1991) or to link data to organizational theory (Rogers and Hough, 1995). However, these designs may strengthen the existing system, in contrast to approaches that result in changes in fundamental assumptions. Leaders in the disability community have called for greater involvement of people with disabilities in policy research (Zola, 1994); they consider lack of involvement by people with disabilities to be a major flaw of policy studies.

Multicultural Analyses and Case Studies

Research data from agencies can be analyzed and reported through a multicultural framework (Pernell-Arnold, 1998) or other frameworks of diversity (Sapon-Shevin, 1996), including mental health's cultural competence. These frameworks may be imposed upon the data as an analytic framework or analyzed through one dimension (e.g., gender, culture,

TABLE 15.1. Excerpts from Case Studies of Agency Family Support Services

"The CITE program is a family support program providing training and education for children with disabilities and their families within the natural home through home-based services. The program was established to prevent residential placement of children and is based on the ideology that the development of children with disabilities can best be facilitated through active support of the natural family."

The case study summarizes themes in creating change in service delivery: moving with the changes in the field; administrative leadership; how do you convince people?; high level of trust; creative redirection of funds; resistance from parents; resistance from within the agency; the struggle with one's own history; and the future. The themes from the visits from the homes and families were time-limited or ongoing support?; a home-based service; helping parents cope; trainers as advocates for the family; the mother is the main caregiver; helping fathers become involved; the mother's point of view; the father's point of view; helping to lead a more normal family life; emotional support; dealing with challenging behaviors; and defining the family to work with.

Source: Traustadottir, R. (1987). *"The Answer to My Prayers": A Case Study of the CITE Family Support Program, Cincinnati, Ohio.* Syracuse, NY: Syracuse University, Center on Human Policy, Research and Training Center on Community Integration.

*   *   *

"A chapter of the Maryland ARC, CARC operates a variety of services: residential, vocational, respite, family support, recreation, etc. CARC is staffed with an Executive Director, and Director of Residential, Vocational, and Family Support Services, as well as clerical support personnel." Major types of services were companions to the family home; child/adult to the respite worker's home; respite at an integrated day care center; parent counselor; parent support group (Share Our Support); financial support; and information referral and coordination.

The family support themes in the case study were involvement with families (different families have different needs), including the frequency of service availability, and the global benefits of the program (prevention and postponement of out-of-home placements, and making life more pleasant while a family waits for out-of-home placement). The major issues (agency) were: making a difference for the family; maximizing resources; problem of disability (retardation) image; being flexible: doing whatever it takes; the future of support services; advocacy versus services; and "what do you do when all you can do is not enough?" Major issues and themes with parents were the mother's role in the families; conflicting interests within the family; expensiveness of basic needs (e.g., adult diapers); unexpected duration; summer without school; parent versus professional relationships; and "parents need all kinds of help." Concluding themes were: the importance of committed leadership, a philosophy of whatever it takes, small size; a commitment to integrated community and family life for everyone regardless of level of disability; and the parents themselves.

Source: Bersani, H. (1987). *Site Visit to Calvert County, Maryland ARC Family Support Services.* Syracuse, NY: Syracuse University, Center on Human Policy, Research and Training Center on Community Integration.

TABLE 15.2. Excerpts from Case Studies of Organizations with Small Group Homes for People with Disabilities

In the late 1970s, a state official pleaded with Sheila to establish a community living organization: "David Walter was the MR director at Fall River. All summer long he followed me around, down to the sand dunes, down to the beach. Finally he said, just come back to Dever [state school] and see some of the people on the waiting list. It was 1980 and a lot of people were waiting. He wanted me to incorporate and serve ten people." Sheila accepted the challenge because of the institution. She thought she could create something better for people outside the institution. The idea of working for herself, controlling her own hours, and, more importantly, the quality of her own program was appealing. But most of all she believed she would enjoy working with and for the ten people.

Source: Biklen, D. (1987). *Small Homes: A Case Study of Westport Associates (Massachusetts).* Syracuse, NY: Syracuse University, Center on Human Policy, Research and Training Center on Community Integration, pp. 3-4.

*   *   *

Boise Group Homes began in 1978 through the joint efforts of two friends interested in working with persons with severe handicaps. One of the two encountered a family who had a son living in an institution in California; the parents wished he would move closer to home so together the group began the first of what is now five homes. Each addition of a new home responded to some new need: George and Tom graduated from high school and had nowhere else to move, the Pattersons needed a place for their daughter whose presence at home threatened the life of her expectant mother. My initial tour recapitulated the organization's evolution from one large twelve-bed nursing home–like facility, through four more homes in increasingly newer, and more expensive looking neighborhood suburbs.

Source: Ferguson, D. (1986). *Site Visit Report: Boise Group Homes.* Syracuse, NY: Syracuse University, Center on Human Policy, Community Integration Project, pp. 2-3.

*   *   *

A local group of parents and interested individuals formed the board and received funding to start the home through a statewide initiative. . . . The Gig Harbor Group Home opened under the auspices of the Neighborhood Living Project (NLP) and still (as of my visit in 1987) operates under this system. Based at the University of Oregon, the NLP provides one way of managing a group home. The model developed by the NLP stipulates the residential program itself as well as a staffing pattern, household management system, and a way of recording the skills taught to the residents.

Source: Lutfiyya, Z. M. (1988, March). *"Going for It": Life At the Gig Harbor Group Home.* Syracuse, NY: Syracuse University, Center on Human Policy, Research and Training Center on Community Integration, pp. 3, 6-7.

TABLE 15.3. Excerpts from a Case Study of an Agency Offering Community-Based Employment Services to People with Severe Disabilities

Community Work Services, Inc., is a private, nonprofit corporation located in Madison, Wisconsin. Started in April 1984, Community Work Services provides community-based vocational services to adults with a wide range of developmental disabilities. They currently serve thirty-three clients, thirty of whom are in community jobs and three of whom still need a place to work. At the time of the October 1985 visit, all people placed in jobs had retained their positions.

Community Work Services believes that all persons should be afforded the option of working in individually arranged and individually meaningful community-based jobs. The mission of Community Work Services is to provide whatever level of training, assistance, and support an individual requires in order to be successful in a community job placement. . . . Services are available as long and as often as needed for each client.

The program is supported primarily through the Dane County Unified Services Board with additional funds from the Department of Vocational Rehabilitation, and donations. The County Unified Services Board provides funding for the long-term support of clients.

The following is a sampling of some of their positive approaches: matching the person to the job (develops jobs only with a specific person in mind); relationships with employers and co-workers (employee productivity is only one factor important to employers; small talk with employers about their business or questions to coworkers about their jobs); flexible, individually designed supports (the amount of job staff support an individual receives may vary from staff on-site at all times to support several times each day to a minimal check on a biweekly basis); commitment to the individual (makes a commitment to the individual); on-site job training (at the integrated site . . . versus being prepared in a segregated environment); and use of individualized and small clustered job sites (for example, two people in the city-county social services department, and two in the city clerk's office).

Source: Racino, J. (1985c, October). *Site Visit Report: Community Work Services.* Syracuse, NY: Syracuse University, Center on Human Policy, Community Integration Project.

ethnicity, disability). For example, Traustadottir (1991) analyzes through the feminist framework of the burden of caregiving to the caregivers, primarily women, and Morris (1991) analyzes through the perspective of housing and personal assistance as forms of empowerment of people with disabilities. Organizations can be methodologically selected for their capacity to highlight aspects of gender, culture, and diversity (O'Connor, 1993), including those which describe themselves in these terms or are of diversity in community (Bogdan, 1991; Racino, 1991b).

Use of Case Studies in Evaluation Research

Case studies may be used to examine variability in local sites and/or people (see Hollister and Hill, 1995). Such studies may be part of a quasi-experimental design (Campbell and Stanley, 1963) with comparative sites with different environmental interventions (e.g., the media, organizing and prevention efforts) (Casswell and Gilmore, 1989). As a formative tool, case studies in evaluation research can highlight the minority perspectives that are blurred by larger qualitative evaluation research studies. Case studies are a manageable method in working with the collection and analysis of large quantities of data, especially with teams of researchers.

Use of Case Studies to Study Support

Case studies are a means of describing phenomena, including the nature of support and support interventions, that may vary by individuals and environmental context (e.g., intermediate care facility in a rural town in northern New York of 15,000 people; playoff hockey match at the local rink in a Midwestern city of 70,000 people). During the 1980s and 1990s, case studies were used to study natural supports, community supports of national research interest, and community sites (for the study of a bakery see Lutfiyya, 1991b; for a study on leisure in everyday life, see Taylor, 1991c).

Use of Case Studies in Communications Research

Case studies can test aspects of communication theory and can be analyzed for communication patterns and discourse analyses (Biklen and Moseley, 1988; Sherman, 1994) and specific concerns that may be related to disability, such as behaviors and behavioral analyses. In early intervention and family support, team meetings may be a focus of study (McWilliams, 1993), together with communication patterns (and communicative intent), the nature of inclusion and exclusion, and the analyses of the language and body of the text. Some case studies, associated with the fields of psychology and psychiatry, may take on a psychoanalytic quality (Hunt, 1989), and those in fields such as social work may appear nearer to case note summaries and clinical descriptions and definitions of the problems.

Use of Case Studies As a Source of Empowerment

Case studies, based upon qualitative research strategies, tend to highlight the perspectives of people who have been underrepresented in social policy (Taylor and Bogdan, 1984), which is consistent with the goals of the Americans with Disabilities Act (Zola, 1994). Case studies make available information on processes, positions, and the status of people in political and managerial roles, opening them up to public scrutiny (see discussion on Jerry Miller, Massachusetts Correctional Reform Commissioner, in Ohlin, Coates, and Miller, 1974), and can be a form of raising expectations and fostering change through this provision of information (see Guba and Lincoln, 1989), a proven change strategy.

Case studies can highlight organizations with philosophies of empowerment and service practices that appear to bear a relationship to empowerment and choice. In contrast, case studies can focus on the lives of people and the process of empowerment (Lord, Schnarr, and Hutchinson, 1987, reporting on Canada). Case studies are congruent with the movement in the United States (Bruyere, 1993) toward greater involvement of service users and consumers, which is of primary concern in the United Kingdom (Jenkins and Gray, 1992).

Case Studies As Illustrations

Case studies can illustrate, for example, certain techniques or approaches (e.g., use of assistive technology); a range of options (e.g., employment sites for people with severe and profound handicaps); functions of job and support roles (e.g., task analyses of jobs); creative solutions to common problems in accommodation and for the worker, other employees, and employers; and ways of understanding how and why people interact in the ways the do, including in diverse environments. Case studies are popular in conjunction with major national studies because they provide concrete examples that are illustrative of findings and generalizable, in the sense of having applicability across a variety of situations and locations (see Wehman and Kregel, 1998).

Case Studies and Organizational Change/Development

Case studies have been used as a primary organizational development tool (Craig, Peer, and Ross, 1987) and as a form of formative assessment and evaluation (Thomas, 1991, a, b), particularly in times of change. They are one basis for organizational developers to work with interested agencies (e.g., housing organizations, realtors, human service agencies) in the process of change. They are especially helpful when what is required is not simply the addition of services or a common approach, but major changes in the nature of the organizations themselves (Gardner et al., 1988; O'Brien and Lyle-O'Brien, 1994; Racino, 1994).

Use of Case Studies As a Form of Policy Development

Case studies are often more difficult to analyze and compare for generalizable policy findings than designs that involve random or assigned selection with a plan for statistical analyses (see Guba and Lincoln, 1989, on transferability). However, as in other forms of qualitative research, they are often excellent methods for identifying major policy and practice concerns and for describing policy and legislative initiatives (Watson, 1993). These policy concerns may include the day-to-day use of technology for communication in the United States, the status of employment of people with severe handicaps, the success and failure of deinstitutionalization efforts, and the interpretation of policies (e.g., Americans with Disabilities Act) on the local levels. Case studies of best practices can identify serious problematic areas across sites, for example, employment concerns in agencies with best practices in community living (Taylor, Bogdan, Racino, 1991).

Case Studies As a Means of Disseminating New Ideas

New ideas, for the time and context of history, can be disseminated through case studies, sometimes counteracting predominant policy decisions. For example, in the 1980s, Medicaid policy supported the development of large day treatment or day habilitation settings for people with severe disabilities (Laski and Shoultz, 1987), in contrast to supported employment, as illustrated in Table 15.3 on Community Work Services in Wisconsin. Yet, supported employment later became an option (Gettings, 1995) for states and communities through this funding mechanism. Case studies can be useful for the transmission or borrowing of ideas across disability fields and in public policy.

Case Studies: Their Public and Private Nature

Case studies may be prepared for public use, which varies from case studies for solely internal, confidential use or analysis. (The reader is cautioned, however, that the latter runs the risk of privacy infringements, via national databases, such as on the Internet). Case studies may or may not use the actual names of people or organizations; one alternative is the use of pseudonyms. Findings are sometimes surprising to the agency and to the informants. Even findings viewed as positive by the researcher may not be perceived as such by the informants. At times, case studies planned for public use may not be made available for that purpose.

Case Studies in Teaching

Case studies have been a traditional form of teaching in the field of public administration, with a gain in prominence in fields such as education, social work, and rehabilitation (Ruckdeschel, Earnshaw, and Firreck, 1994). Case studies of this nature can be combined with news media releases; new research reports on local, state, or national conditions; and national studies of the same phenomena, to engage students in complex problem solving, values clarification, political analyses, and action-research approaches. In addition to formal classroom use, students can prepare descriptive case studies based on observations and interviews which can sharpen observational and presentational skills.

Case Studies in Field Development

As reported elsewhere (Castellani, Bird, and Manning, 1993), case studies from the Center on Human Policy on community integration of people with disabilities (e.g., Taylor, Bogdan, and Racino, 1991) were widely disseminated in the field in the 1980s. Organizational case studies are virtually an ideal method of networking organizations with similar goals, forming working groups for positive change, and encouraging organizational borrowing and sharing of learning (O'Brien and Lyle-O'Brien, 1994). Case studies can be suitable for use and analysis by other than the research team and authors (Biklen and Moseley, 1988). Case studies in the form of evaluations of organizations, such as those conducted by Britain's National Development Team, are a systematic form of organizational development (National Development Team, 1989; Towell, 1989b).

CONCLUSION

Organizational studies is a rich field of study and practice, especially in the agency vendor-based systems that dominate service provision in the United States. Best practices studies within the context of organizational research (e.g., Stone, 1989) continue as a primary form of information dissemination and public research in the United States.

The systemic coordination of evaluations and evaluation research remains sparse, with university emphases often on studies beneath the public reports. Federally funded studies (Messerschmidt, 1981) may diverge from the roots of earlier research studies, thereby providing needed information (e.g., status of nurse practices acts), but without the historical context. Contracting and funding for these evaluations may be conducted and/or paid for by the bodies being evaluated (Joint Committee on Standards for Educational Evaluation, 1981).

Longitudinal organizational studies hold promise in the public policy arena (Rist, 1994), for example, contrasting the roots of organizations in the 1970s with accepted practices in established systems today. Community agencies continue to exclude certain population groups or, conversely, to obtain funding for special programs, with truly integrated efforts still unrealized. Other research focusing on social movements (e.g., independent living movement) and grassroots and activist approaches to organizational studies is needed.

Yet, organizational studies remain primary vehicles for development in disability evaluation research toward community approaches to positive health, well-being, and prevention. They offer promise in realigning organizations to their community roots, instead of an increasing reliance on organizational development driven by available funding categories and sources. As Rossi (1988) explains, good social science research remains controversial, and major changes in organizations through research development remain elusive in moving toward communities that include all people.

Chapter 16

Conclusion:
Toward Better Futures
and Quality Lives

Julie Ann Racino

INTRODUCTION

Since the research in this book was completed, the changes in the fields of disability, as with the rest of the world, continued to evolve. The 1990s remained a time of change, with the independence movements in Africa and Eastern Europe now giving way to unrest and civil strife in other parts of the world. The author herself has experienced the injustices of our current laws and practices in the United States and the continued disparities in the class society of this country.

This chapter highlights the field status of several key areas in the movement toward community acceptance and societies of diversity. It is followed by the support and empowerment paradigm upon which the research has been developed and interpreted and then offers an update on selected policy and practice concerns of interest to evaluators. The author concludes with a brief section on the nature of qualitative evaluation research.

FIELD STATUS

Person-centered approaches, combined with the movements toward community and rights organizing, resulted in changes in support (personal assistance) services. Broadened frameworks based on ecological approaches are still emerging, with scant attention yet being paid to the major, systemic changes needed in our education, employment, recreation, and housing systems.

The disability field followed the world in its movement toward women's rights, ethnic and cultural diversity, and the rights of all people to decent housing, education, employment, income, and recreation. Although moving toward collaboration on the practice level, policy, academia, and management continued to be organized and driven by competition and, in this society, primarily monetary and capitalistic concerns.

From Person-Centered to Better Quality Lives

Person-centered approaches to planning have continued in their initial forms through the 1990s, remaining primarily as group process techniques based on positive roles, images, and expectations (Hagner, Helm, and Butterworth, 1996; Malette et al., 1992; Peterson, 1992). New developments included greater emphasis on career planning (Kregel, 1998), community membership, and diverse lifestyles (Hamer and Martin, 1991). However, diversity in approaches varying by individuals and their desires (see inclusion of typical age peers in educational planning, in Snell, 1994) were minimal, as was movement across disability groups.

Some of these approaches remain targeted at categorical groups (e.g., people with challenging behaviors (e.g., people with challenging behaviors [Smull and Harrison, 1992] or medical needs [Green-McGowan, 1987]), without the incorporation of these aspects into regular planning processes. Also, the critical differences between family-centered and family-directed plans (Summers et al., 1990) and person-centered planning have not yet been addressed.

Financing to allow for more individualized options has occurred, including across several fields of disability (Friedman, 1994; Racino, 1995c), with no evaluation research studies comparing the new financing structures. The person-centered planning approaches were incorporated into Medicaid planning processes (G. Smith, 1994) as part of an effort to demedicalize the process. This reflected a needed overhaul of individual planning in many states and localities (Lakin, Larson, and Prouty, 1994).

Rights, Facilitation, and Organizing

Practices such as facilitated communication with people who were believed incapable of speech or thought (Biklen et al., 1991) entered the services world. People who were thought not to have a right to decide, began to assert their legal rights as adults and to raise their own expectations of the possible. Parents who organized in mental health sought and received foundation funding to work with states across the country to better address their concerns and the needs of their families. Self advocacy became represented regularly at the national levels in the field of mental retardation, and independent living leaders assumed leadership roles in states, localities, and the nation.

Community, Not Institutional, Services

In the field of developmental disabilities, institutions did indeed close, homes became smaller, children did return from out-of-state placements, and new support services (and individual financing) were tested and put in place. People with brain injuries asserted their rights to community services, not solely medical avenues, and renewed efforts at prevention, home services, and employment were developed. The situation in mental health became more complex with the development of new community services for children and heightened local planning. However, despite state challenges to institutions, communities supported the use of segregated treatment and educational facilities, shifts between institutional groups (e.g., construction of prisons replacing sites of institutions for people with mental retardation), and movement of elders to nursing homes (Bauer, 1996). The other sides of consumer control critical to movement from institutional to community access are the continued deprivation of liberty of adolescents and the use of behavior management (e.g., seclusion with children) as abridgements of rights.

Personal Assistance Services

Personal assistance services (PAS), as the next step in translating the Americans with Disabilities Act (ADA) into reality, began to move into mainstream policy and practice. First was the inclusion of PAS in the nation's Health Security Act (White House Domestic Policy Council, 1993), following the broadened recognition of its potential by national organizations (Consortium of Citizens with Disabilities, 1991). In addition, increased innovations by the federal government at the initiative of the states, new research directed toward this development, and political organizing in the context of health care reform occurred in the 1990s.

Individualized and Flexible Support

This author uses a broadened definition of personal assistance services interchangeably with a concept originally called individualized and flexible supports, or individualized and flexible services, in the field of severe disabilities (Knoll and Racino, 1988; Taylor et al., 1987a). Six relevant PAS model development issues (Racino, 1995b) are: model development for children and families; normal growth and development (see Racino, 1997d); user-directed models (Doty, Kasper, and Litvak, 1996); relationship to U.S. health care reform (Buchanan and Alston, 1997); integrated service systems (U.S. Department of Health and Human Services, 1991); community approaches to personalized assistance (Ludlum, 1991); and decision making and people with significant disabilities (Guess, Benson, and Siegel-Causey, 1985).

Toward Recreation, Employment, Education, and Housing

Frameworks of community, whether recreation, employment, education, or housing, were explored in the nondisability worlds, in local communities, and in diverse academic disciplines. Inclusion, as part of a recognition of "all," became an avenue for moving, at the school and classroom levels, toward more collaborative, participatory approaches (Stainback and Stainback, 1996). Housing moved toward more community and grassroots approaches (Wandersman et al., 1996), while at the same time community and community housing translated into bankers, realtors, and the housing industry versus ordinary citizens. Unemployment for people with the most severe disabilities continued to be inordinately high (see Harris and Associates, 1994, for comparison with working-aged adults with disabilities), with support available by federal law at competitive job sites. Recreation continued its struggle between specialized, therapeutic approaches and those which are part of societies (Wetzel, McNabe, and McNaboe, 1995), with all their inequities and diversity, maintaining a continued theme of betterment for all people.

SUPPORT/EMPOWERMENT
AND INDEPENDENT LIVING PARADIGMS

As a guiding framework in disability, the author supports the paradigm of support and empowerment, which varies in several significant ways from the independent living (IL) paradigm (see Figure 1.1). These dimensions include definition of problem, locus of problem, outcomes, social roles, solutions to problems, and control, with three primary service dimensions of degree of consumer control, degree of individualization and personalization, and degree of community membership. Primary outcomes are life quality as defined by individual people and societal change toward pluralistic societies of diversity.

STATUS OF POLICY AND PRACTICE DEVELOPMENT IN FIELD PUBLIC POLICY: IMPLICATIONS OF PAS

As indicated in the quantitative studies based upon normalization community services programs often do not rate very highly on the PASS and PASSING evaluation scales (considerably below what Wolfensberger and Thomas [1983] find minimally acceptable [Flynn et al., 1991]). These ratings include basic aspects of normalization principles in terms of homes and neighborhoods and more complex issues, such as the coherency of the approach or model in all aspects of service design. As described in this article by Flynn and colleagues on 213 programs between 1983 to 1988, "community residential programs were of better quality than community vocational programs, both were superior to institutional residential programs, and Canadian programs scored more highly than U.S. programs" (1991, p. 152). These tools are not as highly rights oriented and may identify as deficiencies areas that can be considered abridgements to the right to regular living and citizenship. These reported findings are consistent with a 1970s qualitative evaluation of forty community residential programs, from 1973 to 1975, using naturalistic observation, identifying barriers to normalization (Bercovici, 1983).

Policy/Services

The Americans with Disabilities Act has been framed as the leading policy legislation that paves the way for the development of personal assistance services in the United States. From a policy perspective, PAS has been framed primarily as a disability issue and as part of national health care reform (Assistant Secretary for Planning and Evaluation, 1994).

Public policy, whether on economics, education, social policy, transportation, health care, housing, and/or employment, has not yet been framed as applying to all citizens. In particular, a stronger public policy focus on youth development is needed in order to shape the environments that affect the futures with youth with disabilities and their families (i.e., an ecological approach), and family policies supporting the capacities of youth.

The legal and planning principle of the least restrictive environment (LRE) and the concept of the continuum of services remain the framework for policy and service design (Taylor et al., 1987a; Taylor, 1988). In its extreme in education, this framework results in institutionalization of children and segregated day care, instead of integrated educational options for all. One implication of LRE is that people with the most significant disabilities are excluded from regular opportunities in the community (e.g., access to twenty-four-hour support services in their own homes) and competitive employment. Significantly, PAS systems remain based upon the legal principles of LRE, whereas emerging support systems are moving toward designs based upon the nonrestrictive environment concept. The latter supports people with the most significant disabilities to live and participate in regular homes and community life.

On a policy basis, the professional framework of prevention broadly interpreted, holds some promise for service systems as distinguished from community forms of assistance. Integrated systems, which are distinctly different from forms of cross-systems collaboration (e.g., child care, child welfare, criminal justice, mental health, developmental disabilities, education) now in place, may be substantially reshaped to support quality lives for all of our citizens.

Access

Accessibility and availability of services are two major criteria used to evaluate support services and programs (Castellani et al., 1986). Access issues are often framed in relationship to services that people may need or want, as program eligibility criteria, or as barriers to outcomes (such as productivity and independence). Access to PAS (defined broadly) has been limited by age group, disability group, household composition, and significance of disability (e.g., with particular exclusions of children, youth, and adults viewed as unable to manage their own care).

Primary types of access and emerging concerns addressed are the following:

- Universal access, primarily in areas such as housing and health care (Alston, 1997)
- As information access (especially by youth, as opposed to access by only parents or legal guardians)
- Service and communication access
- Architectural access (Bowe, 1963)
- Right to refuse access based on principles such as self-determination
- Income access (based on family, agency, and system financial resources)
- Cultural barriers to access (e.g., Malach and Segel, 1990)
- Transportation access (Willer, Linn, and Allen, 1994)
- Cross-disability and intergenerational access

Eligibility and Termination

Universal eligibility and access have tended to be framed within the context of health care reform. Eligibility for services is a major policy tool for controlling the size of the recipient group, and thereby the cost of services or the program. Yet, many of the major problems instead stem from termination of services to people who are eligible for them, and overall costs to the public are not always considered.

In relationship to eligibility with PAS programs, the major problems in the systems as designed were the availability across categorical groups, probably in violation of federal law (G. Smith, 1994), and underfunding for a program serving people across categorical groups and primarily accessed by people with physical disabilities. Other concerns cited were exclusion of youth with mental health needs from insurance; the prohibition of payments in some states to families (Watson, 1993), relatives, or friends; PAS for, by, and with youth with disabilities (e.g., within the family home); state variability (see G. Smith, 1994, for examples in Massachusetts, Maine, New Hampshire, Wisconsin, and Michigan); and the lack of awareness of impact of eligibility within the traditional PAS systems.

One systems barrier to PAS reform is the failure by all categorical and PAS systems to adequately distinguish among the diverse systems, programs, and financing for services in the lives of individual people, their families, and communities and to conduct comprehensive analyses on that basis. On the positive side, person-centered financing approaches have helped to identify some of the primary changes that could pave the way for adequate support.

Assessment

Standardized assessments, based upon thinking similar to that underlying quantitative rather than qualitative methodologies, predominate in this society, emanating from the clinical, behavioral, statistical, and educational worlds. Professional assessments are considered integral to any reform of how, and if, people with disabilities (who are at risk, for example, of being determined incompetent) will have control of their own lives. Assessments are used to determine program eligibility or exclusion/termination, for court determinations and monitoring, and to determine service needs and individual improvement; more progressive forms have been described by Racino and colleagues (1993), as toward quality of life, functional and environmental, and positive life planning focuses. However, none of these developments can address the basic problems with clinical and professional assessments (Biklen, 1988).

Services Limitations

Vast discrepancies exist between eligibility among the states, as well as across federal programs that may include personal assistance services. Most state studies have been directed toward the federal program type or initiative versus study of assistance across disability types and groups. Waiting lists for community services remain a major public policy problem in the states, with financing still shifting from institutional (e.g., nursing homes) to community services (Carmody, 1994). However, in fields such as mental health, waiting lists are not always maintained when the state does not view housing and support as its responsibility. Instead, states may continue to use SROs, room and board homes, and other options that may not be decent or affordable.

The Consortium of Citizens with Disabilities (1991) and the World Institute on Disability (1991b) already use broadened definitions of PAS that include cognitive support and/or child care. Research informants suggested expansion in types of tasks and services, the roles of assistants (e.g., coaches at work, life coaches), the availability of PAS in diverse environments (e.g., leisure and recreation), and assistive technology and adaptations (Enders, 1990; Flippo, Inge, and Barcus, 1995). At the national level, the debate centered, in part, upon whether personal assistance was a social or health service (Nosek and Howland, 1993).

Workforce Issues

Workforce issues have become the major concern of the 1990s (e.g., Petersen and Lippincott, 1993). This is partly due to changing U.S. demographics; the shift to an information-service economy; expectations regarding college education; state downsizing of major governmental departments; civil service systems, the rise in certification, private practice, and reimbursement schemes in related medical (nursing, therapies) and disability (rehabilitation, social work) professions; the diversity in training and background requirements; and the movement from the public, institutional sector to the often private, community services sector.

The major workforces in the states are not mentioned in some federal workforce analyses for training and development in disability (Racino, 1997c). Yet, new alliances of national organizations are forming on the categorical support level (National Alliance for Direct Support Professionals, 1998), without the alliance of management, and across disciplines in the university sectors (Knoll and Racino, 1994). In addition, major studies being released in the 1990s, conducted by categorical service groups, have tended to examine the traditional concerns of turnover, employee wages, and staff training and certification (Braddock and Mitchell, 1992; Larson and Lakin, 1992). States such as Minnesota have pushed certification as the solution (Moore, 1996), with the federal government funding research aimed at certification.

Common problems with PCAs and PCA systems (systems originated for people with medical and physical disabilities) (Racino, 1991e) were the lack of availability of PCAs, turnover of personal assistants, lack of emergency backup systems, personal liability (insurance) with self-directed assistants, qualifications and training of PCAs, lack of career advancement, decent wages and benefits, devaluation of PCAs in professional environments, negotiation of conflict, employee protections of PCAs, and protections of and for PCA users.

Liability Issues

The World Institute on Disability (Sabatino and Litvak, 1995) released a new report on liability concerns in personal assistance services. Other legal concerns were (Racino, 1995c) contractual relationships with teenagers (e.g., for youth approaches to PCAs); the rights of minors and their parents (for example, in health care); guardianship and involuntary commitment; deprivation of youth's liberty; sexual and associational rights of adults; youth legal issues (e.g., emancipated minors, explicit versus presumed consent, youth confidentiality); violations of the ADA and IDEA; advance directives and "values histories"; right to voluntary community services; and experiences of abuse. Common liability issues related to systems risks involved with new programs and between agencies and service users that affect eligibility and termination were not raised (e.g., people being moved to institutional or congregate settings due to perceived agency risk as distinguished from risk for the person).

Service (and Life) Quality

Quality of life (Goode, 1994; Taylor and Bogdan, 1990) and service quality (e.g., Eustis, Kane, and Fischer, 1993) are of primary importance in outcome-based evaluations, with both based on guiding principles and basic philosophical tenets. Service quality is also framed in the context of professional paradigms in rehabilitation medicine, adolescent health care, public health, social work, public administration, psychiatric rehabilitation, and special education, among others.

Services for, and approaches to quality of life (and constitutional rights) are reflected in federal and state laws (e.g., IDEA, ADA), in philosophical frameworks undergirding policies and programs (e.g., community inclusion, youth development, family support and integrity, health and wellness, mutual support and self-help, community [re]integration), and in more explicit principles and outcomes (independence, productivity, personal autonomy, personal choice, universal accessibility, and zero reject). Although quality cannot be assured, systematic quality safeguards, such as evaluation research, can be developed, which include evaluation research (Towell and Beardshaw, 1991).

Service principles of concern today are the movement toward partnerships, alliances, and collaborations (inclusive of service users); grassroots movements by consumers, youth, and parents; ethnic and culturally responsive services; holistic and community approaches (including principles of noninterference); and involving service users in all aspects of service design, planning, implementation, evaluation, and research (with a strong movement toward service-user direction). These principles mean differentiating between outcomes as the person defines them and client outcomes as defined by professionals, and the creation of accessible environments.

Long-Term Services Coordination

Long-term services coordination, as described in Chapter 13 on housing and support services and family support, remains a critical service feature, one which has proven difficult to change. Person-centered planning, although helpful in this regard, has, for example, not necessarily resulted in better allocation of service resources, that is, in ways families and individuals with disabilities would choose. Indeed, recent texts continue to ignore divergent opinions on organization of such resources, expressing unanimous support for case management systems. This support of case management occurs partially because the systems are still in development in some places and in some fields (Richardson and Higgins, 1990), because an empowerment model is still not viewed as feasible (Dunst and Trivette, 1989), and, finally, because some people in long-term care are not well served by current systems (Adler and Nichols, 1990). Other delivery and coordination approaches include single point of entry, cluster groups, and cooperative agreements, "passing the buck on difficult populations" (National Council on State Legislators, 1988), and, in the 1990s, case management as systems change (Surles et al., 1992). Three significant areas associated with long-term services coordination are vouchers and subsidies (i.e., the link to individualized funding), service coordination or brokerage, and community infrastructures.

Vouchers and Subsidies

In relationship to PAS, vouchers and subsidies are often viewed as a way to bypass systems forms of coordination and to move control of financing more directly into the hands of people. On the other hand, they are used as a way to reduce governmental expenditures, with reduced access and availability as one potential outcome. Service brokerage in Canada (e.g., Salisbury, Dickey, and Crawford, 1987) combined access to financing, service brokerage, and advocacy and strengthened community connections, with variations of this model in the United States. Voucher and subsidy approaches are insufficient in themselves to address the major issues of systems reform, with financing, however, moving to more flexible approaches.

Service Coordination

Service coordination and service brokerage are part of the emerging models of agency PAS (e.g., in community living), family support, and natural supports approaches (e.g., employment). Parents, relatives, and sometimes individuals themselves may serve as case managers. However, the management responsibilities of professionals, especially in relationship to people with significant disabilities, still remain problematic. Other divergent ways of thinking about service coordination include the experience of some psychiatric survivors of case management as controlling and new approaches (e.g., case managers having money available for flexible use by their clients) as forms of coercion.

Structures for Coordination

Service integration of any form is a perennial problem that has not been solved and may indeed by exacerbated by increased agency collaboration, which may detract attention from the concerns of service users. Forms may branch out from schools to families and from community agencies to schools at the local levels, with similar models in the business sectors. Individual planning meetings of six or more agencies, sometimes without the person or significant people in their lives involved, are common. At the state levels, departments may indeed be competing for leadership roles in the same area, for instance, with coordination also consisting of competition for contracts at the local levels. Many of the major reform initiatives are based on either modifications of structures as they exist or plans to build a community infrastructure following similar principles to those which resulted in the development of facility-based service systems. Health care delivery (e.g., forms of managed care, health maintenance organizations, and integration of mental health into generic health) that included aspects of choice within managed modes occurred during the past decade.

Consumer Control

Consumer control (Racino and Heumann, 1992b) has been interpreted as the degree of direction (management and coordination) of services (paid and unpaid), the right as an employer to select, hire, and/or terminate (paid or unpaid) assistants, and control of one's own life (e.g., direction, relationships, activities). Most service concepts of consumer control reflected supports or services organized around service users, sometimes framed as collaboration, negotiation, partnerships, or mutuality (mutual support, mutual relationships) within program contexts having different user interpretations (e.g., polarized discussions).

Control or autonomy by people with disabilities remains an organizing concept in independent living and central to user-directed PAS (Doty, Kasper, and Litvak, 1996; Simon-Rusinowitz and Hofland, 1993). However, many models of choice and empowerment are under professional control, with professional decisions, for instance, on "fading" of their involvement and control. Only sporadically are service differentiating between the perspectives of service users and providers, with support in self-direction by providers increasingly problematic. Control and support through communication and community empowerment and relationships emerged beginning in the mid- to late 1980s.

NATURE OF QUALITATIVE EVALUATION RESEARCH

"All qualitative approaches to program evaluation are distinguished by their preference for use of qualitative methods including open-ended interviews, on-site observations, participant observation, and document review" (Greene, 1994, p. 538). Qualitative methods are well suited to the nature of the policy and practice questions that prompt the call for program evaluations and independent evaluations as systematic quality safeguards.

Qualitative Paradigms

Qualitative approaches to program evaluation are guided by interpretive paradigms (e.g., positivism, constructivism) (Guba and Lincoln, 1994) and by theoretical paradigms (e.g., independent living and support/empowerment paradigm) (Racino, 1992a). However, they continue to be used primarily in conjunction with the quantitative methods (Weiss, 1972), prompting repeated calls for the qualitative methods to stand on their own (Bogdan and Lutfiyya, 1992).

"Consumer Voice," Community Membership, and Politics

In the disability fields, the promotion of qualitative research is intimately linked with efforts to promote the voice of the service users and consumers (e.g., Corrigan and Garmon, 1997; Rapp et al., 1994) and to reform movements toward a new generation of services more closely tied to community membership and personal autonomy. Of major interest are the politics of disability evaluation research that closely link funding, policies, and the political positions of organizations, users, and agents (i.e., stakeholders) with the evaluation research agenda (Jenkins and Gray, 1992; Rist, 1994).

Field Use and Evaluations

Qualitative evaluation research faces the traditional problems of the divergence between evaluation findings and field use (Weiss, 1972) and the implications for the reform agendas when the discrepancies between what is known and what is practiced continue in the field (Rossi, 1988; Smith, 1981). Some researchers have suggested a more collaborative approach with administrators, or practitioners as researchers (Goldstein, 1994), which remains problematic (Guba and Lincoln, 1989), with the collaborative approaches of external and internal coalitions being more promising.

Promising Methodological Strategies

A promising strategy for evaluation research is the return to the case study (Stake, 1988) with its in-depth approach to understanding the views of the informants. Case studies have particular power when combined with community studies of the lives, places, and organizations that affect, and are affected by, the lives of all people (or selected group members). As described earlier, case studies can assist in addressing intransigent policy and systems concerns affecting the lives of service users and community members. These insights appear to occur partially by uncovering other sides that have not been made public on these concerns. The methods can be empowering, however, subject to the same forms of misuse, unless understanding, validity, and reliability of these methods are supported on their own terms (Kirk and Miller, 1986; Maxwell, 1992).

Theory-Based Evaluations, Theory Formulation, and Testing

Of particular hope is the emergent linkage with systematic theory formulation (Glaser and Strauss, 1967; Rogers and Hough, 1995; Strauss and Corbin, 1994), raising the long-term promise of more community forms of support and changing societal expectations. Theory-based evaluations (Weiss, 1995) are grounded in a series of assumptions that can be empirically tested, including the focus on urban neighborhoods, neighborhood action, involvement of local citizens, social services without changes in employment conditions, impact with limited funds, and services to adults that confer benefits on children. Community-wide evaluations and increases in the level and regularity of local evaluations are needed in the United States before efforts can be made to coordinate these evaluations in ways that would be useful for public decision making.

A Story of Two Case Studies

For those who believe in comparative sites as the wave of the future or in ethnographic studies of one community, I share with you Hollister's and Hill's (1995) problems in the evaluation of community-wide initiatives at ten sites (cities), one of which had a flood, another a huge, unanticipated volcanic eruption, a third a hurricane, and one simply a major downturn in their primary manufacturing industry. This situation bears some resemblance to my case study of the Berkeley Center for Independent Living (Racino, 1993b), part of a national multisite study of agencies supporting people with disabilities (Racino, 1991c). That area experienced one of the major earthquakes of the decade (with front-page headlines and full newspaper sections devoted to the story in the East) (Herald Journal News Service, 1989) during the referral visits.

The case study that followed, on the Madison Mutual Housing Association (Racino, 1993d), included no such natural disaster. This study involved a community agency that had been introduced over a half a decade earlier (Johnson, 1985) through one of its leading associated disability agencies (Options in Community Living), both national leaders in their own fields (i.e., housing and disability). As with other changes over time, however, the leadership of the housing organization changed shortly there-after, and the support organization began to start new agencies for the people who were moving out of the state institutions back to local commu-nities.

ENDNOTE

As a contribution to the base of qualitative community research, *Policy, Program Evaluation, and Research in Disability: Community Support for All* offers an introduction to a selection of value-based disability evalua-tion and research. Designed to contribute to the incorporation of best practices within the field of evaluation research, the future lies in the extent to which the barriers in society, those which have stood in the way of people who have been excluded and marginalized, can yield, merge, and shift to make way for a new tomorrow for all of us.

Appendix A

Personal Assistance Services: Methodological Considerations

INTRODUCTION

This semistructured interview study was conducted as part of the New Models Research Project that was designed to identify potentially best practices, including consumer-directed program models for particular population groups (e.g., people with combined physical and cognitive disabilities, brain injuries, psychiatric disabilities, technology dependency, communication disabilities, youth, and members of ethnic groups).

The study was designed to address three primary research questions:

1. What are the differences and similarities in service and support needs and preferences among diverse population groups?
2. Why do some groups utilize the existing system more than others? What are the systems barriers to wider access?
3. Are fears regarding safety well-founded? Are there ways to decrease the risks of independent living without also eliminating individual choice and control over one's life?

SELECTION OF INFORMANTS

The nomination process was designed as a variation of a snowballing technique in qualitative research (Bogdan and Biklen, 1982). The primary informants for the study were to be people who have a disability and are considered to be "consumer experts" who could contribute to the design

---

Appendix A describes the methodology for *Part III: Moving Toward Universal Access to Support—Policy Is Personal*, inclusive of Chapters 8 through 11.

and development of new personal assistance (PAS) models. Six to eight key informants were selected for interviews in each categorical group. Selection criteria included personal and/or professional experiences with PAS and familiarity with the experiences of other people who may or do use PAS. The intent was to share the perspectives of people with disabilities and to further the development of personal assistance services).

DATA COLLECTION

An interview guide was developed for use across the categorical groups by this researcher, with review and input by members of the World Institute on Disability (WID) research team. All interviews were conducted by the same person and were varied in length (from one hour and fifteen minutes to a total of two hours). The interviews were semistructured in nature and started with the informants' experiences with PAS and/or their background information. All interviews were conducted over the telephone and audiotaped, with the informants' permission, and transcribed.

INTERVIEW FIELD GUIDE

The semistructured interview field guide was designed to obtain information from experts on their perspectives regarding new conceptual models for each population group. The guide is based upon effectiveness criteria for personal assistance services developed by the World Institute on Disability and elicits information in five major areas: (1) use of personal assistance services; (2) perspectives on accessing such services; (3) needs that are not being met by the existing service system; (4) views on what an effective PAS system means for a particular group; and (5) recommendations on how PAS for their group should be designed.

The field guide, developed by Community and Policy Studies, was reviewed and commented upon by members of the WID research team. It consisted of sample questions in each of the following areas: background (informant, purpose, uses, and outcomes of PAS); universal access (inclusive of access by minorities, disability group, age, and by people with significant disabilities); the consumers' right to know; timing of PAS; types of PAS; consumer input; PAS providers; and additional comments and recommendations.

WORKING DEFINITION
OF PERSONAL ASSISTANCE SERVICES

The working definition of PAS, which was mailed with a copy of the interview field guide to all informants, was developed by the World Institute on Disability (Litvak, Zukas, and Heumann, 1987, p. 1). PAS was defined as tasks performed for a person who has a disability by another person which aim(s) at "maintaining well-being, personal appearance, comfort, safety and interactions within the community and society as a whole." The tasks in the definition were of seven categories: personal maintenance and hygiene, mobility, household maintenance, infant and child-related, cognitive or life management, security-related, and communication services.

DATA ANALYSIS

Each set of interviews was coded in several ways. First, the data for each interview were divided into theme areas. Some of these were predetermined (e.g., universal and information access), whereas others emerged from the data (e.g., vulnerability and abuse). Second, the themes were analyzed across each interview set. Third, the primary themes and subthemes were reviewed and reanalyzed. Fourth, in the process of writing the reports on each of the interview sets, the themes and subthemes were further reorganized. All drafts of the interview summaries (by categorical group) were sent for review by informants and several researchers from the World Institute on Disability.

RESEARCH REPORTS

Research reports were prepared for each categorical group (brain injury, youth with disabilities, mental retardation and physical disabilities, psychiatric survivors/psychiatric disabilities) based on interviews and literature reviews, with a summary report across all categorical groups. Concurrently, an annotated bibliography in this area was prepared. (For all materials, see the edited collection, Racino, 1995c.)

REPORT REFERENCES

Racino, J. (1995). *Edited collection on personal assistance services*. Syracuse, NY, and Boston, MA: Community and Policy Studies.

a. Personal assistance services and people with psychiatric disabilities and psychiatric survivors.
b. Personal assistance services and people with mental retardation and physical disabilities.
c. Personal assistance services and people with brain injuries.
d. Personal assistance services and youth with disabilities.
e. Moving toward integrated approaches in personal assistance services.
f. Annotated bibliography on personal assistance services.

METHODOLOGICAL REFERENCES

Bogdan, R. and Biklen, S. (1982). *Qualitative research for education: An introduction to theory and method.* Boston, MA: Allyn and Bacon.
Litvak, S., Zukas, H., and Heumann, J. (1987). *Attending to America: Personal assistance for independent living.* California: World Institute on Disability.

Appendix B

Policy and Organizational
Research Methodology

INTRODUCTION

The policy research study was designed for two primary purposes. The first was to identify and describe practices and strategies that states use to promote community integration and deinstitutionalization, including how these came about and how they may be applied in other states (Taylor, 1990). The second was to better understand the nature of systems change and its relationship to individual life quality (Racino, 1991). The focus of the organizational study was to identify and examine on the local level practices, issues, and dilemmas facing organizations in attempting to promote community integration and deinstitutionalization (Center on Human Policy, 1991).

The area agency case studies are methodologically a modification of a 1985 to 1990 study of "good" organizations across the United States supporting people with disabilities in the community (for study results and methodology, see Bogdan and Taylor, 1990; Racino, 1991a; Racino, 1993; Taylor, Bogdan, and Racino, 1991). The 1991 interview guide for this study was modified to allow for greater cross-site analyses in four areas: practices and strategies, nature of community life, issues and dilemmas for organizations, and response to minority group populations.

The policy research study reflects a more in-depth and systematic version of state evaluation research studies (Racino et al., 1989; Taylor, Racino, and Rothenberg, 1988; Taylor et al., 1992; Taylor et al., 1987) developed as part of a national technical assistance effort with thirty-five states. The policy research methodology has an interdisciplinary focus that draws on the disciplines of political science, sociology, psychology,

---

Appendix B describes the methodology for *PART II: Community Integration—Policies to Support Community and Systems Change.*

rehabilitation, and other applied disciplines (Majchrzak, 1984; McCrae, 1980). The methodology for both studies builds upon a long history of qualitative research studies, particularly in the field of mental retardation. The studies rely more heavily on in-person semistructured interviewing than on participant observation techniques (Patton, 1980).

FOCUS AREAS FOR THE STUDIES

The focus areas for the studies were refined by an organizational and policy research team and reviewed by a national research advisory committee, which included leading policy researchers, parent leaders, and people with mental retardation. Research field guides (Center on Human Policy, 1991; Racino, 1991b) were developed by a research team to guide the state and local data collection.

The local organizational study guide was organized around four primary research questions:

1. What are specific practices and strategies that these organizations have developed to support people with disabilities in the community?
2. What is the nature of community life for people supported by these organizations?
3. What are the issues and dilemmas these organizations face in trying to promote quality life?
4. How have these organizations responded to members of minority groups and rural populations?

For the policy research guide, key focus areas for the interviews, observations, and review of documents included in the guide are recent history of the (developmental disability) community services system; strengths and weaknesses of the current system; major lawsuits or court cases; legislation, policy, and program initiatives; coalitions, associations, and/or organizations of parents and people with disabilities; local change strategies, such as values-based training; state leadership; national and federal factors; state practices and strategies (including administrative, fiscal, political, human resources, technological, media); and major controversies.

SELECTION OF STATES

A research team developed criteria for the selection of states for study, modifying the original proposal design to include the following three categories of states.

> *Category 1:* States that are considered progressive on deinstitutionalization and community integration measures (e.g., Michigan, New Hampshire).
> *Category 2:* States currently in the process of major systems change toward deinstitutionalization and community integration (e.g., Oklahoma, Illinois).
> *Category 3:* States ranking low on deinstitutionalization and community integration measures, but which have experienced major state efforts for systems change toward deinstitutionalization and community integration (e.g., Arkansas, Louisiana).

The following material includes a listing of the key and additional factors used in the selection of the state of New Hampshire. Two or more of the following key factors must be present, since these reflect primary research areas under investigation: major deinstitutionalization lawsuit; strong state leadership toward community integration and/or deinstitutionalization; major policy and/or legislative initiatives toward community integration and/or deinstitutionalization; strong coalitions, organizations and/or associations of people with disabilities and/or their parents; statewide efforts toward community integration and/or deinstitutionalization through individual and locally applied change strategies (e.g., values-based training).

Additional Factors Identified As Criteria for State Selection

The following factors were also considered in state selection: access to key informants involved in major change efforts; presence of innovative region(s) in community integration and deinstitutionalization within the state that could be studied in-depth as part of the organizational research component (e.g., presence of strong local leadership); presence of innovative local agencies, particularly in areas of housing and supports to families, that could be studied in-depth through the organizational research component; presence and access to information that can aid our current emphases on ethnic and cultural diversity, rural/urban practices, generic strategies, and community/systems/individual change; and applicability and use by other states (e.g., geographical distribution, different types of state structures, size).

Based on these criteria, which were also reviewed by a national policy research advisory committee, the research team recommended the following states for consideration for initial study: Michigan, New Hampshire, Wisconsin, Colorado, and Minnesota. The policy research advisory committee members commented on all proposed states and suggested alternative recommendations (National Advisory Committee, 1991). Based on their recommendations, New Hampshire was selected as the first study site.

SELECTION OF AGENCIES

An in-state panel consisting of the state director in the field of developmental disabilities (Richard Lepore), a parent leader (Sylvia Stanley), a state official knowledgeable about self-advocacy (Jane Hunt), a university disability leader (Jan Nisbet), and a director of a state voluntary association (Chris Nicolletta) selected the local sites for study. The panelists were interviewed by telephone by the study coordinator and asked to recommend two to three local organizations that were good examples of community integration and deinstitutionalization. Panelists were requested to specifically consider organizations that may be particularly responsive to rural/urban issues and/or members of various ethnic or cultural groups.

Based on the recommendation of a national advisory committee, a broad definition of organization was used to encompass those ranging from traditional organizations to less formal groups, such as parents who may have come together to develop a community living situation. With the exception of three special projects, all nominations were of area agencies. Two of the panelists strongly recommended the study of area agencies instead of individual programs to understand how services work in New Hampshire. Five area agencies were nominated, four by two panelists and one by three panelists. From these nominations, a research team made the final decision concerning the research sites based on a number of factors, including match between the team and the study areas, rationales given by panelists for selection, and resource availability. Of the three special projects nominated, self-advocacy efforts and the family leadership institute were incorporated into the case study areas (see Chapters 2 and 5). The third effort, ARC Welders, was already under study by the University of New Hampshire.

DATA COLLECTION AND PRELIMINARY ANALYSES

Eight on-site visits by four researchers were conducted in New Hampshire, including three visits to study the regional area agencies. Six visits took place in fall 1991, with two additional visits in summer 1992. The policy research and organizational visits varied in length from one to three days and consisted of semistructured interviews, participant observation, and document review. Additional telephone interviews were also conducted for more in-depth information on specific thematic areas. The semistructured telephone interviews were from forty to ninety minutes in length and were tape-recorded and transcribed.

Key informants for the policy research were identified through a snowballing technique commonly used in qualitative studies (Bogdan and Biklen, 1982; Taylor and Bogdan, 1984), which was facilitated by this investigator's previous work within the state beginning in 1985. Area agency directors played a primary role in identifying informants for the local site visits, using guidelines suggested by the researcher. The key informants included a wide range of people within and outside New Hampshire, such as people with disabilities, parent leaders, state officials and policymakers in a variety of roles, disability advocates, consultants and planners, lawyers and state guardians, expert witnesses, housing and program consultants, area agency staff and directors, and others.

An initial site visit to New Hampshire was conducted by this investigator to determine areas for further study and to begin interviews with key policy research informants. The visit, conducted in fall 1991, included interviews with the Developmental Disabilities Director, the institutional superintendent (now the Developmental Disabilities Director), Director of the state Division of Mental Health and Developmental Services, Director of the state ARC, member of the state Developmental Disabilities Council familiar with self-advocacy, the state family support coordinator, one of the plaintiff's lawyers in the *Garrity v. Gallen* lawsuit, member of the University of New Hampshire, and a shared staff member between the institution and the Developmental Disabilities Office.

Based on the initial on-site visit to New Hampshire and interviews with key informants, the research team selected the following areas for in-depth case policy studies: *Garrity v. Gallen* (institutional court case), closure of Laconia (state institution for people with developmental disabilities), family support (legislation, councils, task force, and training), self-advocacy (and the role and views of people with disabilities), and the relationship between the area agencies (the regional structures) and the state's Medicaid Home and Community-Based Services waiver program. Specific researchers also were selected to play the primary role in relationship to these substudies.

Two site visits were conducted by one research team member on the development and implementation of New Hampshire's family support legislation in fall 1991. The interviews and observations were conducted with people at various levels within the state, including state officials with in-depth knowledge of the program, the legislator who cochaired the legislative task force set up to study family support needs, three parents who were very involved in the legislative activities that resulted in passage of the Family Support Network Bill, a parent whose daughter was a named plaintiff in the original lawsuit, eleven parents whose families receive services through the Family Support Councils, two Institute on Disability staff members involved in the family leadership series that has trained parents in advocacy skills since 1988, and employees of the Family Support Councils in three regions of the state.

The next two visits were conducted in summer 1992 by another researcher. Specifically, these visits were designed to obtain more detailed information about the institutional lawsuit and closure, the perspectives of people with disabilities involved in self-advocacy efforts in the state, and the state's Medicaid waiver and to visit one additional region in the state. The informants included four people involved with self-advocacy, broadly defined, in the Lakes and Concord regions, the new state coordinator for self-advocacy, a staff member involved internally in the institutional closure, the Director of Mental Health and Developmental Disabilities, the state official responsible for implementing the state's Medicaid waiver program, two lawyers, and two staff members of the state's independent living center. At the Lakes region area agency, the informants included the director, residential director, and a person supported by the agency, together with his home provider.

Area Agency On-Site Visits

The agency on-site visits were conducted by three members of the research team in fall 1991, with each member studying one of the area agencies. In addition to the organizational field guide, the researchers also organized their data collection around the program areas highlighted by the nominations panel:

> *Region IX, Developmental Services of Strafford County, Incorporated Dover, New Hampshire.* This region was nominated particularly for its work in the area of supportive living, with most of the people supported by the agency to live in individualized places.
> *Region VI, Area Agency for Developmental Services, Nashua, New Hampshire.* This region was nominated as one of the overall leading area agencies with a particular emphasis on community supports, including case management, family supports, and housing.

Region V, Monadnock Developmental Services, Keene, New Hampshire. This region was nominated specifically for its work in the area of employment.

DATA ANALYSES

Field data were subsequently recorded and/or transcribed for all site visits and interviews. Over 1,500 pages of field data were collected for analysis, and over fifty documents were identified and reviewed (see Documents Reviewed in this Appendix). The edited collection of case studies reflects an analysis of *over* 1,000 pages of this data, exclusive of the family interviews and Region VI field memorandum. The following are three primary stages of analysis that occurred.

Individual Research Analysis and Case Studies

Each researcher analyzed his or her own and related data, identifying themes for discussion with the broader research team. Case studies were prepared by individual researchers, and the three on the area agencies and the one on family support were commented upon by other members of the research team. These were written with the intent of public distribution and tend to highlight positive practices, issues, and dilemmas within that context. All case studies are available for public use through the federal Educational Resource Information Clearinghouse (ERIC) on Disabilities and Gifted Education.

Cross-Researcher Analysis

In addition to regular research meetings on implementation issues, the research team held four meetings to review research findings, to identify common themes across data, to begin analysis of New Hampshire-specific issues, and to develop the monograph design. The primary researcher completed the final analysis and writing, which are consistent with the full data sets of all researchers involved in the project.

Cross-State Analysis

The policy research study data from the first policy research "framing" visit were coded, analyzed, and prepared for cross-state computer analysis of findings by the study coordinator. The coding and analysis process was similar to that found in traditional in-depth qualitative research studies and involves both the designated study areas (e.g., litigation, state leadership) and critical themes that arose from the data (e.g., "how systems work," "storytelling" by administrators). The secondary data sets were coded and analyzed, but not prepared for computer analysis.

DOCUMENTS REVIEWED

Documents reviewed include selected samples of program materials; newspaper articles and newsletters; national resources (e.g., National Conference of Executives of the Association for Retarded Citizens, National Association of State Mental Retardation Program Directors); administrative samples (e.g., budget, contracts, correspondence, and memorandum); and brochures (e.g., assistive technology centers, family support Lakes Region Community Services Council, Glencliff Home for the Elderly).

Association for Retarded Citizens of New Hampshire (nd). *The rainbow theater project: Mission statement, goals and objectives* (pp. 1-5). Concord, NH: The Concord Center.
Association for Retarded Citizens of New Hampshire (1991, April). Where we have come, where we are going: An interim report of the ARC Welders, *Community Connections,* 1-4.
Biklen, D. (nd). *The AA and other innovations: A case study of Developmental Services of Strafford County, NH.* Syracuse, NY: Center on Human Policy.
Covert, S., MacIntosh, J., and Shumway, D. (1994). Closing the Laconia State School and Training Center: A case study in systems change. Revised version. In V. Bradley, J. Ashbaugh, and B. Blaney (1994). *From vision to reality: Transforming service systems to systems of support for persons with developmental disabilities* (pp. 197-211). Baltimore, MD: Paul H. Brookes.
DiLeo, D. (1991). *Developing individual service plans for persons with disabilities.* Concord, NH: The New Hampshire Division of Mental Health and Developmental Services.
DiLeo, D. and Nisbet, J. (1989). *Enhancing the lives of adults with disabilities: An orientation manual.* Concord, NH: The New Hampshire Division of Mental Health and Developmental Services.
LePore, R. (1991). Laconia Developmental Services. Lawsuit and closure, Draft 1 (Unpublished paper).
LePore, R. (nd). *Historical perspective.* Concord, NH: State of New Hampshire.

LePore, R. and Felix, J. (1991, August). *Alternate means of support and supervision in certified residences. Identical memorandum, Developmental Services.* Concord, NH: State of New Hampshire.

Lutfiyya, Z. M. (1991, April). The importance of friendships between people with and without mental retardation. *ARC FACTS.* Arlington, TX: National Association for Retarded Citizens.

Malloy, J. (1992). *Basic benefit planning: A guide for people with disabilities.* Concord, NH: New Hampshire Developmental Disabilities Council.

The New Hampshire Challenge, Inc. (1991, July). News for families about disability issues. *The New Hampshire Challenge, 3*(4), 1-16.

New England Conference Center (1991). *Forging directions: A New England conference on aging and developmental disabilities.* Durham, NH: New England Conference Center.

New Hampshire Developmental Disabilities Council (1989). *Developmental Disabilities Council: Transitional two-year state plan, Fiscal years 1990-91.* Concord, NH: Author.

New Hampshire Developmental Disabilities Council (1989). *Promises to keep: Supporting people with developmental disabilities, their families and communities in the 1990s.* Concord, NH: Author.

New Hampshire Developmental Disabilities Council (1990). *All people belong: Annual report.* Concord, NH: Author.

New Hampshire Developmental Disabilities Council (1992). *Projects and selected activities for support.* Concord, NH: Author.

New Hampshire Division of Mental Health and Developmental Services (nd). *New Hampshire's components of home and community-based Medicaid waiver program.* Concord, NH: Author.

New Hampshire Division of Mental Health and Developmental Services (1991). *New decade, new decisions: A look at the mission, organization and services of the state supported developmental services system.* Concord, NH: Author.

New Hampshire Division of Mental Health and Developmental Services (1991, Spring). *Profiles: The newsletter for the Association for Retarded Citizens of New Hampshire.* Concord, NH: Author.

New Hampshire Family Support Task Force (nd). *For the love of our families, for the sake of all* (pp. 1-6). Concord, NH: Author.

New Hampshire Transportation Association (nd). *Transportation choices for New Hampshire.* Concord, NH: Author.

People First of New Hampshire (1993, Spring). *New Hampshire Self-Advocacy Newsletter, 5,* 1-6.

Shumway, D. L. (1991). *Independent assessment of New Hampshire's home and community-based waiver services for people with developmental disabilities.* Concord, NH: New Hampshire Division of Mental Health and Developmental Services.

State of New Hampshire (nd). *Evolution and development of family support in New Hampshire.* Concord, NH: Author.

State of New Hampshire (1987). Chapter 171-A, Services for the developmentally disabled.

State of New Hampshire (1989). Family support legislation, 1989 Laws of New Hampshire, Chapter 255.

State of New Hampshire (1989). State Bill No. 147-FN-A.

State of New Hampshire (1989). State Bill No. 195-FN-A.

Twining, J. A. (1990). *Historical issues and future choices: Perspectives on early intervention in New Hampshire.* Concord, NH: New Hampshire Infant and Toddler Project.

Van Keuren, D. (1991, June). *Summary of benefits of community care waiver renewal package: Interpretational communication.* Concord, NH: State of New Hampshire, Bureau of Community Developmental Services.

Van Keuren, D. (1992, January). *FY-92 1st quarter data from the outcome reporting forms.* Concord, NH: New Hampshire Division of Mental Health and Developmental Services.

Watson, D. (1991, March). *Record of Laconia discharges.* Concord, NH: New Hampshire Division of Mental Health and Developmental Services.

Wehmeyer, M. (1991, February). Public Law 94-142: The Individuals with Disabilities Education Act. *ARCFACTS.* Arlington, TX: National Association for Retarded Citizens.

Wehmeyer, M. (1991, March). The education of students with mental retardation: Preparation for life in the community. *ARCFACTS.* Arlington, TX: National Association for Retarded Citizens.

REPORT REFERENCES

Thematic Case Studies: Policy Research

Racino, J. (1993). *An edited collection on deinstitutionalization and community integration in New Hampshire.* Syracuse, NY: Community and Policy Studies.

    a. A qualitative study of self-advocacy and guardianship: Views from New Hampshire.
    b. Critical structural factors in community services development.

c. *Garrity v. Gallen:* The role of the courts in institutional closure.

d. The closing of Laconia: From inside out.

Shoultz, B. (1993). *"Like an angel they came to help us": The origins and workings of New Hampshire's family support network.* Syracuse, NY: Syracuse University, Center on Human Policy, Research and Training Center on Community Integration.

Area Agency Case Studies

Racino, J. (1992). *"People want the same things we all do": The story of the area agency in Dover, New Hampshire.* Syracuse, NY: Center on Human Policy, Syracuse University, Research and Training Center on Community Integration.

Rogan, P. (1992). *Employment for all.* Syracuse, NY: Syracuse University, Center on Human Policy, Research and Training Center on Community Integration.

Walker, P. (1992). *From deinstitutionalization to supporting people in their own homes in Region VI, New Hampshire.* Syracuse, NY: Syracuse University, Center on Human Policy, Research and Training Center on Community Integration.

Related Research Studies

Bogdan, R. and Taylor, S. (1990). Looking at the bright side: A positive approach to qualitative policy and evaluation research. *Qualitative Sociology, 13*(2), 183-192.

Racino, J. (1991a). Organizations in community living: Supporting people with disabilities. *Journal of Mental Health Administration, 18*(1), 51-59.

Racino, J., O'Connor, S., Shoultz, B., Taylor, S., and Walker, P. (1989). *Moving into the 1990s: A policy analysis of community living arrangements for adults with developmental disabilities in South Dakota.* Syracuse, NY: Syracuse University, Center on Human Policy, Research and Training Center on Community Integration.

Taylor, S., Bogdan, R., and Racino, J. (1991). *Life in the community: Case studies of organizations supporting people with disabilities in the community.* Baltimore, MD: Paul H. Brookes.

Taylor, S. J., Racino, J. A., Knoll, J. A., and Lutfiyya, Z. M. (1987). *The non-restrictive environment: On community integration for people with the most severe disabilities.* Syracuse, NY: Human Policy Press.

Taylor, S., Racino, J., and Rothenberg, K. (1988). *A policy analysis of private community living arrangements in Connecticut.* Syracuse, NY: Syracuse University, Center on Human Policy.

Taylor, S., Racino J., Walker, P., Lutfiyya, Z., and Shoultz, B. (1992). *Permanency planning for children with developmental disabilities in Pennsylvania: The lessons of PROJECT STAR.* Syracuse, NY: Syracuse University, Center on Human Policy, Research and Training Center on Community Integration.

Methodological References

Bogdan, R. and Biklen, S. (1982). *Qualitative research for education: An introduction to theory and methods.* Boston: Allyn and Bacon.

Center on Human Policy (1991). *Guides for data collection, organizational studies and policy research.* Syracuse, NY: Syracuse University, Center on Human Policy.

Majchrzak, A. (1984). *Methods for policy research (Applied research methods series, Vol. 3).* Beverly Hills, CA: Sage.

McCrae, D. (1980). Policy analysis methods and government functions. In S. Nagel (Ed.), *Improving policy analysis* (pp. 129-151). Beverly Hills, CA: Sage.

National Advisory Committee. (1991). *Summary of recommendations: Policy research on deinstitutionalization and community integration.* Syracuse, NY: Syracuse University, Center on Human Policy.

Patton, M.Q. (1980). *Qualitative evaluation methods.* Newbury Park, CA: Sage.

Racino, J. (1991b). *Policy research interview guide.* Syracuse, NY: Syracuse University, Center on Human Policy.

Taylor, S. (1990). *A proposal for a Research and Training Center on Community Integration.* Syracuse, NY: Syracuse University, Center on Human Policy.

Taylor, S. and Bogdan, R. (1984). *An introduction to qualitative research methods* (Second Edition). New York: John Wiley.

Yin, R. (1989). *Case study research: Design and methods.* Newbury Park, CA: Sage.

Bibliography

Aber, J.L. (1983). The role of state government in child and family policy. In E.F. Zigler, S.L. Kagan, and E. Klugman (Eds.), *Children, families and government: Perspectives on American social policy* (pp. 96-116). New York: Cambridge University Press.

Aberbach, J., Putnam, R., and Rockman, B. (1981). Roles and styles of policy making. In *Bureaucrats and politicians in Western Democracies* (pp. 84-114). London and Cambridge, MA: Harvard University Press.

Abery, B. and Fahnestock, M. (1994). Enhancing the social inclusion of persons with developmental disabilities. In M. Hayden and B. Abery (Eds.), *Challenges for a service system in transition* (pp. 83-119). Baltimore, MD: Paul H. Brookes.

Abery, B. and Stancliffe, R. (1996). The ecology of self determination. In D.J. Sands and M.L. Wehmeyer (Eds.), *Self-determination across the lifespan: Independence and choice for people with disabilities* (pp. 111-145). Baltimore, MD: Paul H. Brookes.

Abeson, A. (1976). Litigation. In F.J. Weintraub, A. Abeson, J. Ballard, and M. LaVor (Eds.), *Public policy and the education of exceptional children* (pp. 240-258). Reston, VA: Council on Exceptional Children.

Able-Boone, H., Sandall, S., and Loughry, A. (1989). Preparing family specialists in early childhood special education. *Teacher Education and Special Education, 12*(3), 96-102.

Abrams, P. (1992). *Historical sociology.* Somerset, Great Britain: Open Books Publishing Company.

Abt, C.C. (1979). *Perspectives on the costs and benefits of applied social research.* Cambridge, MA: Abt Books.

Achtenberg, E.P. (1989). Subsidized housing-at-risk: The social costs of private ownership. In S. Rosenberry and C. Hartmann (Eds.), *Housing issues in the 1990s* (pp. 227-267). New York: Praeger Publishing Company.

Adler, D. (1993). Perspectives of a support worker. In J. Racino, P. Walker, S. O'Connor, and S. Taylor (Eds.), *Housing, support and community* (pp. 217-231). Baltimore, MD: Paul H. Brookes.

Adler, D. and Nichols, N. (1990). *The Onondaga adult intensive casemanagement program: An evaluation of the first year of service.* Syracuse, NY: Onondaga Casemanagement Services, Inc.

Adler, P.A. and Adler, P. (1994). Observational techniques. In N.K. Denzin and Y.S. Lincoln (Eds.), *Handbook of qualitative research* (pp. 377-392). Thousand Oaks, CA: Sage.

Agosta, J., Smith, P., Deatherage, M. (1991). How families can organize for change: educating policymakers. *Exceptional Parent, 21*(2), 79.

Aharoni, C. (1991). *Akim Hadera (Israel): What did we do in 30 years?* Unpublished manuscript. Hadera, Israel.

Aiken, M. and Hage, J. (1971). *The organic organization and innovation.* London: Oxford University Press.

Albin, J. (1992). A case study in quality improvement and organizational change to community-based employment. In *Quality improvement in employment and other human services* (pp. 291-307). Baltimore, MD: Paul H. Brookes.

Albin, J., Ross, K., Renes, D., Rhodes, L., and Sandow, D. (1993, May). *Quality and supported employment: A bibliography.* Eugene, OR: Specialized Training Program, University of Oregon.

Allen, G.E., Fitts, J., and Glatt, E. (1981). The experimental housing allowance program. In K. Bradbury and A. Downs (Eds.), *Do housing allowances work?* (pp. 1-31). Washington, DC: Brookings Institution.

Allen, Shea and Associates and Forrest, C. (1993). *Patterns of supportive living: A resource catalog.* Napa, CA: Author.

Alston, R. (1997). Disability and health care reform: Principles, practices and politics. *Journal of Rehabilitation, 63*(3), 5-9.

Altshuler, A. and Thomas, N. (1977). III: Administrative decisionmaking. In *The politics of the federal bureaucracy* (pp. 113-146). New York: Harper & Row Publishers.

American Association on Mental Retardation (nd, a). Homeownership or control. *AAMR policy positions on legislative and social issues: Executive summary.* Washington, DC: Author.

American Association on Mental Retardation (nd, b). Personal assistance. *AAMR policy positions on legislative and social issues.* Washington, DC: Author

American Association on Mental Retardation (1992). *Mental retardation: Definition, classification, and systems of support.* Washington, DC: Author.

American Bar Association (1995). *Guide to homeownership.* New York: Random House/Times Books.

American Evaluation Association, Task Force on Guiding Principles for Evaluators (1995). Guiding principles for evaluators. *New Directions for Program Evaluation, 66,* 19-26.

Americans with Disabilities Act (1990). PL 101-336, 42 U.S.C., section 12101 et seq.

Andersson, S. and Carlsson, I. (1987). *Special services for intellectually handicapped persons act and Act concerning the implementation of special services for intellectually handicapped persons act.* Swedish Statute Book. Stockholm, Sweden: Ministry of Health and Social Affairs, International Secretariat.

Andrews, H., Barker, J., et al. (1992). National trends in vocational rehabilitation: A comparison of individuals with physical and psychiatric disabilities. *Journal of Rehabilitation, 58*(1), 7-16.

Anthony, W.A. and Blanch, A. (1987). Supported employment for persons who are psychiatrically disabled: A historical and conceptual perspective. *Psychosocial Rehabilitation Journal, 11*(2), 5-23.

Antonak, R., Livneh, H., and Antonak, C. (1993). A review of research on psychosocial adjustment to impairment in persons with traumatic brain injury. *Journal of Head Trauma Rehabilitation, 8*(4), 87-100.

Apolloni, T. (1989). Guardianships, trusts and protective services. In G. Singer and L. Irvin (Eds.), *Support for caregiving families* (pp. 283-294). Baltimore, MD: Paul H. Brookes.

Applebaum, P.S. (1986, October). Editorial. Outpatient commitment: The problems and the promise. *American Journal of Psychiatry, 143*(10), 1270-1272.

Apter, D. (1994). From dream to reality: A participant's view of the implementation of Part H of the PL 99-457. *Journal of Early Intervention, 18*(2), 131-140.

ARC-Ohio (1989). *On closing an institution*. ARC-Ohio, pp. 6-9.

Argyris, C. (1978). The individual and organization: Some problems of mutual adjustment. In W. Natemeyer (Ed.), *Classics of organizational behavior* (pp. 253-266). Oak Park, IL: Moore Publishing Company.

ARISE Independent Living Center (1988). *Meetings on attendant care services*. Syracuse, NY: ARISE.

Arnold, M. and Case, T. (1993). Supporting providers of in-home care: The needs of families with relatives who are disabled. *Journal of Rehabilitation, 59*(1), 55-59.

Arokiasamy, C., McMorrow, D., and Moss, G. (1994). *The tbi (traumatic brain injury) annual research index: Volume one*. Orlando, FL: Paul M. Deutsch.

Arranda-Coddou, P. (1992, April). *Twelve years of law review commentary on the fair housing law: A bibliography of selected articles (1980-1991)*. Washington, DC: HUD Law Library.

Ashbaugh, J. and Nerney, T. (1990). Costs of providing residential and related support services to individuals with mental retardation. *Mental Retardation, 28*(5), 269-273.

Assistant Secretary for Planning and Evaluation, U.S. Department of Health and Human Services (1994, December). *Research agenda: Personal assistance services and related supports*. Washington, DC; Author.

Austerberry, H. and Watson, S. (1985). A woman's place: A feminist approach to housing in Great Britain. In C. Ungerson (Ed.), *Women and social policy: A reader* (pp. 91-108). London: Macmillan Education Ltd.

Austin, M., Ahearn, F., and English, R. (1997). Guiding organizational change. *New Directions and Higher Education, 98*(2), 31-56.

Bachrach, L. (1976). *Deinstitutionalization: An analytical review and sociological perspective*. Rockville, MD: U.S. Department of Health, Education and Welfare, Public Health Service, ADMHA, NIMH.

Bachrach, L. (1994). Residential planning: Concepts and themes. *Hospital and Community Psychiatry, 45*(3), 202-203.

Balser, R. and Harvey, B. (1993). Using hospitals as job-training and employment sites for people with disabilities: A ten year experience. *Journal of Vocational Rehabilitation, 3*(4), 46-50.

Bank-Mikkelsen, N. (1969). A metropolitan area in Denmark, Copenhagen. In R. B. Kugel and W. Wolfensberger (Eds.), *Changing patterns in residential services for the mentally retarded* (pp. 227-254). Washington, DC: President's Committee on Mental Retardation.

Barker, C., Hambleton, R., and Hoggett, P. (1987). Decentralisation in Birmingham: A case study. In P. Hoggett and R. Hambleton (Eds.), *Decentralisation and democracy: Localising public services*. Bristol, UK: University of Bristol, School for Advanced Urban Studies.

Barr, D. and Cochran, M. (1992). Understanding and supporting empowerment: Redefining the professional role. *Networking Bulletin: Empowerment and Family Support, 2*(3), 1-8.

Bartlett, S.N. (1997). Housing as a factor in the socialization of children: A critical review of the literature. *Merrill-Palmer Quarterly, 43*(2), 169-198.

Batavia, A. (1992). *The failure of disability policy research*. Paper prepared for the National Council on Disability's Policy Research conference, December 7, 1992, Washington, DC.

Bath, H.I. and Haapala, D.A. (1994). Family preservation services: What does the outcome research really tell us? *Social Services Review, 68*, 386-404.

Bauer, E.J. (1996). Transitions from home to nursing home in a capitated long-term care program: The role of individualized support systems. *Health Services Research, 31*(3), 309-326.

Baumgart, D., Brown, L., Pumpian, I., Nisbet, J., Ford, A. Sweet, M., Messina, R., and Schroeder, J. (1982). Principle of partial participation and individualized adaptations in educational programs for severely handicapped students. *Journal of the Association of Persons with Severe Handicaps, 7*(2), 17-27.

Beare, P., Severson, S., and Lynch, E. (1992). Small agency conversion to community-based employment: Overcoming the barriers. *Journal of the Association of Persons with Severe Handicaps, 17*(3), 170-178.

Beatty, L. and Seeley, M. (1980). Characteristics of operators of adult psychiatric foster homes. *Hospital and Community Psychiatry, 31*, 774-776.

Becker, H.S. (1960). "Notes on the concept of commitment." *American Journal of Sociology, 66*, 32-40.

Becker, H.S. (1963). *Outsiders: Studies in the sociology of deviance*. New York: The Free Press.

Becker, H.S. and Geer, B. (1957). Participant observation and interviewing: A comparison. *Human Organization, 16*(3), 28-32.

Behar, L. (1995). Changing patterns of state responsibility: A case study of North Carolina. *Journal of Clinical Child Psychology, 14*(3), 188-195.

Benne, K.D. (1976). The current state of planned changing in persons, groups, communities and societies. In W. G. Bennis, K.D. Benne, R. Chin, and K.E. Corey (Eds.), *The planning of change* (Third Edition) (pp. 68-83). NY: Holt, Rinehart, and Winston.

Benshoff, J., Kroeger, S., and Scalia, V. (1990). Career maturity and academic achievement in college students with disabilities. *Journal of Rehabilitation, 56*(2), 40-44.

Ben-Yishay,Y. and Diller, L. (1993, February). Cognitive remediation in traumatic brain injury: Update and issues. *Archives of Physical Medicine, 74,* 204-213.

Bercovici, S. (1983). *Barriers to normalization: The restrictive management of retarded persons.* Baltimore, MD: University Park Press.

Bergland, M. and Thomas, K. (1991). Psychosocial issues following severe head injury in adolescence: Individual and family perceptions. *Rehabilitation Counseling Bulletin, 35*(1), 5-21.

Bergman, A. and Singer, G. (1996). The thinking behind new public policy. In G. Singer, L. Powers, and A. Olson (Eds.), *Redefining family support: Innovations in public-private relationships* (pp. 435-460). Baltimore, MD: Paul H. Brookes.

Berkman, K. and Meyer, L.H. (1988). Alternative strategies and multiple outcomes in the remediation of self injury. Going "all out" nonaversively. *Journal of the Association of Persons with Severe Handicaps, 13*(2), 76-86.

Bersani, H. (1987). *Site visit to Calvert County, Maryland ARC Family Support Services.* Syracuse, NY: Syracuse University, Center on Human Policy, Research and Training Center on Community Integration.

Bersani, H. (1990). Family monitoring: Making sure a house is still a home. In V. Bradley and H. Bersani (Eds.), *Quality assurance for individuals with developmental disabilities: It's everybody's business* (pp. 77-91). Baltimore, MD: Paul H. Brookes.

Bersani, H. and Nerney, T. (1988). Legal and legislative initiatives in disability. In V. Van Hasselt, P.S. Strain, and M. Hersen (Eds.), *Handbook of developmental and physical disabilities* (pp. 159-173). New York: Permagon Press.

Bertsch, E. (1992, November). A voucher system that enables persons with severe mental illness to purchase community services. *Hospital and Community Psychiatry, 43*(11), 1109-1113.

Betts, H. (1994). *Community living issues in brain injury planning.* Chicago: Midwest Regional Head Injury Prevention Center for Rehabilitation and Prevention.

Biklen, D. (1974). *Let our children go: An organizing manual for advocates and parents.* Syracuse, NY: Human Policy Press.

Biklen, D. (1977). Advocacy comes of age. In B. Blatt, D. Biklen, and R. Bogdan (Eds.), *Alternative textbook in special education* (pp. 391-402). Denver, CO: Love Publishing Company.

Biklen, D. (1985). *Achieving the complete school: Strategies for effective mainstreaming.* Baltimore, MD: Paul H. Brookes.

Biklen, D. (1987). *Small homes: Westport Associates.* Syracuse, NY: Syracuse University, Center on Human Policy, Research and Training Center on Community Integration.

Biklen, D. (1988). The myth of clinical judgment. *Journal of Social Issues, 44*(1), 127-140.

Biklen, D. (1992). *Schooling without labels: Parents, educators and inclusive education.* Philadelphia, PA: Temple University Press.

Biklen, D. and Baker, M. (1979). *Principles of whistleblowing.* Syracuse, NY: Center on Human Policy.

Biklen, D. and Knoll, J. (1987a). The community imperative revisited. In J. Mulick and R. Antonak (Eds.), *Transitions in mental retardation, Volume 3: The community imperative revisited* (pp. 1-27). Norwood, NJ: Ablex.

Biklen, D. and Knoll, J. (1987b). The disabled minority. In S.J. Taylor, D. Biklen, and J. Knoll (Eds.), *Community integration for people with severe disabilities* (pp. 3-24). New York: Teachers College Press.

Biklen, D., Morton, M.W., Gold, D. Berrigan, C., and Swaminathan, S. (1992). Facilitated communication: Implications for individuals with autism. *Topics in Language Disorder, 12*(4), 1-28.

Biklen, D., Morton, M.W., Saha, S.N., Duncan, J., Gold, D, Hardardottir, M., Karna, E., O'Connor, S., and Rao, S. (1991). "I amn not a utistive on thje typ" ("I'm not Autistic on the Typewriter"). *Disability, Handicap and Society, 6*(3), 161-180.

Biklen, S.K. and Moseley, C. (1988). "Are you retarded?" "No, I'm Catholic": Qualitative methods in the study of people with severe handicaps. *Journal of the Association of Persons with Severe Handicaps, 13*(3), 155-162.

Birnebaum, A. and Cohen, H. (1993). On the importance of helping families: Policy implications from a national study. *Mental Retardation, 31*(2), 67-74.

Biscup, K. (1990). Survival, struggle, and success: Comprehensive rehabilitation of traumatic brain injury. *Journal of Rehabilitation, 56*(1), 11-13.

Bittner, S. (1991). PAS from a teenage perspective. In J. Weissman, J. Kennedy, and S. Litvak (Eds.), *Personal perspectives on personal assistance services* (pp. 31-35). Oakland, CA: Research and Training Center on Public Policy and Independent Living, World Institute on Disability, InfoUse, and Western Public Health Consortium.

Bittner, S. (1993). Language: Bridge or barrier between cultures. In C.M. Wade (Ed.), *Range of motion: An anthology of disability poetry, prose and art* (pp. 22-24). Berkeley, CA: KIDS Project, Squeaky Wheels Press.

Blanch, A. (1992). *Proceedings of roundtable discussion of the use of involuntary interventions,* Washington, DC, October 1-2, 1992.

Blanchard, K. (1988). *The power of ethical management.* New York: Fawcett Crest.

Blank, M. (1992). *Leadership for collaboration: A national dialogue.* Washington, DC: The Institute for Educational Leadership.

Blatt, B. (1976). *Revolt of the idiots.* Glen Ridge, NJ: Exceptional Press.

Blatt, B., Bogdan, R., Biklen, D., and Taylor, S. (1977). From institution to community: A conversion model—Educational programming for the severely/ profoundly handicapped. In E. Sontag, J. Smith, and N. Certo (Eds.), *Educational programming for the severely and profoundly handicapped* (pp. 40-52). Reston, VA: Council for Exceptional Children.

Blatt, B. and Kaplan, F. (1974). *Christmas in Purgatory: A photographic essay on mental retardation.* Syracuse, NY: Human Policy Press.

Blum, H. (1974). *Planning for health: Development and application of social change theory.* New York: Human Science Press.

Blum, R.W., Garell, D., Hodgman, C., Jorrissen, T., Okinow, N., Orr, D., and Slap, G. (1993). Transitions from child-centered to adult-health care systems for adolescents with chronic conditions. *Journal of Adolescent Health, 14,* 570-576.

Bogdan, R. (1980, February). What does it mean when a person says, "I am not retarded"? *Education and Training of the Mentally Retarded, 15,* 74-79.

Bogdan, R. (1986). *It's a nice place to live: Professional foster homes and supervised apartments in Washington County, Vermont.* Syracuse, NY: Syracuse University, Center on Human Policy, Research and Training Center on Community Integration.

Bogdan, R. (1991). We care for our own: Georgia Citizen Advocacy. In S. Taylor, R. Bogdan, and J. Racino (Eds.), *Life in the community: Case studies of organizations supporting people with disabilities* (pp. 215-225). Baltimore, MD: Paul H. Brookes.

Bogdan, R. and Biklen, S. (1982). *Qualitative research for education: An introduction to theory and methods.* Boston: Allyn and Bacon.

Bogdan, R. and Knoll, J. (1988). The sociology of disability. In E.L. Meyen and T.M. Sktric (Eds.), *Exceptional children and youth: An introduction* (pp. 449-477). Denver, CO: Love Publishing Company.

Bogdan, R. and Ksander, M. (1980). Policy data as a social process: A qualitative approach to quantitative data. *Human Organization, 39*(4), 302-309.

Bogdan, R. and Lutfiyya, Z.M. (1992). Standing on its own: Qualitative research in special education. In S. Stainback, and W. Stainback (Eds.), *Controversial issues in special education* (pp. 243-251). Boston: Allyn and Bacon.

Bogdan, R. and Taylor, S. (nd). *Observing in institutions.* Syracuse, NY: Syracuse University, Center on Human Policy, School of Education.

Bogdan, R. and Taylor, S. (1982). *Inside out: The social meaning of mental retardation.* Toronto: University of Toronto Press.

Bogdan, R. and Taylor, S. (1987). Toward a sociology of acceptance: The other side of the study of deviance. *Social Policy, 18*(2), 34-39.

Bogdan, R. and Taylor, S. (1990). Looking at the bright side: A positive approach to qualitative policy and evaluation research. *Qualitative Sociology, 13*(2), 183-192.

Bogdan, R., Taylor, S., De Grandpre, B., and Haynes, S. (1974). Let them eat programs: Attendants' perspectives and programming on wards in state schools. *Journal of Health and Social Behavior, 15,* 142-151.

Boggs, E., Hanley-Maxwell, C., Lakin, K.C., and Bradley, V. (1988). Federal policy and legislation: Factors that have constrained and facilitated community integration. In L.W. Heal, J.I. Haney, and A.R. Novak Amado (Eds.), *Integration of developmentally disabled individuals in the community* (Second Edition) (pp. 245-271). Baltimore, MD: Paul H. Brookes.

Boles, S., Horner, R., and Bellamy, G. (1988). Implementing transition programs for supported living. In B. Ludlow, A. Turnbull and R. Luckasson (Eds.), *Transitions to adult life for people with mental retardation: Principles and practices* (pp. 101-117). Baltimore, MD: Paul H. Brookes.

Borthwick-Duffy, S., Widaman, K.F., Little, T., and Eyman, R. (1992). *Foster family care for persons with mental retardation*. Washington, DC: American Association on Mental Retardation.

Bowe, F. (1963). *Rehabilitation America: Toward independence for disabled and elderly people*. New York: Harper & Row.

Bowen, J. (1994). The power of self advocacy. In V. Bradley, J. Ashbaugh, and B. Blaney (Eds.), *Creating individual supports for people with developmental disabilities* (pp. 335-345). Baltimore, MD: Paul H. Brookes.

Bowes, G., Sinnema, G., Suris, J.C., and Buhlmann, U. (1995). Transition health services for youth with disabilities: A global perspective. *Journal of Adolescent Health Care, 17,* 23-31.

Boyjian, J. (1990). *Minnesota adult protection guide*. Minneapolis, MN: Department of Human Services.

Bradbury, K. and Downs, A. (Eds.) (1981). *Do housing allowances work?* Washington, DC: The Brookings Institution.

Braddock, D. (1977a). A national deinstitutionalization study. *State Government, 50*(4), 220-226.

Braddock, D. (1977b). *Opening closed doors: The deinstitutionalization of disabled individuals*. Reston, VA: The Council for Exceptional Children.

Braddock, D. (1985). *Federal financial assistance for mental retardation and developmental disabilties II: The modern era 1962-84*. Chicago: University of Illinois at Chicago, Institute for the Study of Developmental Disabilities, Evaluation and Public Policy Program.

Braddock, D. (1987). *Federal policy toward mental retardation and developmental disabilities*. Baltimore, MD: Paul H. Brookes.

Braddock, D., Bachelder, L., Hemp, R., and Fujiura, G. (1995). *The state of the states in developmental disabilities* (Fourth Edition.). Washington, DC: American Association on Mental Retardation.

Braddock, D., Fujiura, G., Hemp, R., Mitchell, D., and Bachelder, L. (1991). Current and future trends in state-operated mental retardation institutions in the United States. *American Journal of Mental Retardation, 95*(4), 451-462.

Braddock, D. and Heller, T. (1985). The closure of mental retardation institutions. *Mental Retardation, 23*(4), 156-176 and *23*(5), 222-229.

Braddock, D., Hemp, R., Fujiura, G., Bachelder, L., and Mitchell, D. (1990). *The state of the states in developmental disabilities*. Baltimore, MD: Paul H. Brookes.

Braddock, D. and Mitchell, D. (1992). *Residential services and developmental disabilities in the United States: A national survey of staff compensation, turnover and related issues*. Washington, DC: American Association on Mental Retardation.

Bradley, V. (1978). *Deinstitutionalization of developmentally disabled persons: A conceptual analysis guide.* Baltimore, MD: University Park Press.

Bradley, V. (1985). Implementation of court and consent decrees: Some current lessons. In R. Bruininks and K. C. Lakin (Eds.), *Living and learning in the least restrictive environment.* Baltimore, MD: Paul H. Brookes.

Bradley, V. (1986). *Rights and resources: The impact of litigation on the mental retardation system in Massachusetts.* Boston: Human Services Research Institute.

Bradley, V. and Bersani, H. (Eds.) (1990). *Quality assurance for individuals with developmental disabilities* (pp. 345-354). Baltimore, MD: Paul H. Brookes.

Bradley, V. and Knoll, J. (1993). Shifting paradigms in services to people with developmental disabilities. In O. Karan, and S. Greenspan (Eds.), *New direction in community support for people with a disability.* Andover.

Bradley, V and Knoll, J. (1995). Shifting paradigms in services to people with developmental disabilities. In O. Karan and S. Greenspan, *Community rehabilitation services for people with disabilities* (pp. 5-19). Boston: Butterwork-Heinemann. Press.

Bradley, V., Knoll, J., and Agosta, J. (1992). *Emerging issues in family support.* Washington, DC: American Association on Mental Retardation.

Bragg, R., Klockars, A., and Berninger, V. (1992). Comparison of families with and without adolescents with traumatic brain injury. *Journal of Head Trauma Rehabilitation, 7*(3), 94-108.

Braisby, D., Echlin, R., Hill, S., and Smith, H. (1988). *Changing futures: Housing and support services for people discharged from psychiatric hospitals (Project paper #76).* London: King Edwards' Hospital Fund.

Brandon, D. and Economu, B.C. (1973). State housing programs. In D.J. Reeb and J. T. Kirk Jr. (Eds.), *Housing the poor* (pp. 72-85). New York: Praeger.

Braun, P., Kochansky, G., Shapiro, R., Greenberg, S., Gudeman, J., Johnson, S., and Shore, M. (1981). Overview: Deinstitutionalization of psychiatric patients, a critical review of outcome studies. *American Journal of Psychiatry, 138*(6), 736-749.

Brightman, A. (1985). *Ordinary moments: The disabled experience.* Syracuse, NY: Human Policy Press.

Bronfenbrenner, U. (1974). Developmental research, public policy and the ecology of childhood. *Child Development, 45,* 1-5.

Bronfenbrenner, U. (1979). Childrens' institutions as contexts of human development. In U. Bronfenbrenner (Ed.), *The ecology of human development* (pp. 132-163). Cambridge, MA: Harvard University Press.

Bronfenbrenner, U. (1986). Ecology of the family as a context for human development: Research perspectives. *Developmental Psychology, 22*(6), 723-742.

Brooke, V., Barcus, M., and Inge, K. (1992, May). *Consumer advocacy and supported employment: A vision for the future.* Richmond, VA: Virginia Commonwealth University, Research and Training Center on Supported Employment.

Brooks-Gunn, J., Duncan, G., Klebanov, P.K., and Seland, N. (1993). Do neighborhoods influence child and adolescent development? *American Journal of Sociology, 99*(2), 353-395.

Brophy, B. (1991, July). Things change: Final chapter for Laconia. *TASH Newsletter, 17*(4), 1-2.

Brost, T. and Johnson, T. (1982). *Getting to know you: One approach to service assessment and planning for individuals with disabilities.* Madison, WI: DHSS-DCS.

Browder, J., Ellis, L., and Neal, J. (1974, December). Foster homes: Alternatives to institutions? *Mental Retardation, 12*(6), 33-36.

Brown, L., Pumpian, I., Baumgarat, D., Van Deventer, P., Ford, A., Nisbet, J., Schroeder, J., and Gruenwald, L. (1981). Longitudinal transition plans in programs for severely handicapped students. *Exceptional Children, 47*, 624-631.

Bruininks, R. (1990). There is more than a zipcode to changes in services. *American Journal on Mental Retardation, 95*(1), 13-15.

Bruininks, R., Thurlow, M., Thurman, S. Kenneth, and Fiorelli, J. (1980). Deinstitutionalization and community services. In J. Wortis (Ed.), *Mental retardation and developmental disabilities: An annual review* (Volume XI, pp. 55-101). New York: Brunner/Mazel.

Brunk, G. (1991). *Supporting the growth of the self advocacy movement: What we can learn from its history and activists.* Lawrence, KS: University of Kansas, Beach Center on Families and Disability.

Bruyere, S. (1993). Participatory action research: Overview and implications for family members of persons with disabilities. *Journal of Vocational Rehabilitation, 3*(2), 62-68.

Bruyn, S.T. (1966). *The human perspective in sociology: The method of participation observation.* Englewood Cliffs, NJ: Prentice-Hall.

Buchanan, R. and Alston, R. (1997). Medicaid policies and home health care provisions for persons with disabilities. *Journal of Rehabilitation, 63*(3), 20-34.

Budde, J. and Bachelder, J. (1986). Independent living: The concepts of the model and methodology. *Journal of the Association of Persons with Severe Handicaps, 11*(4), 240-245.

Bulmer, M. (1987). Interweaving formal and informal care. In M. Bulmer (Ed.), *The social basis of community care* (pp. 172-209). Winchester, MA: Allen and Unwin, Inc.

Burd, L., Randall, T., Martsolf, J. T., and Kerbeshian, J. (1991). Rett's syndrome symptomology of institutionalized adults with mental retardation: Comparison of males and females. *American Journal of Mental Retardation, 95*(5), 596-601.

Burke, W., Wesolowski, M., Buyer, D., and Zawlocki, R. (1989). The rehabilitation of adolescents with traumatic brain injury: Outcome and followup. *Brain Injury, 4*(4), 371-378.

Burkhauser, R. (1991). United States public policy and the elderly: The disproportionate risk to the well-being of women. *Journal of Population Economics, 4,* 217-221.

Burkhauser, R.V., Haveman, R.H., and Wolfe, B. (1993). How people with disabilities fare when public policies change. *Journal of Policy Analysis and Management, 12*(2), 251-269.

Callahan, M. J. and Garner, J. B. (1997). *Keys to the workplace: Skills and supports for people with disabilities.* Baltimore, MD: Paul H. Brookes.

Calvez, M. (1993). Social interactions in the neighborhood: Cultural approach to social integration of individuals with mental retardation. *Mental Retardation, 31*(6), 418-423.

Campbell, D.T. and Stanley, J.C. (1963). *Experimental and quasi-experimental designs for research.* Chicago: Rand McNally College Publishing.

Canadian Association for Community Living (1990, Summer). Self-advocate elected President. *Newsbreak,* p. 2.

Carabello, B. and Siegel, J.F. (1996). Self-advocacy at the crossroads. In G. Dybwad and H. Bersani (Eds.), *New voices: Self-advocacy by people with disabilities* (pp. 237-239). Cambridge, MA: Brookline Books.

Carling, P. (1984, October). *Developing family foster care programs in mental health: A resource guide.* Rockville, MD: National Institute on Mental Health.

Carling, P. (1993). Housing and supports for persons with mental illness: Emerging approaches to research and practice. *Hospital and Community Psychiatry, 44*(5), 439-449.

Carling, P. (1995). *Return to community: Building supports for people with psychiatric disabilities.* New York: Guilford Press.

Carling, P.J., Randolph, F.L., Blanch, A.K., and Ridgway, P. (1988). A review of the research on housing and community integration for people with psychiatric disabilities. *NARIC Quarterly, 1*(3), 1, 6-18.

Carmody, K. (1994). Creating individual supports for people moving out of nursing facilities: Supported placements in integrated community environments (SPICE). In V. Bradley, J. Ashbaugh, and B. Blaney (Eds.), *Creating individual supports for people with developmental disabilities* (pp. 465-479). Baltimore, MD: Paul H. Brookes.

Caro, F. and McKaig, F. (1987). *Family partnership program: The first year experience.* New York: Community Service Society of New York.

Carrier, J. (1992, December). Gatekeepers of the Himalaya: Nepal's Sherpa people prosper amid dizzying change as climbers and trekkers descend upon their mountain home. *National Geographic, 182*(6), 70-89.

Casswell, S. and Gilmore, L. (1989). An evaluated community action project on alcohol. *Journal of Studies on Alcohol, 50*(4), 339-347.

Castellani, P., Bird, W., and Manning, B. (1993). *Supporting individuals with developmental disabilities in the community.* Albany, NY: New York State Office of Mental Retardation and Developmental Disabilities.

Castellani, P., Downey, N.A., Tausig, M., and Bird, W.A. (1986). Availability and accessibility of family support services. *Mental Retardation, 24,* 71-79.

Center for Community Change through Housing and Support (1990, August). *National evaluation of National Institute for Mental Health Housing Demonstration Project.* Burlington, VT: University of Vermont, Department of Psychology.

Center on Human Policy (1979). *The community imperative: A refutation of all arguments in support of institutionalizing anyone because of mental retardation.* Syracuse, NY: Syracuse University, Center on Human Policy.

Center on Human Policy (1985-1992). *Site visits to technical assistance sites in the United States.* Syracuse, NY: Syracuse University, Center on Human Policy, Community Integration Project and RTC on Community Integration.

Center on Human Policy (1987). *A statement in support of children and their families.* Syracuse, NY: Syracuse University, Center on Human Policy.

Center on Human Policy (1989a). *A statement in support of adults living in the community.* Syracuse, NY: Syracuse University, Center on Human Policy.

Center on Human Policy (1989b). *Housing and support strategies: Practices and strategies—A proposal for a Research and Training Center on Community Integration.* Syracuse, NY: Syracuse University, Center on Human Policy.

Center on Human Policy (1991). *Organizational field guide* (revised, 1986). Syracuse, NY: Syracuse University, Center on Human Policy.

Central New York Traumatic Brain Injury Coalition (1994). *Mission statement.* Syracuse, NY: Author.

Centre for Research and Education in Human Services (1983). *Closing institutions: Implications for policy development, human services and community planning—The case of Ontario.* Kitchener, Ontario: Author.

Chamberlin, J. (1978). *On my own.* New York: McGraw-Hill.

Chamberlin, J. (1990). The ex-patients' movement: Where we've been and where we are going. *The Journal of Mind and Behavior, II(3-4),* 323(77)-336 (90).

Chamberlin, J. (1992, Summer). Psychiatric survivors and other disabilities. In A. Enders (Ed.), Special Issue: The politics of disability. *Disability Studies Quarterly, 12*(3), 24-27.

Chamberlin, J. and Rogers, J. (1990). Planning a community mental health system: Perspectives of service recipients. *American Psychologist, 45*(11), 1241-1244.

Chamberlin, J. and Unzicker, R. (1991). Psychiatric survivors, expatients and users: An observation of organizations in Holland and England. *IDEAS Portfolio II,* 3-5.

Chamberlin, P. (1990, Fall). Comparative evaluation of specialized foster care for seriously delinquent youth: A first step. *Community Alternatives: International Journal of Family Care, 2*(2), 21-36.

Chamberlin, P. and Reid, J. (1991, July). Using a specialized foster care community treatment model for children and adolescents leaving the state mental hospital. *Journal of Community Psychology, 19,* 266-276.

Chambler, N., Beverly, C., and Beck, C.K. (1997). Rural older adults' likelihood of receiving a personal response system: The Arkansas Medicaid waiver program. *Evaluation and Program Planning, 20*(2), 117-127.

Chelimsky, E. (1995, Fall). Preamble: New dimensions in evaluations. In R. Picciotto and R.C. Crist (Eds.) *New directions for evaluation* (pp. 3-23). San Francisco, CA: Jossey-Bass Publishers.

Child Welfare League of America (1989a). *Standards for independent living.* Washington, DC: Author.

Child Welfare League of America (1989b). *Standards for services to strengthen and preserve families with children.* Washington, DC: Author.

Child Welfare League of America (1993). *Independent living services for youth in out-of-home care.* Washington, DC: Author.

Children's Defense Fund (1992). *The state of America's children.* Washington, DC: Author.

Christian, G. and Whitmer, J. (1988, July). *Foster care in Idaho and twelve other states.* Boise, Idaho: Idaho State Council on Developmental Disabilities.

Christiansen, C., Schwartz, R., and Barnes, K. (1993). Self care: Evaluation and management. In J. DeLisa and B. Gans (Eds.), *Rehabilitation medicine: Principles and practices* (pp. 178-200). Philadelphia, PA: Lippincott.

Clark, H. B. and Foster-Johnson, L. (1996). Serving youth in transition to adulthood. In B. Stroul (Ed.), *Children's mental health* (pp. 533-551). Baltimore, MD: Paul H. Brookes.

Cline, D.H. (1990, May). A legal analysis of policy initiatives to exclude handicapped/disruptive students from special education. *Behavioral Disorders, 15*(3), 159-173.

Coalition for the Closure of the Syracuse Developmental Center (1989, November). *Community for all: Closure of the Syracuse Developmental Center.* Syracuse, NY: Author.

Cobb, S. (1976). Social support as a moderator of life stress. *Psychosomatic Medicine, 38,* 300-310.

Cochran, M. (1990a). *Extending families: The social networks of parents and their children.* New York: Cambridge University Press.

Cochran, M. (1990b). The transforming role. *Networking Bulletin: Empowerment and Family Support, 1*(3), 25.

Cochran, M. (Ed.) (1991). Evaluation and the empowerment process (Topical issue). *Networking Bulletin: Empowerment and Family Support, 2*(2).

Cohen, S. and Warren, R. (1985). *Respite care: Principles, programs and policies.* Austin, Texas: PRO-ED, Inc.

Coleman, J. (1973). Conflicting theories of social change. In G. Zaltman (Ed.), *Processes and phenomenon of social change* (pp. 61-74). New York: John Wiley and Sons, Inc.

Coleman, J.C. (1980). *The nature of adolescence.* London: Metheun.

Colligan, F. (1986). The role of reasonable accommodation in employing disabled persons in private industries. In M. Berkowitz and M. Hill, *Disability and the labor market.* Itaca, NY: Cornell University.

Commission on the Accreditation of Rehabilitation Facilities (1985). *Standards manual for facilities serving people with disabilities.* Tucson, AZ: Author.

Commission on the Mentally Disabled, Commission of the Elderly and American Bar Association (1989). *Guardianship: An agenda for reform.* Washington, DC: Authors.

Complair, P.S., Kreutzer, J.S., and Doherty, K.S. (1991). Family outcome following adult traumatic brain injury: A critical review of the literature. In J. Kreutzer and P. Wehman (Eds.), *Community integration following traumatic brain injury* (pp. 207-233). Baltimore, MD: Paul H. Brookes.

Condeluci, A. (1991). *Interdependence: The route to community.* Orlando, FL: PMD Press.

Condeluci, A. (1996). *Beyond difference.* Delray Beach, FL: Lucie Press, Inc.

Condeluci, A., Ferris, L., and Bogdan, A. (1992). Outcome and value: The survivor perspective. *Journal of Head Trauma Rehabilitation, 7*(4), 37-45.

Cone, A. (1998). Self advocacy in the United States: Historical overview and future vision. In P. Wehman and J. Kregel (Eds.), *More than a job: Securing satisfying careers for people with disabilities* (pp. 25-45). Baltimore, MD: Paul H. Brookes.

Congressional Research Service (1993). *Medicaid source background: Background data and analysis.* Washington, DC: Author.

Congressional Review (1990). The 101st Congress in review. *Word from Washington.* Washington, DC: United Cerebral Palsy Associations, Governmental Affairs Office.

Conroy, J. and Bradley, V. (1985). *The Pennhurst longitudinal study: A report of five years of research and analysis.* Philadelphia, PA: Temple University, Developmental Disabilities Center.

Consortium of Citizens with Disabilities (1991). *Recommended federal policy directions on personal assistance services for Americans with disabilities.* Washington, DC: CD Personal Assistance Task Force, CCD.

Consortium of Citizens with Disabilities (1992). *Report of a housing task force.* Washington, DC: CD, Housing Task Force.

Cook, J. (1992). *Outcome assessment in psychiatric rehabilitation services for persons with severe and persistent mental illness.* Chicago, IL: Thresholds National Research and Training Center on Rehabilitation and Mental Illness.

Cook, J., Lefley, H., Pickett, S., and Cohler, B. (1994, July). Age and family burden among parents of offspring with severe mental illness. *American Journal of Orthopsychiatry, 64*(3), 435-447.

Cooley, E.A., Glang, A., and Voss, J. (1997). Making connections: Helping children with ABI build friendships. In A. Glang, G.H. Singer, and B. Todis (Eds.), *Students with acquired brain injury* (pp. 255-275). Baltimore, MD: Paul H. Brookes.

Copeland, A. and White, K. (1991). *Studying families. Applied social research methods series* (Volume 27). Newbury Park, CA: Sage Publications.

Corrigan, P. and Garmon, A. (1997). Considerations for research on consumer empowerment and psychosocial interventions. *Psychiatric Services, 48*(3), 347-352.

Covert, S. (1992). Supporting families. In J. Nisbet (Ed.), *Natural supports in school, at work and in the community for people with severe disabilities* (pp. 121-163). Baltimore, MD: Paul H. Brookes.

Covert, S., MacIntosh, J., and Shumway, D. (1994). Closing the Laconia State School and Training Center: A case study of systems change. In V. Bradley, J. Ashbaugh, and B. Blaney (Eds.), *Creating individual supports for people with developmental disabilities* (pp. 197-211). Baltimore, MD: Paul H. Brookes.

Craig, T., Peer, S., and Ross, M. (1987). Psychiatric rehabilitation in a state hospital transitional residence: The cottage program at Greystone Park Psychiatric Hospital, Greystone Park, New Jersey. In M. Farkas and W.A. Anthony (Eds.), *Psychiatric rehabilitation programs: Putting theory into practice* (pp. 57-80). Baltimore, MD: Johns Hopkins University Press.

Cress, D.M. (1997). Non-profit incorporation among movements of the poor: Pathways and consequences for homeless social movement organizations. *The Sociological Quarterly, 38*(2), 343-360.

Crisp, R. (1992). Return to work after traumatic brain injury. *Journal of Rehabilitation, 58*(4), 27-33.

Crittiden, P. (1990). Toward a concept of autonomy in adolescents with a disability. *Children's Health Care, 19*(3), 162-168.

Crossmaker, M. and Merry, D. (1990). *Stigma, stereotypes and scapegoats.* Columbus, OH: Ohio Legal Rights Service.

Crowley, J. and Miles, M. (1991). Cognitive remediation in pediatric head injury: A case study. *Journal of Pediatric Psychology, 16*(5), 611-627.

Cunningham, M. with Schumer, F. (1984). *Powerplay: What really happened at Bendix.* NY: Fawcett Gold Medal.

Cuomo, M. (1994). *The New York idea: An experiment in democracy.* New York: Random House, Inc.

Danielson, L. and Bellamy, G.T. (1989). State variation in placement of children with handicaps in segregated environments. *Exceptional Children, 55*(5), 448-455.

Danzy, J. and Jackson, S. (1997). Family preservation and support services: A missed opportunity for kinship care. *Child Welfare, LXXXVI,* 31-44.

Davidson, P.W. and Fifield, M.G. (1992). Quality assurance and impact measurement of university-affiliated programs. *Mental Retardation, 30*(4), 205-213.

Davis, P. and May, J. (1991). Involving fathers in early intervention and family support programs: Issues and strategies. *Children's Health Care, 20*(2), 87-92.

Davis, S. and Berkobien, R. (1994, August). *Meeting the needs and challenges of at-risk, two generation, elderly families.* Arlington, TX: The ARC.

DeBuono, B. and Glass, M.E. (1985). *A proposal for reforming the New York State Medicaid Program.* Albany, NY: New York State Department of Health and New York State Department of Social Services.

Deegan, P. (1988). Recovery: The lived experience of rehabilitation. *Psychosocial Rehabilitation Journal, 11*(4), 11-19.

Deegan, P. (1992). The independent living movement and people with psychiatric disabilities: Taking back control of our own lives. *Psychosocial Rehabilitation Journal, 15*(3), 3-19.

DeJong, G. (1978). *The movement for independent living: Origins, ideology, and implications for disability research.* Boston: Tufts-New England Medical Center, Medical Rehabilitation Institute.

DeJong, G. (1979). Independent living: From social movement to analytic paradigm. *Archives of Physical Medicine and Rehabilitation, 60,* 435-446.

DeJong, G. (1983). Defining and implementing the independent living concept. In N. Crewe and I. Zola (Eds.), *Independent living for physically disabled people* (pp. 4-27). San Francisco, CA: Jossey-Bass.

DeJong, G., Batavia, A., and McKnew, L. (1992). The independent living model of personal assistance in national long-term care policy. *Generations, 16*(1), 89-95.

DeJong, G., Branch, L., and Corcoran, P. (1984). Independent living outcomes in spinal cord injury: Multivariate analysis. *Archives of Physical Medicine and Rehabilitation, 65,* 66-73.

DeJong, G. and Hughes, J. (1982). Independent living: Methodology for measuring long-term outcomes. *Archives of Physical Medicine, 63,* 68-73.

DeJong, G. and Lifchez, R. (1983). Physical disability and public policy. *Scientific American, 248*(6), 40-49.

DeJong, G. and Wenker, T. (1983). Attendant care. In N.M. Crewe and I. Zola (Eds.), *Independent living for physically disabled people* (pp. 157-170). San Francisco, CA: Jossey-Bass.

Dencker, K. and Gottfries, C. (1990). The closure of a mental hospital in Sweden: Characteristics of patients in long-term care facing relocation in the community. *European Archives of Psychiatry and Neuroscience, 240,* 325-330.

Denzin, N. (1997). *Interpretive ethnography: Ethnographic practices for the 21st Century.* London: Sage.

Denzin, N.Z. and Lincoln, Y.S. (1994). *Handbook of qualitative research.* Thousand Oaks, CA: Sage.

De Paiva, S. and Lowe, K. (1986). *Patterns of service useage and degree of satisfaction amongst consumers of services for people with mental handicaps.* Cardiff, Wales: The Mental Handicap in Wales Applied Research Unit.

Dickenson, M. (1987). *Thumbs up: The life and courageous comeback of White House Press Secretary Jim Brady.* New York: Morrow.

Diehl, S., Moffitt, K., and Wade, S. (1991). Focus group interviews with parents of children with medically complex needs: An intimate look at their perceptions and feelings. *Children's Health Care, 20*(3), 150-161.

Dilworth-Andersen, P., Burton, L., and Turner, W. (1993, July). The importance of values in the study of culturally diverse families. *Family Relations, 42,* 238-242.

Dion, G. and Anthony, W. (1987). Research in psychiatric rehabilitation: A review of experimental and quasi-experimental studies. *Rehabilitation Counseling Bulletin, 30,* 177-203.

DiStaso, J. (1990). NH mental health system leads U.S. *The Union Leader,* (Manchester, NH), December 17, pp. 1, 5.

Divers, C.S. (1979). The judge as political powerbroker: Superintending structural changes in public institutions. *Virginia Law Review, 65,* 43-106.

Doherty, J., Braun, W., Kelly, L., and Libman, R. (1984, July). *Residential services implementation plan for developmentally disabled and chronically mentally ill persons: 1985-1987.* Milwaukee, WI: Milwaukee County Combined Community Services Board, Housing and Residential Services Committee.

Doty, P., Kasper, J. and Litvak, S. (1996). "Consumer-directed models" of personal care: Lessons from Medicaid. *Milbank Quarterly, 74*(3), 377-409.

Drucker, P.F. (1995). *Managing a time of great change.* New York: Truman Talley Books/Dutton.

Dryfoos, J. (1991). Adolescents at risk: A summation of work in the field—Programs and policies. *Journal of Adolescent Health Care, 12,* 630-637.

Duchonowski, A. and Friedman, R. (1990). Children's mental health: Challenges for the 90s. *Journal of Mental Health Administration, 17*(1), 3-12.

Dunst, C. and Trivette, C.M. (1989). An enablement and empowerment perspective on casemanagement. *Topics in Early Childhood Special Education: Families in Special Education, 8*(4), 87-102.

Dvoskin, J. and Steadman, H. (1994, July). Using intensive case management to reduce violence by mentally ill persons in the community. *Hospital and Community Psychiatry, 45*(7), 679-684.

Dybwad, G. (1989, March). Empowerment means power sharing. *International TASH Newsletter, 5,* 8.

Dybwad, G. and Bersani, H. (1996). *New voices: Self advocacy by people with disabilities.* Cambridge, MA: Brookline Books.

Dybwad, R. (1990). *Perspectives on a parent movement: The result of parents of children with intellectual disabilities.* Brookline, MA: Brookline Books.

Ebert, G. (1990). *Panel presentation on "What are the meaning, characteristics and dimensions of support?"* Policy Institute on Support, sponsored by the Center on Human Policy, Syracuse University.

Edgerton, R.B. (1979). *Mental retardation.* Cambridge, MA: Harvard University Press.

Edgerton, R.B. (1988). Aging in the community: A matter of choice. *American Journal on Mental Retardation, 92,* 331-335.

Edinger, B., Schultz, B., and Morse, M. (1984). Final report: Issues relevant to respite services for people with a developmental disability. Part One: The research. In J. Racino (Ed.), *Final report of the Respite Project of CNY.* Syracuse, NY: Respite Project of Central New York, Transitional Living Services, and Syracuse Developmental Services Office.

Egley, L. (1994). *Program models providing personal assistance services (PAS) for independent living* (Table 1). Oakland, CA: World Institute on Disability.

Ellis, J.W. (1988). Residential placement of "dual diagnosis" clients: Emerging legal issues. In J.A. Stark, F. J. Menolascino, M.H. Albarelli, and V.C. Gray

(Eds.), *Mental retardation and mental health: Classification, diagnosis, treatment and services* (pp. 326-337). New York: Springer-Verlag.

Enders, A. (1990). Funding for assistive technology and related services: An annotated bibliography. *Physical and Occupational Therapy in Pediatrics, 10(2),* 147-173.

England, S., Linsk, N., Simon-Rusinowitz, L., and Keigher, S. (1990). Paid family caregiving and market view of home care: Agency perspectives. *Journal of Health and Social Policy, 1*(2), 31-53.

English, D. (1993). Research in a public welfare agency: Integrating research and practice. In C. Liberton, K. Kutash, and R.M. Friedman (Eds.), *A system of care for children's mental health: Expanding the research base* (pp. 321-324). Tampa, FL: University of Florida, Research and Training Center for Children's Mental Health, Florida Mental Health Institute.

Erikson, E. (1965). *The challenge of youth.* Garden City, NJ: Doubleday and Company, Inc.

Estroff, N. (1981). *Making it crazy.* Berkeley, CA: University of California Press.

Etzioni, A. (1961). *Complex organizations: A sociological reader.* New York: Holt, Reinhart and Winston, Inc.

Etzioni, A. (1993). *The spirit of community: Rights, responsibilities, and communitarian agenda.* New York: Crown Publishers, Inc.

Eustis, N., Kane, R., and Fischer, L. (1993). Home care quality and the home care workers: Beyond quality assurance as usual. *The Gerontologist, 33*(1), 64-73.

Evans, B., Martinez, C., and Hopkins, T. (1991). PAS for people with cognitive disabilities. In J. Weissman, J. Kennedy, and S. Litvak (Eds.), *Personal perspectives on personal assistance services* (pp. 43-51). Oakland, CA: Research and Training Center on Public Policy in Independent Living, World Institute on Disability, InfoUse, and Western Consortium for Public Health.

Everett, B. and Boydell, K. (1994). A methodology for including consumer opinions in mental health evaluation research. *Hospital and Community Psychiatry, 45*(1), 76-77.

Everett, T. H. and Collignon, F.C. (1975). Transportation. In *Cost and policy considerations in improving the capacity for independent living of the most severely handicapped* (pp. 11-53). Berkeley, CA: Berkeley Planning Associates.

Everitt, A. (1989). The new Swedish guardianship law. In K. Grunewald (Ed.), *Current Sweden* (pp. 1-6). Unpublished papers. Stockholm, Sweden: Svenska Institute.

Fanning, R., Judge, J., Weihe, F., and Emener, W. (1991). Housing needs of individuals with severe mobility impairments: A case study. *Journal of Rehabilitation, 57,* April/May/June, 7-13.

Farkas, M. and Anthony, W.A. (1987). Outcome analysis in psychiatric rehabilitation. In M.J. Fuhrer (Ed.), *Rehabilitation outcomes: Analysis and measurement* (pp. 43-69). Baltimore, MD: Paul H. Brookes.

Fay, G., Jaffe, K., Polissar, N., and Liao, S. (1993, September). Mild pediatric traumatic brain injury: A cohort study. *Archives of Physical Medicine, 74,* 895-901.

Felce, D. (1988). Evaluating the extent of community integration following the provision of staffed residential alternatives to institutional care. *The Irish Journal of Psychology, 9*(2), 346-360.

Felce, D. (1989). *Staffed housing for adults with severe or profound mental handicaps: The Andover Project—Summary report of a Department of Health and Social Security funded project.* Kidderminster, UK: BIMH Publications.

Feldman, M. (1994). Parents with intellectual disabilities. *Network News, New Zealand, 4*(1), 41-47.

Ferguson, D. (1986). *Site visit report: Boise Group Homes.* Syracuse, NY: Syracuse University, Center on Human Policy, Community Integration Project.

Ferguson, D. and Ferguson, P. (1986). The New Victors: A progressive policy analysis of work reform for people with severe handicaps. *Mental Retardation, 24*(6), 331-338.

Ferguson, D.L., Ferguson, P., and Bogdan, R. (1987). If mainstreaming is the answer, what is the question? In V. Richardson-Koehler (Ed.), *Educator's handbook: A research perspective* (pp. 394-419). New York: Longnen.

Ferguson, D., Ferguson, P., and Taylor, S. (1992). *Interpreting disability.* New York: Teachers College Press.

Ferguson, P. and Ferguson, D. (1993). The promise of adulthood. In M. Snell (Ed.), *Systematic instruction of persons with severe disabilities* (pp. 588-607). Columbus, OH: Charles E. Merrill.

Ferguson, P.M., Ferguson, D., and Taylor, S. (1992). The future of interpretivism in disability studies. In P.M. Ferguson, D. Ferguson, and S. Taylor (Eds.), *Interpreting disability: A qualitative reader* (pp. 295-302). New York: Teachers College Press.

Fields, T., Lakin, K.C., Seltzer, B., and Wobschall, R. (1995, September). *A guidebook on consumer controlled housing for Minnesotans with developmental disabilities.* Minneapolis, MN: ARC of Minnesota and the Research and Training Center on Residential Services and Community Living, College of Education and Human Development, University of Minnesota.

Fink, A., Kosecoff, J., Chassin, M., and Brook, R.H. (1984). Consensus methods: Characteristics and guidelines for use. *American Journal of Public Health, 74*(9), 979-983.

Flanagan, S.A. and Green, P. (1997, October). *Consumer-directed personal assistance services: Key operational issues for state CD-PAS programs using intermediary service organizations.* Appendixes. Cambridge, MA: The Medstat Group.

Flippo, K., Inge, K., and Barcus, M. (1995). *Assistive technology: A resource for school, work, and community.* Baltimore, MD: Paul H. Brookes.

Floden, R. and Weiner, S. (1982). Rationality to ritual: The multiple roles of evaluation in governmental processes. In F. Leyden and E. Miller (Eds.),

Public budgeting: Program planning and implementation (pp. 366-377). Englewood Cliffs, NJ: Prentice-Hall.

Florio, D.H., Behrmann, M., and Goltz, D.L. (1979). What do policymakers think of educational research and evaluation? Or do they? *Educational Evaluation and Policy Analysis, 1,* 61-87.

Flower, C.D. (1994). Legal guardianship: The implications of law, procedure, and policy for the lives of people with developmental disabilities. In M. Hayden, and B. Abery (Eds.), *Challenges for a service system in transition* (pp. 427-447). Baltimore, MD: Paul H. Brookes.

Flynn, M. (1989a). *An overview of Barnardo residential services for young people with a handicap.* Barkingside, UK: Barnardo's Research and Development Section, Child Care Department.

Flynn, M. (1989b). The social environment. In A. Brechinn, and J. Walmsley (Eds.), *Making connections.* Toronto: Open University.

Flynn, R.J., LaPointe, N., Wolfensberger, W., and Thomas, S. (1991). Quality of institutional and community human service programs in Canada and the United States. *Journal of Psychiatry and Neurosciences, 16*(3), 146-153.

Ford, M. (1991). Personal assistance services for people with mental retardation: One person's perspectives. In J. Weissman, J. Kennedy, and S. Litvak (Eds.), *Personal perspectives on personal assistance services* (pp. 15-18). Oakland, CA: Research and Training Center on Public Policy in Independent Living, World Institute on Disability, InfoUse, Western Consortium for Public Health.

Forest, M. (1991). It's about relationships. In L.H. Meyer, C.A. Peck, and L. Brown (Eds.), *Critical issues in the lives of people with severe disabilities* (pp. 399-407). Baltimore, MD: Paul H. Brookes.

Foster, P.M. (1976). The theory and practice of action research in work organizations. In A.W. Clark (Ed.), *Experimenting with organizational life: The action research approach* (pp. 59-75). New York: Plenum Press.

Fratangelo, P. (1994, March). Creating supports based on the person versus the organization: The story of an organizational change. *The TASH Newsletter, 20*(3), 1-6.

Freedman, R. and Fesko, S. (1996, July-September). The meaning of work in the lives of people with significant disabilities: Consumer and family perspectives. *Journal of Rehabilitation, 62*(3), 49-55.

Freeman, H.E. and Solomon, M. (1979). The next decade in evaluation research. *Evaluation and Program Planning, 2,* 255-262.

Frieden, L. and Nosek, M. (1985). *The efficacy of the independent living program model based on descriptive and evaluative studies.* Washington, DC: D:ATA Institute.

Friedenberg, E. (1959). *The vanishing adolescent.* New York: Dell Publishing Company.

Friedman, H. (1993). Promoting the health of adolescents in the USA: A global perspective. *Journal of Adolescent Health Care, 14,* 509-519.

Friedman, J. and Weinberg, D.H. (1982). *The economics of housing vouchers.* New York: Academic Press.

Friedman, R. (1988, January). *The role of therapeutic foster care in an overall system of care: Issues in service delivery and program evaluation.* Tampa, FL: University of South Florida, Research and Training Center for Children's Mental Health.

Friedman, R. (1994). Restructuring of systems to emphasize prevention and family support. *Journal of Clinical Child Psychology, 23* (Suppl.), 40-47.

Friedman, R.M., Kutash, K., and Duchnowski, A. (1996). The population of concern: Defining the issues. In B. Stroul (Ed.), *Children's mental health* (pp. 69-96). Baltimore, MD: Paul H. Brookes.

Friesen, B. (1993). *Family support in child and adult mental health.* Portland, OR: Research and Training Center on Family Support and Children's Mental Health, Portland State University.

Furman, M. (1987, September). *The Madison Mutual Housing Cooperative: Resident handbook.* Madison, WI: Madison Mutual Housing Association.

Gallant, R. (1993). People with disabilities need buses on nights and weekend. *The Concord Monitor,* April 13, p. B6.

Gannon, J. and Burke, E. (1994, September). The National Council on Disability: Recommendations for the Reauthorization of the Individuals with Disabilities Education Act. *TASH Newsletter, 20*(9), 8-9.

Gans, H.J. (1962). *The urban villagers: Group and class in the life of Italian-Americans.* New York: The Free Press.

Garbarino, J. and Sherman, D. (1980). High-risk neighborhoods and high-risk families: The human ecology of child maltreatment. *Child Development, 51,* 188-198.

Gardner, J.F. (1986). Implementation of the home and community-based waiver. *Mental Retardation, 24*(1), 18-26.

Gardner, J., Chapman, M.S., Donaldson, G., and Jacobsen, S.G. (1988). *Toward supported employment: A process guide for planned change.* Baltimore, MD: Paul H. Brookes.

Gardner, J. and Parsons, C. (1990). Accreditation as synthesis. In V. Bradley and H. Bersani (Eds.), *Quality assurance for individuals with developmental disabilities* (pp. 207-220). Baltimore, MD: Paul H. Brookes.

Garrity v. Gallen, 522F, Supp.171 (D.N.H. 1981) aff'd sub.nom. *Garrity v. Sununu,* 697F. ad 452 (1st Cir. 1983) and 752F. ad 272 (1st Cir. 1984).

Gartner, A., Lipsky, D., and Turnbull, A. (1991). *Supporting families with a child with a disability: An international outlook.* Baltimore, MD: Paul H. Brookes.

Gavazzi, S., Alford, K., and McHenry, P. (1996). Culturally specific programs for foster care youth: The sample of African-American rites of passage program, *Family Relations, 45,* 166-174.

General Accounting Office (1993). *Health care: Rochester's community approach yields better access, lower costs.* Washington, DC: Author

Gerry, M.H. and McWhorter, C. (1991). A comprehensive analysis of federal statutes and programs for persons with severe disabilities. In: L.H. Meyer, C.A. Peck, and L. Brown (Eds.), *Critical issues in the lives of people with severe disabilities* (p. 495-525). Baltimore, MD: Paul H. Brookes.

Gettings, R. (1977). Hidden impediments to deinstitutionalization. *State Government, 50*(4), 214-219.

Gettings, R. (1994). The link between public financing and systemic change. In V.J. Bradley, J. W. Ashbaugh, and B. C. Blaney (Eds.), *Creating individual supports for people with developmental disabilities* (pp. 155-170). Baltimore, MD: Paul H. Brookes.

Gettings, R. (1995). Supported employment and the Medicaid home and community-based waiver authority: Current status and unresolved issues. *Journal of Vocational Rehabilitation, 5*(3), 249-254.

Gilgun, J. (1994, July)., A case for case studies in social work research. *Social Work, 39*(4), 371-380.

Gillis, L.S., Koch, A., and Joyi, M. (1989). The value and cost effectiveness of a home-visiting programme for psychiatric patients. *South Africa Medical Journal, 77,* 309-310.

Gilman, B., Spangler, P., and Meadows, S. (1990). Residential placement of individuals with mental retardation: Factors influencing court decisions. *Mental Retardation, 28*(4), 241-244.

Gitlin, A., Siegel, M. and Boru, K. (1989). The politics of method: From leftist ethnography to educative research. *Qualitative Studies in Education, 2*(3), 237-253.

Glaser, B. and Strauss, A. (1967). *The discovery of grounded theory: Strategies for qualitative research.* New York: Aldine de Gruyter.

Goffman, E. (1961). *Asylums: Essays on the social situation of mental patients and other inmates.* New York: Doubleday.

Gold, M. (1980). *Try another way training manual.* Champaign, IL: Research Press.

Golden, T., Smith, S., and Golden, J. (1993). A review of current strategies and trends for the enhancement of vocational outcomes following brain injury. *Journal of Rehabilitation, 59*(4), 55-60.

Goldstein, H. (1994). Ethnography, critical inquiry, and social work practice. In E. Sherman, and W.J. Reid (Eds.), *Qualitative research in social work.* New York: Columbia University Press.

Goodall, P., Groah, C., Sherron, P., Kreutzer, J., and Wehman, P. (1991). *Supported employment services for individuals with traumatic brain injury: A guide for service providers.* Richmond, VA: Virginia Commonwealth University.

Goodall, P., Lawyer, H., and Wehman, P. (1994). Vocational rehabilitation and traumatic brain injury: A legislative and public policy perspective. *Journal of Head Trauma Rehabilitation, 9*(2), 61-81.

Goode, D. (1994). Towards an understanding of holistic quality of life in people with profound intellectual and multiple disabilities. In D. Goode (Ed.), *Quality of life for persons with disabilities: International perspectives and issues* (pp. 197-207). Cambridge, MA: Brookline Books.

Goodrick, D. (1989). State and local collaboration in the development of Wisconsin's mental health system. *Journal of Mental Health Administration, 16,* 37-43.

Gordon, W. (1993). A model system approach to the rehabilitation of people with traumatic brain injury. *American Rehabilitation, 19*(2), 24-28.

Gordon, W., Hibbard, M., and Kreutzer, J. (1989). Cognitive remediation: Issues in research and practice. *Journal of Head Trauma Rehabilitation, 4*(3), 76-84.

Granberg, O. (1989). Municipal housing allowance for the handicapped. *Care and service: A brochure of the Stockholm County Council Care Committee.* Unpublished manuscript. Omsorgsnämnden, Sweden: County Council Care Committee.

Graney, P. (1988). *Status report: Special education in South Dakota.* Pierre, SD: Department of Education and Cultural Affairs.

Grant, G. (1989). Letting go: Decisionmaking among family carers of people with a mental handicap. *Australia and New Zealand Journal of Developmental Disabilities, 15*(3/4), 189-200.

Grant, G. and McGrath, M. (1990). Need for respite-care services for caregivers of persons with mental retardation. *American Journal of Mental Retardation, 94*(6), 638-648.

Greene, J. (1994). Qualitative program evaluation. In N.K. Denzin and Y.S. Lincoln (Eds.). *Handbook of qualitative research* (pp. 530-544). Thousand Oaks, CA: Sage.

Greene, J. and McClintock, C. (1985). Triangulation in evaluation: Design and analysis issues. *Evaluation Review, 9*(5), 523-545.

Green-McGowan, K. (1987). *Functional life planning for persons with complex needs.* Peachtree City, GA: KGM Seminars.

Griffin, R., Skivington, K., and Moorhead, G. (1987). Symbolic and international perspectives on leadership: An integrative framework. *Human Relations, 40*(4), 199-218.

Grimes, S. and Vitello, S. (1990). Followup study of family attitudes toward deinstitutionalization: Three to seven years later. *Mental Retardation, 28*(4), 219-225.

Groce, N. (1985). *Everyone here spoke sign language: Hereditary deafness in Martha's vineyard.* Cambridge, MA: Harvard University Press.

Groce, N. (1992). *The US role in international disability activities: A history and a look towards the future.* Oakland, CA: World Institute on Disability, International Disability Exchanges and Studies (IDEAS) Project.

Grodin, M.A. (1993). Religious advance directives: The convergence of law, religion, medicine and public health. *American Journal of Public Health, 83*(6), 899-903.

Guba, E. (1984). The effect of definitions of policy on the nature and outcomes of policy analysis. *Educational Leadership, 42*(2), 63-70.

Guba, E.G. and Lincoln, Y.S. (1989). *Fourth generation evaluation.* Newbury Park, CA: Sage.

Guba, E. and Lincoln, Y. (1994). Competing paradigms in qualitative research. In N.K. Denzin and Y.S. Lincoln (Eds.), *Handbook of qualitative research*. Thousand Oaks, CA: Sage.

Guess, D., Benson, H., and Siegel-Causey, E. (1985). Concepts and issues related to choice-making and autonomy among persons with severe disabilities in classroom settings. *Journal of the Association of Persons with Severe Handicaps, 12*(1), pp. 79-86.

Gustavsson, A. (nd, circa 1989). *Difficulties and opportunities for people with disabilities living in an integrated society: Scandinavian experiences.* Unpublished manuscript. Stockholm, Sweden: Stockholm College of Health and Caring Sciences.

Gwin, L. (1994, September/October). The myth of rescue. *Mouth: The voice of disability rights, V*(3) 4-5.

Häfner, H. and an der Heiden, W. (1991). Evaluating cost-effectivness and cost of community care for schizophrenic patients. *Schizophrenia Bulletin, 17,* 441-451.

Hagedorn, J.M. (1995). *Forsaking our children: Bureaucracy and reform in the child welfare system.* Chicago: Lake View Press.

Hagner, D. and Helm, D. (1994). Qualitative methods in rehabilitation research. *Rehabilitation Counseling Bulletin, 37,* 290-330.

Hagner, D., Helm, D., and Butterworth, J. (1996). "This is my meeting": A qualitative study of person-centered planning. *Mental Retardation, 34*(3), 159-171.

Hahn, H. (1985). Toward a politics of disability: Definitions, disciplines and policies. *The Social Science Journal, 22,* 87-105.

Haimon, T.Z. (1991, January). Americans with Disabilities Act of 1990: Its significance for people with mental illness. *Hospital and Community Psychiatry, 42*(1), 23-24.

Hallenbeck, B.A., Kauffman, J.M., and Lloyd, J.W. (1993, April). When, how, and why educational placement decisions are made: Two case studies. *Journal of Emotional and Behavioral Disorders, 1*(2), 109-117.

Halpern, A.S., Nave, G., Close, D.W., and Nelson, W. (1986). An empirical analysis of the dimensions of community adjustment for adults with mental retardation in semi-independent living programs. *Australia and New Zealand Journal of Developmental Disabilities, 12*(3), 147-157.

Hamer, D. and Martin, P. (1991). Lifestyle planning. *New Zealand Network News, 1*(2), 8-13.

Hanley-Maxwell, C., Whitney-Thomas, J., and Pogoloff, S.M. (1995). The second shock: A qualitative study of parents' perspectives and needs during their child's transition from school to adult life. *Journal of the Association of Persons with Severe Handicaps, 20*(1), 3-15.

Hanna, J. (1978). Advisor's role in self advocacy groups. *American Rehabilitation, 4*(2), 31-32.

Hannan, M. and Freeman, J. (1984). Structural inertia and organizational change. *American Sociological Review, 49,* 149-164.

Harp, H. (1990). Independent living with support services: The goal and future for mental health consumers. *Psychosocial Rehabilitation Journal, 13*(4), 85-90.

Harp, H. (1993). Taking a new approach to independent living. *Hospital and Community Psychiatry, 44*(5), 413.

Harrington, C. and Swan, J. (1990). State Medicaid ICF-MR utilization and expenditures in 1980-84. *Mental Retardation, 28*(1), 15-27.

Harris, L. and Associates (1994). *N.O.D. survey of Americans with Disabilities.* Washington, DC: National Organization on Disability.

Hasenfeld, Y. (1980). Implementation of change in human service organizations: A political economic perspective. *Social Service Review, 54*(4), 508-520.

Haveman, R.H. (1987). Policy analysis and evaluation research after twenty years. *Policy Studies Journal, 16*(2), 191-218.

Hayden, M., DePaepe, P. (1994). Waiting for community services. In M. Hayden and B. Abery (Eds.), *Challenges for a service system in transition* (pp. 173-206). Baltimore, MD: Paul H. Brookes.

Hayden, M., DePaepe, P., Solen, T., and Polister, B. (1995). *Deinstitutionalization and community integration of adults with mental retardation: Summary and comparison of the baseline and one year followup of residential data for the Minnesota longitudinal study.* Minneapolis, MN: University of Minnesota, Research and Training Center on Residential Services and Community Living.

Hayden, M., Lakin, K.C., Braddock, D., and Smith, G. (1995, October). Growth in self advocacy organizations. *Mental Retardation, 33*(5), 342.

Hayman, H.M. (1954). *Interviewing in social research.* Chicago: University of Chicago Press.

Hayman, R. (1990). Presumptions in justice, law and politics and the mentally retarded parent. *Harvard Law Review, 103*, 1202-1271.

Heckler, S. (1994). Facilitated communication: A response by child protection. *Child Abuse and Neglect, 18*(6), 495-503.

Heidenheimer, A.J., Heclo, H., and Adams, C.T. (1990). Housing policy. *Comparative public policy: The politics of social choice in America, Europe and Japan* (pp. 97-131). New York: St. Martin's Press.

Heller, J. and Factor, A. (1991). Permanency planning for adults with mental retardation living with their family caregivers. *American Journal of Mental Retardation, 96*(2), 163-176.

Hemp, R. (1994). State agency and community provider perspectives on financing community services (pp. 265-288). In M. Hayden and B. Abery (Eds.), *Challenges for a service system in transition.* Baltimore, MD: Paul H. Brookes.

Herald Journal News Service (1989). Quake toll rises: Northern California staggered by devastation, injuries, deaths. *Syracuse Herald-Journal*, City edition, October 18, p. 1.

Herr, S. (1993). The ADA in international and developmental disabilities perspectives. In L.O. Gostin and H.A. Beyer (Eds.), *Implementing the Americans with Disabilities Act* (pp. 229-249). Baltimore, MD: Paul H. Brookes.

Hess, G.A., Flinspach, S.L., and Ryan, S.P. (1993, Fall). Case studies of Chicago schools under reform. *New Directions for Program Evaluation, 59*, 43-55.

Heumann, J. (1993). A disabled woman's reflections: Myths and realities of integration. In J. Racino, P. Walker, S. O'Connor, and S. Taylor (Eds.), *Housing, support and community: Choices and Strategies for Adults with Disabilities* (pp. 233-249). Baltimore, MD: Paul H. Brookes.

Heuman, J. (1994). Clinton appointee talks about growing up with a disability. *Exceptional Parent, 24*(2), 30-32.

Heumann, J. and Racino, J. (1988). *Panel presentation: Advocacy and integration: National developments.* Hartford, CT: Connecticut Protection and Advocacy Agency.

Hibbard, M., Ferguson, P., Leinen, J., and Schaff, S. (1989). Supported community life and mediating structures in disability policy reform. In P. Ferguson and D. Olson (Eds.), *Supported community life: Connecting policy to practice in disability research* (pp. 1-21). Eugene, OR: University of Oregon, Specialized Training Program.

High, D. (1991). A new myth about families of older people? *The Georontologist, 31*(5), 611-618.

Hildebrand, A.J. (1992). Asking for citizen advocates in Beaver Co. In D. Schwartz (Ed.), *Crossing the river.* Boston: Brookline Books.

Hill, B., Lakin, K.C., Bruininks, R., Amado, A., Anderson, D., and Copher, J. (1989). *Living in the community: A comparative study of foster homes and small group homes for people with mental retardation.* Minneapolis, MN: University of Minnesota.

Hill, B.K., Lakin, K.C., Novak, A., and White, G. (1987). *Foster care for children and adolescents with handicaps: Child welfare and adult social services.* Minneapolis, MN: University of Minnesota, Institute on Community Integration.

Hogan, M.F., Johnson, P.J., and Jones, P. (1989). Who can provide new community services? A case study in provider agency development. *Administration and Policy in Mental Health, 16*(3), 131-139.

Holburn, C.S. (1992). Rhetoric and realities in today's ICF/MR: Control out of control. *Mental Retardation, 30*(3), 133-141.

Hollister, R.G. and Hill, J. (1995). Problems in the evaluation of community-wide initiatives. In J. Connell, A. Kubish, L. Schorr, and C.H. Weiss (Eds.), *New approaches to evaluating community initiatives: Concepts, methods and contexts* (pp. 127-172). Washington, DC: Aspen.

Holohan, J., Rowland, D., Feder, J. and Heslam, D. (1993). *Explaining the recent growth in Medicaid expenditures.* Washington, DC: The Urban Institute, Department of Health Policy and Management of the Johns Hopkins School of Hygiene, and Public Health, and the U.S. Department of Health and Human Services.

Horner, R.H., Close, D., Fredericks, H.D., O'Neill, R., Albin, R., Sprague, J., Kennedy, C., Folannery, K.B., and Heathfield, L. (1996). Supported living for people with profound disabilities and severe behavioral problems. In D. Lehr and F. Brown (Eds.), *People with disabilities who challenge the system:* Baltimore, MD: Paul H. Brookes.

Horner, R., Dunlap, G., Koegel, R., Carr, E., Sailor, W., Anderson, J., Albin, R., and O'Neill, R. (1990). Toward a technology of "nonaversive" behavioral support. *Journal of the Association of Persons with Severe Handicaps, 15*(3), 125-132.

Housing and Intellectual Disability Project (1988). *The need for coordination between the Ministry of Housing (MOH) and Community Services Victoria-Office of Intellectual Disability Services.* Collingwood, Victoria, Australia: Author.

Howe, J., Horner, R.H., and Newton, J.S. (1998). Comparison of supported living and traditional residential services in the state of Oregon. *Mental Retardation, 36*(1), 1-11.

Hudley, C. (1995). Assessing the impact of separate schooling for African American male adolescents. *Journal of Early Adolescence, 15*(1), 38-57.

Hughes, C., Hwang, B., Kim, J., Eisenman, L., and Killian, D.J. (1995). Quality of life in applied research: An analysis of empirical measures. *American Journal of Mental Retardation, 99*(6), 623-641.

Hunt, J.C. (1989). *Psychoanalytic aspects of fieldwork (Qualitative research methods series 18).* Thousand Oaks, CA: Sage.

Hunt, P., Haring, K., Farron-Davis, F., Staub, D., Rogers, J., Beckstead, S., Karasoff, P., Goetz, L., and Sailor, W. (1993). Factors associated with the integrated educational placement of students with severe disabilities. *Journal of the Association of Persons with Severe Handicaps, 18*(1), 6-15.

Intagliata, J., Crosby, N., and Neider, L. (1981). Foster family care for mentally retarded people: A qualitative review. In R. Bruininks, C. E. Meyers, B. Sigford, and K. C. Lakin (Eds.), *Deinstitutionalization and community adjustment of mentally retarded people* (pp. 233-259). Washington, DC: American Association on Mental Deficiency.

Intagliata, J. and Willer, B. (1981). A review of training programs for providers of foster family care to mentally retarded persons. In R. Bruininks, C.E. Meyers, B. Sigford, and K. C. Lakin (Eds.), *Deinstitutionalization and community adjustment of mentally retarded people* (pp. 282-315). Washington, DC: American Association on Mental Deficiency.

Jablonski, J.R. (1991). Implementing total quality management: An overview. San Diego, CA: Pfeiffer and Company. In M.C. Wetzel, J.R. Patterson, and W.C. Dobias (1994). Provider network for mission centered enhancement of service quality, *Journal of Rehabilitation Administration, 18*(2), 111-126.

Jackson, A., Felner, R., Milstein, S., Pittman, K., and Selden, R. (1993). Adolescent development and educational policy: Strengths and weaknesses in the knowledge base. *Journal of Adolescent Health, 14*(3), 172-189.

Jacobs, H., Blatnick, M., and Sandborst, J. (1990). What is lifelong living, and how does it relate to quality of life? *Journal of Head Trauma Rehabilitation, 5*(1), 1-8.

Jacobson, J.W. and Otis, J.W. (1992). Limitations of regulations as a means of social reform in developmental services. *Mental Retardation, 30*(3), 163-171.

Jenkins, B. and Gray, A. (1992). Evaluation and the consumer: The UK experience. In J. Mayne, J. Hudson, M.L. Bemelmans-Videc, and R. Conner (Eds.), *Advancing public policy evaluations* (pp. 226-299). Amsterdam, Netherlands: Elsevier Science Publishers, Inc.

Johnson, A. (1990). *Out of bedlam: The truth about deinstitutionalization.* New York: Basic Books.

Johnson, B.S. (1946, January). A study of cases discharged from the Laconia State School from July 1, 1924 to July 1, 1934. *American Journal of Mental Deficiency, 1*(3), 437-445.

Johnson, T.Z. (1985). *Belonging in the community.* Madison, WI: Options in Community Living.

Joint Committee on Standards for Educational Evaluation (1981). *Standards for evaluations of educational programs, projects and materials.* New York: McGraw-Hill.

Jones, M.A. (1991). Measuring outcomes. In K. Wells and D.E. Biegel (Eds.), *Family preservation services* (pp. 159-186). Newbury Park, CA: Sage.

Jones, M.L., Patrick, P., Evans, R., and Wulff, J. (1991). The life coach model of community re-entry. In B. McMahon and L. Shaw (Eds.), *Work worth doing.* Orlando, FL: Paul M. Deutsch Press, Inc.

Jones, M.L., White, G.W., Ulciny, G.R., and Mathews, R.M. (1988). A survey of service by independent living centers for people with cognitive disabilities. *Rehabilitation Counseling Bulletin, 31,* 244-248.

Judson Center (1990). *L.I.F.E. Program: Living in a family environment.* Unpublished manuscript. Royal Oak, MI: Author.

Kagan, S., Powell, B., Weissbourd, B., and Zigler, E.F. (Eds.) (1987), *America's family support programs: Perspectives and prospects.* New Haven, CT: Yale University Press.

Kahkonen, P. (1997, May-June). From the child welfare trap to the foster care trap. *Child Welfare, 86*(3), 429-445.

Kailes, J. (1988). *Putting advocacy rhetoric into practice: The role of the independent living center.* Houston, TX: Independent Living Research Utilization-Research and Training Center on Independent Living.

Kandel, D.B. (1986). Processes of peer influences in adolescence. In R.K. Silbereisen, K. Eyferth, and G. Rudinger (Eds.), *Development as action in context: Problem behavior and normal youth development* (pp. 203-227). New York: Springer-Verlag.

Kapp, M. (1994, April). Implications of the patient self-determination act for psychiatric practice. *Hospital and Community Psychiatry, 45*(4), 355-358.

Kappel, B. and Wetherow, D. (1986, Autumn). People caring about people: The Prairie Housing Cooperative. *Entourage, 1*(4), 37-42.

Karan, O.C. and Gardner, W.I. (1984). Planning community services using the Title XIX waiver as a catalyst for change. *Mental Retardation, 22*(5), 240-247.

Kauffmann, J. and Smucker, K. (1995). The legacies of placement: A brief history of placement options and issues with commentary on their evolution. In J.M. Kauffmann, J.W. Lloyd, D.P. Hallahan, and T.A. Astuto (Eds.), *Issues in educational placement: Students with emotional and behavioral disorders.* Hillsdale, NJ: Lawrence Erlbaum Associates, Inc.

Kaufmann, C., Ward-Colasante, C., and Farmer, J. (1993). Development and evaluation of drop-in centers operated by mental health consumers. *Hospital and Community Psychiatry, 44*(7), 675-678.

Kay, T. (1993). Selection and outcome criteria for community-based employment: Perspectives, methodological problems and options. In T.F. Menz and D. McAlees (Eds.), *Community-based employment following traumatic brain injury* (pp. 29-80). Menomonie, WI: University of Wisconsin-Stout, Research and Training Center.

Kaylanpur, M. and Rao, S. (1991). Empowering low-income black families of handicapped children. *Journal of Orthopsychiatry, 61*(4), 523-532.

Keefe, J. (1994). Long term care and support services for persons with traumatic brain injury. *Journal of Head Trauma Rehabilitation, 9*(2), 49-60.

Keller, M.J. and Wilhite, B. (1995). The case study approach in therapeutic recreation: Educational implications. *Therapeutic Recreation Journal, 29*(4), 270-280.

Kelley, J.D. and Frieden, L. (1989). *Go for it: A book on sport and recreation for persons with disabilities.* Orlando, FL: Harcourt Brace Jovanovich.

Kelly, K. and Van Vlaendern, H.V. (1995). Evaluating participation processes in community development. *Evaluation and program planning, 18*(4), 371-383.

Kemper, P., Applebaum, R., and Harrigan, M. (1987). Community care demonstrations: What have we learned? *Health Care Financing Review, 8*(4), 87-100.

Kenefich, B. (1981). Court decisions: The impact of litigation. In J. Wortis (Ed.), *Mental retardation and developmental disabilities* (pp. 20-54). New York: Elsevier.

Kennedy, J. (1993). Policy and program issues in providing personal assistance services. *Journal of Rehabilitation, 59*(3), 17-23.

Kennedy, J. and Litvak, S. (1991). *Case studies of six state personal assistance programs funded by the Medicaid personal care option.* Oakland, CA: World Institute on Disability.

Kennedy, M. (1993). Turning the pages of life. In J. Racino, P. Walker, S. O'Connor, and S. Taylor (Eds.), *Housing, support and community: Choices and strategies for adults with disabilities* (pp. 205-216). Baltimore, MD: Paul H. Brookes.

Kennedy, M., Killius, P., and Olson, D. (1987). Living in the community: Speaking for yourself. In S. Taylor, D. Biklen, and J. Knoll (Eds.), *Community integration for people with severe disabilities* (pp. 202-208). New York: Teachers College Press.

Kiesler, C.A. (1982). Mental hospitals and alternative care: Noninstitutionalization as potential public policy for mental patients. *American Psychologist, 37*(4), 349-360.

King, R.D., Raynes, N.V., and Tizard, J. (1971). *Patterns of residential care: Sociological studies in institutions of handicapped children.* London: Routledge and Kegan Paul.

Kingdon, J. (1984). *Agendas, alternatives and public policies.* Boston: Little, Brown and Company.

Kiracofe, J. (1994). Strategies to help agencies shift from services to support. In V. Bradley, J. Ashbaugh, and B. Blaney (Eds.), *Creating individual supports for people with developmental disabilities* (pp. 281-298). Baltimore, MD: Paul H. Brookes.

Kirk, J. and Miller, M. (1986). *Reliability and validity in qualitative research: Qualitative research methods series 1.* Newbury Park, CA: Sage Publications.

Kirshbaum, M. (1996). Mothers with physical disabilities. In D. Krotoski, M.A. Nosek, and M. Turk (Eds). *Women with physical disabilities. Achieving and maintaining health and well-being.* Baltimore, MD: Paul H. Brookes.

Kishi, G., Teelucksingh, B., Zollers, N., Park-Lee, S., and Meyer, L. (1988). Daily decision-making in community residences: A social comparison of adults with and without mental retardation. *American Journal of Mental Retardation, 92*(5), 430-435.

Kittrie, N. (1971). *The right to be different.* Baltimore, MD: John Hopkins Press.

Klein, J. (1992). Get me the hell out of here: Supporting people with disabilities to live in their own home. In J. Nisbet (Ed.), *Natural supports in school, at work, and in the community for people with severe disabilities* (pp. 277-339). Baltimore, MD: Paul H. Brookes.

Kliewer, C. and Biklen, D. (1996). Labeling: Who wants to be called retarded? In W. Stainback and S. Stainback (Eds.), *Controversial issues confronting special education* (pp. 83-95). Boston: Allyn and Bacon.

Knisley, M. and Fleming, M. (1993). Implementing supported housing in state and local mental health systems. *Hospital and Community Psychiatry, 44*(5), 456-460.

Knitzer, J. (1982). *Unclaimed children.* Washington, DC: Children's Defense Fund.

Knoll, J. (1992). Being a family: The experience of raising a child with a disability or chronic illness. In V.J. Bradley, J. Knoll, and J. Agosta (Eds.), *Emerging issues in family support* (pp. 9-56). Washington, DC: American Association on Mental Retardation.

Knoll, J., Covert, S., Osuch, R., O'Connor, S., Agosta, J., and Blaney, B. (1992a). *Family support services in the United States: An end of the decade status report.* Cambridge, MA: Human Services Research Institute.

Knoll, J., Covert, S., Osuch, R., O'Connor, S., Agosta, J., and Blaney, B. (1992b). Supporting families: State family support efforts. In V. Bradley, J. Knoll, and J. Agosta (Eds.), *Emerging issues in family support* (pp. 57-97). Washington, DC: American Association on Mental Retardation.

Knoll, J. and Ford, A. (1987). Beyond caregiving: A reconceptualization of the role of the residential services provider. In S.J. Taylor, D. Biklen, and J. Knoll (Eds.), *Community integration for people with severe disabilities* (pp. 129-146). New York: Teachers College Press.

Knoll, J. and Meyer, L. (1987). Integrated schooling and educational quality: Principles and effective practices. In M. Berres and P. Knoblock (Eds.), *Pro-*

gram models for mainstreaming: Integrating students with moderate to severe disabilities (pp. 41-59). Rockville, MD: Aspen Publications.

Knoll, J. and Racino, J. (1988). *Community supports for people labeled by the mental retardation and mental health systems.* Syracuse, NY: Syracuse University, Center on Human Policy, Community Integration Project.

Knoll, J. and Racino, J. (1994). Field in search of a home: An exploration of the need for support personnel to develop a distinct professional identity. In V.J. Bradley, J. Ashbaugh, and B. Blaney (Eds.), *Creating supports for individuals with developmental disabilities.* Baltimore, MD: Paul H. Brookes.

Kofman, F. and Senge, P. (1993, Autumn). Communities of commitment: The heart of learning organizations. *Organizational dynamics: Special issue of learning organizations, 22*(2), 5-22.

Koroloff, N.M., Friesen, B., Reilly, L., and Rinkin, J. (1996). The role of family members in systems of care. In B. Stroul (Ed.), *Children's mental health* (pp. 409-426). Baltimore, MD: Paul H. Brookes.

Krauss, M.W. (1993, April). On the medicalization of family caregiving. *Mental Retardation, 31*(2), 78-79.

Krefting, L. and Groce, N. (1992). Anthropology in disability research and rehabilitation. *Practicing Anthropology, 14*(1), 3-4.

Kregel, J. (1993) Public accommodations and housing reforms. In P. Wehman (Ed.), *The ADA Mandate for Social Change* (pp. 199-215). Baltimore, MD: Paul H. Brookes.

Kregel, J. (1998). Developing a career path: Application of person-centered planning. In P. Wehman and J. Kregel (Eds.), *More than a job: Securing satisfying careers for people with disabilities* (pp. 71-91). Baltimore, MD: Paul H. Brookes.

Kregel, J. and Wehman, P. (1989). Supported employment: Promises deferred for persons with severe disabilities. *Journal of the Association of Persons with Severe Handicaps, 14*(4), 293-303.

Kregel, J., Wehman, P., Sayfarth, J., and Marshall, K. (1986, March). Community integration of young adults with mental retardation: Transition from school to adulthood. *Education and Training of the Mentally Retarded, 21*(1), 35-43.

Kreutzer, J., Conder, R., Wehman, P., and Morrison, C. (1989). Compensatory strategies for enhancing independent living and vocational outcomes following traumatic brain injury. *Cognitive Rehabilitation, 7*(1), 30-35.

Kreutzer, J. and Harris, J. (1990). Model systems of treatment for alcohol abuse following traumatic brain injury. *Brain Injury, 4*(1), 1-5.

Kreutzer, J. and Wehman, P. (1991). *Cognitive rehabilitation for persons with traumatic brain injury: A functional approach.* Baltimore, MD: Paul H. Brookes.

Kutash, K. and Rivera, V.R. (1996). *What works in children's mental health: Uncovering answers to critical questions.* Baltimore, MD: Paul H. Brookes.

Lachat, M.A. (1988). *The independent living service model: Historical roots, core elements, and current practices.* South Hampton, NH: Center for Resource Management in collaboration with the National Council on Disability.

Lakin, K.C. (1988). *An overview of the concept and research on community living.* Minneapolis, MN: University of Minnesota, Research and Training Center on Residential Services and Community Living.

Lakin, K.C. (1991). Foreword. In S. Taylor, R. Bogdan, and J. Racino (Eds.), *Life in the community: Case studies of organizations supporting people with disabilities in the community* (pp. xiii-xv). Baltimore, MD: Paul H. Brookes.

Lakin, K.C. (1995). Places of residence of Medicaid HCBS recipients. *Mental Retardation, 33*(6), 406.

Lakin, K.C., Braddock, D., and Smith, G. (1994). Trends and milestones: State institution closures. *Mental Retardation, 32*(1), 77.

Lakin, K.C., Bruininks, R.H., Chen, T., Hill, B., and Andersen, D. (1993). Personal characteristics and competence of people with mental retardation living in foster homes and small group homes. *American Journal of Mental Retardation, 97*(6), 616-627.

Lakin, K.C., Bruininks, R.H., and Larson, S.A. (1992). The changing face of residential services. In L. Rowitz (Ed.), *Mental Retardation in the Year 2000* (pp. 197-247). New York: Springer-Verlag.

Lakin, K.C., Hill, B., and Bruininks, R.H. (1985, September). *An analysis of Medicaid's intermediate care facility for the mentally retarded (ICF-MR) program.* Minneapolis, MN: University of Minnesota, Center for Residential and Community Services.

Lakin, K.C., Larson, S.A., and Prouty, R. (1994). Assessment and enhancement of quality services for persons with mental retardation and other developmental disabilities. In M. Hayden and B. Abery (Eds.), *Challenges to a service system in transition* (pp. 207-230). Baltimore, MD: Paul H. Brookes.

Lakin, K.C. and Prouty, R. (1995/1996). Trends in institutional closure and Leaving institutions: Effects on those who move. *IMPACT, 9*(1), 4-5.

Lakin, K.C., White, C., Prouty, R.W., Bruininks, R., and Kimm, C. (1991). *Medicaid institutional (ICF-MR) and home and community based services for people with mental retardation and related conditions (Project Report #35).* Minneapolis, MN: University of Minnesota.

Lamb, R.K. (1952). Suggestions for a study of your hometown. *Human Organization,* 11(2), 29-32. (As reprinted in Cox, F.M., Erlich, J.L., Rothman, J., and Tropman, J. [1977]. *Tactics and techniques of community practice* [pp. 17-23]. Itasca, IL: F.E. Peacock Publications.)

Langer-Ellison, M.L., Bersani, H. Jr., Blaney, B., and Freud, E. (1992). Family empowerment: Four case studies. In V. Bradley, J. Knoll, and J. Agosta, (Eds.) *Emerging issues in family support* (pp. 151-174). Washington, DC: American Association on Mental Retardation.

Larson, S. and Lakin, K.C. (1991). Parent attitudes about residential placement before and after deinstitutionalization: A research synthesis. *Journal of the Association of Persons with Severe Handicaps, 16*(1), 25-38.

Larson, S.A. and Lakin, K.C. (1992). Direct care staff stability in a national sample of small group homes. *Mental Retardation, 30,* 13-22.

LaRue, A. (1990). Rare Rett Syndrome afflicts only girls. *Herald American/ Herald Journal,* Syracuse, NY.

Laski, F. (1991). Achieving integration during the second revolution. In L.H. Meyer, C.A. Peck, and L. Brown (Eds.), *Critical issues in the lives of people with severe disabilities* (pp. 409-421). Baltimore, MD: Paul H. Brookes.

Laski, F. and Shoultz, B. (1987). Supported employment: What about those Medicaid-funded day treatment and day activity centers? *Word from Washington,* 12-14.

LeCompte, M.D. and Goetz, J.P. (1982). Problems in reliability and validity in ethnographic research. *Review of Educational Research, 52*(1), 31-60.

Lehman, K. (1988). Beyond Oz: The path to regeneration. *Social Policy, 18*(4), 56-58.

Leismer, J. (nd, circa 1985). *Prevention of institutional admissions and returns (especially those due to client behavioral difficulties).* Unpublished paper. Michigan.

Lepore, R. (1989). Promises for New Hampshire to keep: Three perspectives. In F. Setter (Ed.), (1990, November). *Historical issues and future choices: Perspectives on early intervention in New Hampshire.* Concord, NH: The New Hampshire Infant and Toddler Project.

Levy, S., Perhats, C., Nash-Johnson, M., and Welter, J. (1992). Reducing the risk in pregnant teens who are very young and those with mild mental retardation. *Mental Retardation, 30*(4), 195-203.

Lewin, K. (1947). Group decision and social change. In T.M. Newcombe and E.L. Hartley (Eds.), *Readings in social psychology* . New York: Holt, Rinehart, and Winston.

Lewis, D. and Bruininks, R. (1994). Costs of community-based residential and related services to individuals with mental retardation and other developmental disabilities (pp. 231-263). In M. Hayden and B. Abery, *Challenges for a services system in transition.* Baltimore, MD: Paul H. Brookes.

Lewis, O. (1959). *Five families: Mexican case studies in the culture of poverty.* New York: New American Library.

Lindsay, J.W. (1987). *Open adoption: A caring option.* Buena Park, CA: Morning Glory Press.

Lindsey, D. (1991, April). Factors affecting the foster care placement decision: An analysis of national survey data. *American Journal of Orthopsychiatry, 61*(1), 272-281.

Lindstrom, B. (1997). A sense of place: Housing selection in Chicago's north shore. *The Sociological Quarterly, 38*(1), 19-39.

Linn, M.W., Caffey, E.M., Klett, J., and Hogarty, G. (1977). Hospital versus community (foster) care for psychiatric patients. *Archives of General Psychiatry, 34,* 78-83.

Linn, R., Allen, K., and Willer, B. (1994). Affective symptoms in the chronic stage of traumatic brain injury: A study of married couples. *Brain Injury, 8*(2), 135-147.

Linton, R. (1954). The problem of universal values. In R.F. Spencer (Ed.), *Method and perspective in anthropology* (pp. 145-168). Minneapolis, MN: The University of Minnesota Press.

Linton, S. (1998). Disability studies/Not disabilitity studies. *Disability and Society, 13*(4), 525-540.

Litvak, S. and Heumann, J. (1993). Where do we go from here and how do we get there? *International Rehabilitation Gazette, 33*(2), 6-8.

Litvak, S., Zukas, H., and Brown, S. (1991, Spring). A brief economy of personal assistance services. *Spinal Cord Life Injury*, 3-5. (As reprinted in World Institute on Disability (1991). *Personal assistance services: A guide to policy and action* (Second Edition). Oakland, CA: The Research and Training Center on Public Policy in Independent Living at the World Institute on Disability, World Institute on Disability, InfoUse, and the Western Public Health Consortium.)

Litvak, S., Zukas, H., and Heumann, J. (1987). *Attending to America: Personal assistance for independent living*. Berkeley, CA: World Institute on Disability.

Livingston, J. and Srebnik, D. (1991, November). States' strategies for promoting supported housing for persons with psychiatric disabilities. *Hospital and Community Psychiatry, 42*(11), 1116-1119.

Longhurst, N. (1994). *The self advocacy movement by people with developmental disabilities: A demographic study and directory of self-advocacy groups in the United States*. Washington, DC: American Association on Mental Retardation, People First of Illinois, and Illinois University Affiliated Program on Developmental Disabilities.

Longmore, P. (1987, September). Uncovering the hidden history of people with disabilities. *Reviews in American History, 15*, 355-364.

Lord, J. (1984). The context of human services planning. In N. Marlett, R. Gail, and A. Wight-Felske (Eds.), *Dialogue in disability: A Canadian perspective* (Volume I: *The service system*). Calgary, Alberta, Canada: The University of Calgary Press.

Lord, J. (1985). *Creating responsive communities: Reflections on a process of social change*. Kitchener, Ontario, Canada: Centre for Research and Education in Human Services.

Lord, J. and Hearn, C. (1987). *The process of closing an institution*. Kitchener, Ontario, Canada: Centre for Research and Education in Human Services.

Lord, J. and Pedlar, A. (1991). Life in the community: Four years after the closure of an institution. *Mental Retardation, 24*(4), 213-221.

Lord, J., Schnarr, A., and Hutchinson, P. (1987). The voice of the people: Qualitative research and the needs of the consumers. *Canadian Journal of Community Mental Health, 25*, 25-36.

Lottman, M.S. (1990). Quality assurance and the courts. In V. Bradley and H. Bersani (Eds.), *Quality assurance for individuals with developmental disabilities: It's everybody's business* (pp. 149-169). Baltimore, MD: Paul H. Brookes.

Lourie, I.S., Katz-Leavy, J., and Stroul, B. (1996). Individualized services. In B. Stroul (Ed.), *Children's mental health* (pp. 429-452). Baltimore, MD: Paul H. Brookes.

Lovett, H. (1996). Some notes on positive approaches for students with difficult behaviors. In S. Stainback and W. Stainback (Eds.), *Inclusion: A guide for educators* (pp. 349-358). Baltimore, MD: Paul H. Brookes.

Lowe, K., DePaiva, S., and Humphreys, S. (1986). *Long-term evaluation of services for people with mental handicaps in Cardiff: Clients' views.* Cardiff, Wales: Mental Handicap in Wales-Applied Research Unit, Department of Psychological Medicine, University of Wales, College of Medicine.

Ludlum, C. (1991, May). Cathy's story: The power of a circle of support. In B. Mount (Ed.), *Dare to dream: An analysis of the conditions leading to personal change for people with disabilities* (pp. 20-26). Manchester, CT: Communitas.

Ludlum, C., Beeman, P., and Ducharme, G. (1991). *Dare to dream: An analysis of the conditions leading to personal change with people with disabilities.* Manchester, CT: Communitas.

Luecking, B. (1986, April). *Adult foster care handbook.* Oshkosh, WI, and Neenah, WI: Winnebago County Department of Social Services. In R. Luecking (1981). *Resource handbook for group homes.* Oshkosh, WI: Winnebago County Association for Retarded Citizens.

Lutfiyya, Z.M. (1988, March). *"Going for it": Life at the Gig Harbor Group Home.* Syracuse, NY: Syracuse University, Center on Human Policy, Research and Training Center on Community Integration.

Lutfiyya, Z.M. (1991a, April). Tony Santi and the bakery. In Z.M. Lutfiyya (Ed.), *Personal relationships and social networks: Facilitating the participation of individuals with disabilities in community life* (pp. 1-14). Syracuse, NY: Syracuse University, Center on Human Policy, Research and Training Center.

Lutfiyya, Z.M. (1991b). The Orion community: Prophets of the future. In S. Taylor, R. Bogdan, and J. Racino (Eds.), *Life in the community: Organizations supporting people with disabilities in the community* (pp. 227-241). Baltimore, MD: Paul H. Brookes.

Lutfiyya, Z.M. (1992). When "staff" and "clients" become friends. In A.N. Amado (Ed.), *Friendships and community connections between people with and without disabilities* (pp. 97-108). Baltimore, MD: Paul H. Brookes.

Lutfiyya, Z.M., Hagner, D., O'Connor, S., and Racino, J. (1991). Qualitative research: Its value and role in policymaking. *Policy research bulletin: University of Minnesota, 3*(1), 1-8.

Mackas, F., Marshall, C., and Wehman, P. (1997). Cultural diversity and disability: Developing respect for difference. In P. Wehman (Ed.), *Exceptional individuals in school, work and community* (pp. 83-108). Baltimore, MD: Paul H. Brookes.

Macklin, E. (1974). *Adolescents in society.* Ithaca, NY: Cornell University, College of Human Development.

Macomb-Oakland Regional Center (nd). *Community training home informational booklet.* Clement, MI: Author.

Majchrzak, A. (1984). *Methods for policy research* (Applied research methods series, Volume 3). Beverley Hills, CA: Sage Publications.

Malette, P., Mirenda, P., Kandborg, J., Jones, P., Bunz, J., and Rogow, S. (1992).

402   *Policy, Program Evaluation, and Research in Disability*

Application of a lifestyle development process for persons with severe intellectual disabilities. *Journal of the Association of Persons with Severe Handicaps, 17*(3), 179-191.

Mallory, B. and Herrick, S. (1987). The movement of children with mental retardation from institutional to community care. *Journal of the Association of Persons with Severe Handicaps, 12*(4), 297-305.

Mamula, R. (1970). Developing a training program for family caretakers. *Mental Retardation, 8*(2), 30-37.

Mamula, R. (1971). The use of developmental plans for mentally retarded children in foster family care. *Children, 18*(2), 65-68.

Mancuso, L. (1993, June). *Case studies on reasonable accommodations for workers with psychiatric disabilities.* Sacramento, CA: California Departmenet of Health.

Mandeville, H. (1992). *Building the foundation: Public policy in supported parenting.* Madison, WI: Supported Parenting Project, Wisconsin Council on Developmental Disabilities.

Manning, P. (1970). Talking and becoming: A view of organizational socialization. In J. Douglas (Ed.), *Everyday life: Toward the reconstruction of sociological knowledge* (pp. 239-256). Chicago: Aldine Publishing.

Mansell, J. and Ericsson, K. (1996). *Deinstitutionalization and community living: Intellectual disability services in Britain, Scandinavia, and the USA.* London: Chapman Hall.

Marafino, K. (1990). The right to marry and parental rights of persons with mental retardation. In B. Whitman and P. Accardo (Eds.), *When a parent is mentally retarded.* Baltmore, MD: Paul H. Brookes.

Marcuse, P. (1989). The pitfalls of specialism: Special groups and the general problem of housing. In S. Rosenberry and C. Hartmann (Eds.), *Housing issues in the 1990s* (pp. 67-82). New York: Praeger Publishers.

Marshall, C., Johnson, S., and Lonetree, G. (1993). Acknowledging our diversity: Vocational rehabilitation and American Indians. *Journal of Vocational Rehabilitation, 3*(1), 12-19.

Marshall, C., Johnson, M., Martin, W., and Saravanhabhaven, R. (1992). The rehabilitation needs of American Indians with disabilities in an urban setting. *Journal of Rehabilitation, 58*(2), 13-21.

Martin, P. (1990, June). Rethinking feminist organizations. *Gender and Society, 4*(2), 182-206.

Martin, P., Harrison, D., and Dinitto, D. (1983). Advancement of women in hierarchical organizations: A multi-level analysis of problems and prospects. *The Journal of Applied Behavioral Sciences, 19*(1), 19-33.

Maxwell, J.A. (1992). Understanding and validity in qualitative research. *Harvard Educational Review, 62*(3), 279-300.

Mayo, J.K. (1995, Fall). The housing indicators program: A model for evaluation research and policy analysis? In R. Picciotto and R. Rist, *New directions for evaluation: Evaluating country development policies and programs—New ap-*

proaches for a new agenda (pp. 67, 119-131). San Francisco: Jossey-Bass Publishers.

McCamant, K. and Durnett, C. (1991). Building a cohousing community. *Co-op America Quarterly, 3*(1), 17-20.

McCrae, D. (1980). Policy analysis methods and government functions. In S. Nagel (Ed.), *Improving policy analysis* (pp. 129-151). Beverly Hills, CA: Sage.

McGee, J. (1988). *Position statements on serving persons with behavioral difficulties.* Unpublished manuscript. Brussels, Belgium: The International League of Societies for the Mentally Handicapped, Task Force on Behavioral Difficulties.

McKnight, J. (1987). Regenerating community. *Social Policy, 17*(3), 54-58.

McKnight, J. (1989a, April). *Beyond community services.* Evanston, IL: Northwestern University. Center for Urban Affairs and Policy Research.

McKnight, J. (1989b, Summer). *Do no harm: A policymaker's guide to evaluating human services and their alternatives. Social Policy, 20*(1), 5-14.

McNamara, R.D. (1994, June). The Mansfield training school is closed: The swamp is finally drained. *Mental Retardation, 32*(3), 239-242.

McWhorter, A. (1986). *Mandate for quality.* (Volume III: *Changing the system*). Philadelphia, PA, and Cambridge, MA: Temple University and Human Services Research Institute.

McWilliams, P.J. (1993). The team meeting Case 16. In P. J. McWilliams and D.B. Bailey (Eds.), *Working together with children and families: Case studies of early intervention* (pp. 219-225). Baltimore, MD: Paul H. Brookes.

McWilliams, P.J. and Bailey, D.B. (1993). *Working together with children and families: Case studies of early intervention.* Baltimore, MD: Paul H. Brookes.

Means, B. and Bolton, B. (1992). A national survey of employment services by independent living programs. *Journal of Rehabilitation, 58*(4), 22-26.

Menolascino, F. and Stark, J. (1990). Research versus advocacy in the allocation of resources: Problems, causes, solutions. *American Journal of Mental Retardation, 95*(1), 21-25.

Messerschmidt, D.A. (1981). Constraints in government research: The anthropologist in a rural school district. In D.A. Messerschmidt (Ed.), *Anthropologists at work in North America: Methods and issues in the study of one's own society* (pp. 185-201). London: Cambridge University Press.

Meyers, J. (1994). Financing strategies to support innovations in service delivery to children. *Journal of Clinical Child Psychology, 23* (Suppl.), 48-54.

Michaels, R. (1989). *Title VII, Part A: A survey of state independent living programs: Issues in independent living.* Houston, TX: Independent Living Research Utilization- Research and Training Center on Independent Living at the Training Institute for Rehabilitation Research.

Miller, A.B. and Keys, C.B. (1996, October). Awareness, action and collaboration: How the self-advocacy movement is empowering for persons with developmental disabilities. *Mental Retardation, 34*(5), 312-319.

Miller, C. (1994, June). Harvard student athlete talks about growing up. *Exceptional Parent, 24*(6), 18-21.

Miller, J. and Yelton, S. (1991, June). *The child welfare/children's mental health partnership: A collaborative agenda for strengthening families.* Tampa, FL: National Association of Public Child Welfare Administrators and the State Mental Health Representatives for Children and Youth.

Miller, R.D. and Fiddleman, P.B. (1984, February). Outpatient commitment: Treatment in the least restrictive environment? *Hospital and Community Psychiatry, 35*(2), 147-151.

Millman, L.J. (1992). Issues in housing. In *Legal issues for older adults* (pp. 79-95). Santa Barbara, CA: ABC-CLIO.

Mills, P., Turk, T., and Marguiles, N. (1987). Value structures, formal structures, and technology for lower participants in service organizations. *Human Relations, 40*(4), 177-198.

Milstein, B. and Hitov, S. (1993). Housing and the ADA. In L.O. Gostin and H.A. Beyer (Eds.), *Implementing the Americans with Disabilities Act* (pp. 137-153). Baltimore, MD: Paul H. Brookes.

Minnesota Department of Human Services (1987a). *Minnesota home and community-based medicaid waiver services renewal request to the Health Care Financing Administration (HCFA).* St. Paul, MN: Author.

Minnesota Department of Human Services (1987b). *Minnesota state plan for services to people with mental retardation and related conditions.* St. Paul, MN: Author, Mental Retardation Division.

Mitchell, D. and Braddock, D. (1994). Compensation and turnover of direct care staff: A national survey. In M. Hayden, and B. Abery (Eds.), *Challenges for a service system in transition* (pp. 289-312). Baltimore, MD: Paul H. Brookes.

Mittler, P. and Mittler, H. (Eds.). (1995). *Innovations in family support for people with learning disabilities.* Lancashire, England: Lisieux Hall, Whittle-le-Woods, Chorley.

Monroe, T.J. (1996, April). We need to educate the professionals. *Mental Retardation, 34*(2), 122-123.

Moore, M. (Ed.) (1996, July). National voluntary credentialing for direct service workers. *Policy research brief: University of Minnesota, 8*(2), 1-8.

Morgan, D. (1988). *Focus groups as qualitative research* (Qualitative research methods series 16). Thousand Oaks, CA: Sage.

Morgan, S. (1990, January). Determinants of family treatment choice and satisfaction in psychiatric emergencies. *American Journal of Orthopsychiatry, 60*(1), 96-107.

Morris, C.D., Niederbuhl, J.M., and Mahr, J. (1993). Determining the capability of individuals with mental retardation to give informed consent. *American Journal of Mental Retardation, 98*(2), 263-272.

Morris, J. (1991). Feminist research and "community care." *Pride against prejudice: Transforming attitudes to disability* (pp. 146-168). Philadelphia, PA: New Society Publisher.

Morrissey, J.R. (1966). Status of family care programs. *Mental Retardation, 4,* 8-11.

Morse, M.T. (1990). P.L. 94-142 and P.L. 99-457: Considerations for coordination between the health and the education systems. *Children's Health Care, 19*(4), 213-218.

Mount, B. (1994). Benefits and limitations of personal futures planning. In V. Bradley, J. Ashbaugh, and B. Blaney (Eds.), *Creating individual supports for people with developmental disabilities* (pp. 97-108). Baltimore, MD: Paul H. Brookes.

Mount, B., Ludlum, C., Beeman, P., Ducharme, G., DeMarasse, R., Meadows, L., and Riley, E. (1990). *Imperfect change: Embracing the tensions of person-centered work.* Manchester, CT: Communitas Publications.

Mowbray, C. and Herman, S. (1991, Summer). Using multiple sites in mental health evaluations: Focus on program theory and implementation issues. *New Directions in Program Evaluation, 50,* 45-57.

Moynihan, D.P. (1993). *Pandaemonium: Ethnicity in international politics.* Oxford, England: Oxford University Press.

Muenchow, S. and Gilfillan, S.S. (1983). Social policy and the media. In E. F. Zigler, S.L. Kagan, and E. Klugman (Eds.), *Children, families and government: Perspectives in American social policy* (pp. 223-245). London: Cambridge University Press.

Mulroy, E. and Ewalt, P. (1996, May). Affordable housing: A basic need and a social issue: Editorial. *Social Work, 41*(3), 245-249.

Murphy, S.T. and Rogan, P.M. (1995). *Closing the shop: Conversion from sheltered to integrated work.* Baltimore, MD: Paul H. Brookes.

National Advisory Committee (1991). *Summary of recommendations: Policy research on deinstitutionalization and community integration.* Syracuse, NY: Syracuse University, Center on Human Policy.

National Alliance for Direct Support Professionals (1998). *Frontline Initiative: A Quarterly Newsletter, 2*(1), 1-12.

National Association of Developmental Disabilities Councils (1990). Forging a new era: The 1990s reports on people with developmental disabilities. *Journal of Disability Policy Studies, 1*(4), 15-42.

National Center for Youth with Disabilities (1992, March). *CYDLINES reviews: Recreation and leisure—Issues for adolescents with chronic illnesses and disabilities.* Minneapolis, MN: University of Minnesota.

National Center for Youth with Disabilities (NCYD) (1993, Winter). *Teenagers at risk: A national perspective of state level services for adolescents with chronic illness and disability.* Minneapolis, MN: Author.

National Council on Disability (1996). *Achieving independence: The challenge for the 21st Century.* Washington, DC: Author

National Council on State Legislators (1988). *Mental health financing and programming.* Colorado: Author.

National Council on the Handicapped (1988). Housing, personal assistance services. *On the thresholds of independence* (pp. 71-76, 85-87). Washington, DC: Author.

National Development Team (1989). *Services for people with learning difficulties living in Hereford and Worcester.* London: Author and Health, Local Authority and Voluntary Agencies.

National Institute on Mental Retardation (1975). *Residential services: Community housing options for handicapped people.* Toronto: Author.

Neilson Associates Ply. Ltd. (1987). *Ten year plan for the redevelopment of intellectual disability services: Interim report—Community Services, Victoria, Australia.* Victoria, Australia: Author.

Nelis, T. (1994). Self advocate's perspective. In President's Committee on Mental Retardation (Ed.), *The national reform agenda and people with mental retardation: Putting people first* (pp. 11-12). Washington, DC: U.S. Department of Health and Human Services, Administration of Children and Families, Editor.

Nelkin, B. (1987). *Family-centered health care for medically fragile children: Principles and practices.* Washington, DC: The National Center for Networking Community-Based Services, Georgetown University Child Development Center.

New England Conference Center (1991). *Forging directions: A New England conference on aging and developmental disabilities.* Durham, NH: Author.

New Hampshire Division of Mental Health and Developmental Services (1991). *New decade, new decisions: A look at the mission, organization and services of the state supported developmental services system.* Concord, NH: Author.

New Hampshire Office of the Legislative Budget Assistant (199, April). *New Hampshire developmental disabilities services performance audit.* Concord, NH: Author.

Newman, S.J. (1994). The effects of independent living on persons with chronic mental illness: An assessment of the Section 8 certificate program. *Milbank Quarterly, 72*(1), 171-199.

Newman, S.J. (1995). Housing policy and home-based care. *Milbank Quarterly, 73*(3), 407-437.

Newton, J.S., Horner, R., Ard, W., LeBaron, N., and Sappington, G. (1994). A conceptual model for improving the social life of individuals with mental retardation. *Mental Retardation, 32*(6), 393-402.

New York State Department of Health (1992). *Workplan for improving the delivery of services for persons with head injuries.* Albany, NY: Author.

New York State Department of Health and New York State Department of Social Services (1993). *Home and community-based Medicaid waiver for individuals with traumatic brain injury.* Albany, NY: Author.

New York State Department of Health Traumatic Brain Injury Program (1997, January). Tbi Medicaid waiver increases living options. *Special Report: NYS Department of Health Traumatic Brain Injury Program,* 13A.

New York State Office of Mental Retardation and Developmental Disabilities (NYSOMRDD) (1985). *Respite services.* Albany, NY: Author.

New York State Office of Mental Retardation and Developmental Disabilities. (1990a). *Family reimbursement program.* Albany, NY: Author.

New York State Office of Mental Retardation and Developmental Disabilities (NYSOMRDD) (1990b, January). *The closure of developmental centers in New York State.* Albany, NY: Author.

Nirje, B. (1969). A Scandinavian visitor looks at the US institutions. In R. Kugel, and W. Wolfensberger (Eds.), *Changing patterns in residential services for the mentally retarded* (pp. 52-57). Washington, DC: President's Committee on Mental Retardation.

Nirje, B. (1976). The normalization principle and its human service management implications. In M. Rosen, G. Clark, and M. Kivitz, (Eds.), *History of mental retardation*, Volume 2 (pp. 361-376). Baltimore, MD: University Park Press.

Nirje, B. (1980). The normalization principle. In R.J. Nitsch and K.E. Nitsch (Eds.), *Normalization, social integration and community services* (pp. 31-49). Baltimore, MD: University Park Press.

Nirje, B. (1985). The basis and logic of the normalization principles. *Australia and New Zealand Journal of Developmental Disabilities, 11*(2), 65-68.

Nisbet, J., Rogan, P., and Hagner, D. (1989). Squeezing long-term supports out of a short-term program: Independence issues and supported employment. *Journal of Applied Rehabilitation Counseling, 20*(3), 21-25.

Noble, J., Conley, R.W., Laski, F., and Noble, F. A. (1990, Summer). Issues and problems in the treatment of brain injury. *Journal of Disability Policy Studies, 1*(2), 19-45.

Nolan, M.R., Grant, C., and Ellis, N.C. (1990). Stress is in the eye of the beholder: Reconceptualizing the measurement of carer burden. *Journal of Advanced Nursing, 15*, 544-555.

Nosek, M. (1991). Personal assistance services: A review of the literature and analysis of policy implications. *Journal of Disability Policy Studies, 2*(2), 1-16.

Nosek, M. (1992). Independent living. In R.M. Parker, and E. Szymanski (Eds.), *Rehabilitation counseling* (pp. 103-133). Austin, TX: PRO-ED.

Nosek, M. and Howland, C. (1993). Personal assistance services: The hub of the policy wheel for community integration of people with severe physical disabilities. *Policy Studies Journal, 21*(4), 789-799.

Nosek, M., Roth, P., and Zhu, Y. (1990). Independent living programs: The impact of program age, consumer control, and budget on program operation. *Journal of Rehabilitation, 56*(4), 28-35.

O'Brien, C. (1992). *To boldly go: Individualized supports for Georgians with severe disabilities.* Atlanta, GA: Responsive Systems Associates (for the Georgia Planning Council on Developmental Disabilities).

O'Brien, J. (nd). *Signs of community building.* Atlanta, GA: Responsive Systems Associates.

O'Brien, J. (1987). A guide to personal futures planning. In G. T. Bellamy and B.

Wilcox (Eds.), *A comprehensive guide to the activities catalog: An alternative curriculum* (pp. 175-190). Baltimore, MD: Paul H. Brookes.

O'Brien, J., Forest, M., Snow, J., and Hasbury, D. (1989). *Action for inclusion: How to improve schools by welcoming children with special needs into regular classrooms.* Toronto: Centre for Integrated Education, Frontier College Press.

O'Brien, J. and Lyle O'Brien, C. (1991a, October). Making a move: Advice from People First members about helping people move out of institutions and nursing homes. *TASH newsletter, 17*(10), 8-9.

O'Brien, J. and Lyle-O'Brien, C. (1991b). Sustaining positive changes: The future development of the residential support program of Centennial Developmental Services. In S. Taylor, R. Bogdan, and J. Racino (Eds.), *Life in the community: Case studies of organizations supporting people with disabilities* (pp. 153-168). Baltimore, MD: Paul H. Brookes.

O'Brien, J. and Lyle-O'Brien, C. (1992). *Remembering the soul of our work: Stories by staff of Options in Community Living, Madison, Wisconsin.* Madison, WI: Options in Community Living.

O'Brien, J. and Lyle-O'Brien, C. (1994). More than just a new address: Images of supported living agencies. In V. Bradley, J. Ashbaugh, and B. Blaney (Eds.), *Creating individual supports for people with developmental disabilities* (pp. 109-140). Baltimore, MD: Paul H. Brookes.

O'Brien, J. and Mount, B. (1991). Telling new stories: The search for capacity among people with severe handicaps. In L.H. Meyer, C.A. Peck, and L. Brown (Eds.), *Critical issues in the lives of people with severe disabilities* (pp. 84-92). Baltimore, MD: Paul H. Brookes.

O'Connor, S. (1992). *Supporting families: What they want versus what they get.* Unpublished manuscript. Syracuse, NY: Syracuse University, Center on Human Policy, Research and Training Center on Community Integration and Research and Training Center on Community Living, University of Minnesota.

O'Connor, S. (1993). "I'm not Indian anymore": The challenge of providing culturally sensitive services to American Indians. In J. Racino, P. Walker, S. O'Connor, and S. Taylor (Eds.), *Housing, support and community: Choices and strategies for adults with disabilities* (pp. 313-331). Baltimore, MD: Paul H. Brookes.

O'Connor, S. (1995). More than they bargained for: The meaning of support to families. In S. Taylor, R. Bogdan, and Z.M. Lutfiyya (Eds.), *The variety of community experiences: Qualitative studies of family and community life* (pp. 193-210). Baltimore, MD: Paul H. Brookes.

O'Connor, S. and Racino, J.A. (1993). "A home of my own": Community housing options and strategies. In J. A. Racino, P. Walker, S. O'Connor, and S. Taylor (Eds.), *Housing, support and community: Choices and strategies for adults with disabilities* (pp. 137-160). Baltimore, MD: Paul H. Brookes.

Office of the Legislative Auditor, State of Minnesota (1987). *Evaluation of residential programs for mentally retarded persons: Final report.* St. Paul, MN: Author.

Ohlin, L., Coates, R., and Miller, A. (1974). Radical correctional reform: A case study of the Massachusetts youth-correctional system. *Harvard Educational Review, 44*(1), 74-111.

O'Neill, J., Brown, M., Gordon, W., Orazen, J., Hoffman, C., and Schonhorn, R. (1990). Medicaid versus state funding of community residences: Impact on daily life of people with mental retardation. *Mental Retardation, 28*(3), 183-188.

Options in Community Living (1987). *Options policy on quality of life.* Madison, WI: Author and the Wisconsin Developmental Disabilities Planning Council.

Orfield, G., Eaton, S., and the Harvard Project on School Desegregation (1996). *Dismantling desegregation.* New York: The New Press.

Owen, M.J. (1992). PASS: Plan for Achieving Self Support. *Exceptional Parent, 22*(1), 24-26.

Padgett, W. and Raymer, R. (1989). Diagnosis and treatment of Rett's Syndrome. *Psychiatric Aspects of Mental Retardation Reviews, 8*(9), 59-62.

Parette, H.P. and Van Biervliet, A. (1992). Tentative findings of a study of the technology needs and use patterns of persons with mental retardation. *Journal of International Disability Research, 36,* 7-27.

Patton, M.Q. (1980). *Qualitative evaluation methods.* Newbury Park, CA: Sage.

Patton, M.Q. (1997). *Utilization-focused evaluation: The new century text.* Thousand Oaks, CA: Sage.

Pedersen, E.L., Chaikin, M., Koehler, D., Campbell, A., and Arcand, M. (1993). Strategies that close the gap between research, planning and self advocacy. In E. Sutton, A.R. Factor, B.A. Hawkins, T. Heller, and G.B. Seltzer (Eds.), *Older adults with developmental disabilities: Optimizing choice and change* (pp. 277-326). Baltimore, MD: Paul H. Brookes.

Pelton, L.H. (1991). Beyond permanency planning: Restructuring the public child welfare system. *Social Work, 36*(4), 337-343.

Pennsylvania Developmental Disabilities Planning Council (1997). *RFP, Parents with disabilities.* Harrisburg, PA: Author.

People First of Washington (nd). *Officer handbook.* Tacoma, WA: Author.

Perlin, M. (1994, April). Law and the delivery of mental health services in the community. *Journal of Orthopsychiatry, 64*(2), 194-208.

Pernell-Arnold, A. (1998). Multiculturalism: Myths and miracles. *Psychiatric Rehabilitation Journal, 21*(3), 224-229.

Perry, A. (1991). Rett's Syndrome: A comprehensive review of the literature. *American Journal of Mental Retardation, 96*(3), 275-290.

Perry, G.J. and Ullman, C. (1987). *Planning issues of deinstitutionalization: A selected and annotated bibliography.* Chicago, IL: Council of Planning Librarians.

Perry-Varner, E. (1996). Seizure disorders. In P. McLaughlin and P. Wehman (Eds.), *Mental retardation and developmental disabilities.* Austin, TX: PRO-ED.

Perske, R. (1988). *Circles of friends: People with disabilities and their friends enrich the lives of one another.* Nashville, TN: Abingdon Press.

Peter, D. (1991). We began to listen (TSSR, California). In S. Taylor, R. Bogdan, and J. Racino, *Life in the community: Case studies of organizations supporting people with disabilities* (pp. 129-151). Baltimore, MD: Paul H. Brookes.

Peters, T.J. and Waterman, R.H. (1982). *In search of excellence: Lessons from America's best run companies.* New York: Harper & Row.

Petersen, P. and Lippincott, R. (1993). State mental health directors' priorities for human resource development. *Psychiatric Services, 44*(8), 788-790.

Peterson, M. (1992, revised). *Life assessment and planning: Supporting self-determination and community contributions of people with special needs.* Detroit, MI: Developmental Disabilities Institute, Wayne State University.

Petr, C., Zollars-White, J., Garlow, J., Turnbull, H.R., and Roesler, J. (1990, April). *Annotated bibliography: Permanency planning (PL 96-272).* Lawrence, KS: University of Kansas, Beach Center on Families and Disability.

Phelps, L.A., and Hanley-Maxwell, C. (1997). School-to-work transitions for youth with disabilities: A review of outcomes and practices. *Review of Educational Research, 67*(2), 197-226.

Pieper, B. (nd). *In-home family supports: What families of youngsters with traumatic brain injury really need.* Unpublished manuscript. New York: NYS Head Injury Council, pp. 1-21.

Pinderhughes, E.E. (1996). Alternate paths to family status and implications for mental health service delivery and policy: Adoptive and foster families. In A. Heflinger and C.T. Dixon (Eds.), *Families and the mental health system for children and adolescents: Policy services and research* (pp. 191-216). Thousand Oaks, CA: Sage.

Pine, B., Warsh, R., and Maluccio, A.N. (1993). *Together again: Family reunification in foster care.* Washington, DC: Child Welfare League of America.

Pollitt, C. (1988). Bringing consumers into performance measurement: Concepts, consequences and constraints. *Policy and Politics, 16*(2), 77-87.

Pollock, H. M. (1936). *Family care of mental patients: A review of systems of family care in America and Europe.* Utica, NY: State Hospital Press.

Price, J.A. (1972). Reno, Nevada: The city as a unit of study. *Urban Anthropology, 1,* 14-28.

Prouty, K.C., Lakin, K.C., Braddock, D., and Smith, G. (1996, April). Trends and milestones: Growth in residential settings of 6 or fewer individuals with MR/DD. *Mental Retardation, 34*(2), 130.

Pulice, T., McCormick, L., and Dewees, M. (1995). A qualitative approach to assessing the effects of systems change on consumers, families, and providers. *Psychiatric Services, 46*(6), 575-579.

Rabice, J. (1990). *The Rome experience: A chronicle of events that guided the Rome DDSO through closure.* Rome, NY: Rome Developmental Disabilities Services Office.

Racino, J. (1985a, April). Respite program models: A new focus—Use of generic service agencies and family subsidy. In J. Racino, *Respite services in New York State: An analysis of program models, policies, and issues* (pp. 27-30). Paper prepared for completion of master's program in public administration, Maxwell School of Public and International Affairs. Syracuse, NY: Author.

Racino, J. (1985b). *Site visit report: Seven Counties Services, Louisville, Kentucky.* Syracuse, NY: Center on Human Policy, Syracuse University, Community Integration Project.

Racino, J. (1985c). *Site visit report: Community Work Services, Madison, Wisconsin.* Syracuse, NY: Syracuse University, Center on Human Policy, Community Integration Project.

Racino, J. (1985-1992). *Technical assistance agreements in states and localities.* Syracuse, NY: Syracuse University, Center on Human Policy, Community Integration Project, and Research and Training Center on Community Integration.

Racino, J. (1987). *Memorandum, case study: From staff-client to a family relationship.* Syracuse, NY: Syracuse University, Center on Human Policy, Community Integration Project.

Racino, J. (1988a). *An evaluation of the adult family home program: Milwaukee, Wisconsin.* Syracuse, NY: Syracuse University, Center on Human Policy, Community Integration Project.

Racino, J. (1988b). *Consultation to Milwaukee Combined Community Service Board on use of the home and community-based Medicaid services waiver.* Syracuse, NY: Syracuse University, Center on Human Policy, Community Integration Project.

Racino, J. (1988c). *Individualized family support and community living for adults: A case study of a for-profit agency in Minnesota.* Syracuse, NY: Syracuse University, Center on Human Policy, Research and Training Center on Community Integration.

Racino, J. (1989). *National issues in housing: Report from the National Research and Training Center on Community Integration, Syracuse University.* Prepared for the national policy institute on housing: Covert, S. (1990). *A facility is not a home.* Durham, NH: University of New Hampshire.

Racino, J. (1989-1991). *Case studies and field memos on families.* Syracuse, NY: Syracuse University, Center on Human Policy (confidential case study field memos).

Racino, J. (1990a, June). *Brief case study memo: Byron family.* Syracuse, NY: Syracuse University, Center on Human Policy.

Racino, J. (1990b, October). *A case study of the Jeffries family.* Syracuse, NY: Syracuse University, Center on Human Policy, Research and Training Center on Community Living.

Racino, J. (1991a). Individualized supportive living arrangements: Pride Industries, North Dakota. In S. Taylor, R. Bogdan, and J. Racino (Eds.), *Life in the community: Case studies of organizations supporting people with disabilities in the community* (pp. 113-127). Baltimore, MD: Paul H. Brookes.

Racino, J. (1991b). *Madison Mutual Housing Association and Cooperative: Learnings from the disability field.* Syracuse, NY: Syracuse University. Center on Human Policy, Syracuse University, Research and Training Center on Community Integration.

Racino, J. (1991c). Organizations in community living: Supporting people with disabilities. *Journal of Mental Health Administration, 18*(1), 51-59.

Racino, J.A. (1991d). *Policy research interview guide.* Syracuse, NY: Syracuse University, Center on Human Policy.

Racino, J. A. (1991e). *Thoughts and reflections on personal assistance services: Issues of concern to people with mental retardation.* Syracuse, NY: Syracuse University (prepared for International Personal Symposium in Oakland, CA).

Racino, J. (1992a). Living in the community: Independence, supporta nd transition. In F.R. Rusch, L. DeStefano, J. Chadsey-Rusch, L.A. Phelps, and E. Szymanski (Eds.), *Transition from school to adult life for youth and adults with disabilities* (pp. 131-148). Sycamore, IL: Sycamore Press.

Racino, J. (1992b). *"People want the same things we all do". The story of the area agency in Dover, New Hampshire.* Syracuse, NY: Syracuse University, Center on Human Policy, Research and Training Center on Community Integration.

Racino, J. (1993a). *An edited collection on community integration and deinstitutionalization in New Hampshire.* Syracuse, NY: Community and Policy Studies.

Racino, J. (1993b). Center for independent living: Disabled people take the lead for full community lives. In J. Racino, P. Walker, S. O'Connor, and S. Taylor (Eds.), *Housing, support and community* (pp. 333-354). Baltimore, MD: Paul H. Brookes.

Racino, J. (1993c). *Living in the community: Toward supportive policies in housing and community services.* Syracuse, NY: Community and Policy Studies.

Racino, J. (1993d). The Madison Mutual Housing Association: "People and housing building communities." In J. Racino, S. Taylor, S. O'Connor, and P. Walker (Eds.), *Housing, support and community* (pp. 253-280). Baltimore, MD: Paul H. Brookes.

Racino, J. (1993e). "There if you need and want them": Changing roles of support organizations. In J. Racino, P. Walker, S. O'Connor, and S. Taylor (Eds.), *Housing, support and community: Choices and strategies for adults with disabilities* (pp. 107-135). Baltimore, MD: Paul H. Brookes.

Racino, J. (1993f). *Monograph on deinstitutionalization and community integration in New Hampshire.* Syracuse, NY: Community and Policy Studies, draft.

Racino, J. (1994a). Creating change in states, agencies and communities: Moving toward a people first approach. In V. Bradley, J. Ashbaugh, and B. Blaney (Eds.), *Creating individual supports for people with developmental disabilities* (pp. 171-196). Baltimore, MD: Paul H. Brookes.

Racino, J. (1994b, draft). *Personal assistance services: People with mental retardation and physical disabilities: Consumer expert interviews.* Syracuse, NY: Community and Policy Studies.

Racino, J. (1994c, draft). *Personal assistance services: Psychiatric survivos and people with psychiatric disabilities: Consumer expert interviews.* Syracuse, NY: Community and Policy Studies.

Racino, J. (1995a). Community living for adults with developmental disabilities: A housing and support approach. *Journal of the Association of Persons with Severe Handicaps, 20*(4), 300-310.

Racino, J. (1995b). Personal assistance services and personal support services for, by and with adults, youth and children with disabilities. *Journal of Vocational Rehabilitation, 9*(2), 35-48.

Racino, J. (1995c). *Toward universal access to support: An edited collection on personal assistance services.* Syracuse, NY, and Boston, MA: Community and Policy Studies.

Racino, J. (1997). Youth and community life. In S. Pueschel, and M.Sustrova (Eds.), *Adolescents with Down Syndrome: Toward a more fulfilling life* (pp. 433-449). Baltimore, MD: Paul H. Brookes.

Racino, J. (1998). "Innovations" in family support: What are we learning? *Journal of Child and Family Studies, 7*(4), 433-449.

Racino, J. and Heumann, J. (1992a). Independent living and community life: Building coalitions among elders, people with disabilities and our allies. *Generations: Journal of the American Society on Aging, XVI*(1), 43-47.

Racino, J. and Heumann, J. (1992b). Whose life is it? The issue of control of personal assistance services. *Disability Studies Quarterly, 12*(3), 22-24.

Racino, J. and Lutfiyya, Z.M. (1988). *Region VI AC/DC, Pocatello, Idaho: Consultation on personal futures planning.* Syracuse, NY: Syracuse University, Center on Human Policy, Research and Training Center on Community Integration.

Racino, J. and Merrill, D. (1988). *Residential supports for children with severe disabilities in northeast South Dakota.* Syracuse NY: Syracuse University, Center on Human Policy.

Racino, J. and O'Connor, S. (1994). "A home of our own": Homes, neighborhoods and personal connections. In M. Hayden, and B. Abery (Eds.), *Challenges for a service system in transition: Ensuring quality community experiences for persons with developmental disabilities* (pp. 381-403). Baltimore, MD: Paul H. Brookes.

Racino, J., O'Connor, S., Shoultz, B., Taylor, S.J., and Walker, P. (1989). *Moving into the 1990s: A policy analysis of community living arrangements for adults with developmental disabilities in South Dakota.* Syracuse, NY: Syracuse University, Center on Human Policy, Research and Training Center on Community Integration.

Racino, J., O'Connor, S., Shoultz, B., Taylor, S., and Walker, P. (1991, April/May). Housing and support services: Some practical strategies. *TASH Newsletter,* 9-11, 16-19.

Racino, J., O'Connor, S., Walker, P., and Taylor, S. (1991). *A study of innovative family support programs in central New York.* Syracuse, NY: Syracuse University, Center on Human Policy.

Racino, J. and Taylor, S. (1993). "People First": Approaches to housing and support. In J. Racino, P. Walker, S. O'Connor, and S. Taylor (Eds.), *Housing, support and community: Choices and strategies for adults with disabilities* (pp. 33-56). Baltimore, MD: Paul H. Brookes.

Racino, J., Walker, P., and Lutfiyya, Z. (1987). *Adult foster homes: A national perspective.* Chicago: International Association of Persons with Severe Handicaps Annual Conference.

Racino, J., Walker, P., O'Connor, S., and Taylor, S. (1993). *Housing, support and community: Choices and strategies for adults with disabilities.* Baltimore, MD: Paul H. Brookes.

Racino, J. with Whittico, P. (1998). The promise of self advocacy and community employment. In P. Wehman and J. Kregel (Eds.), *More than a job: Securing satisfying careers for people with disabilities* (pp. 47-69). Baltimore, MD: Paul H. Brookes.

Racino, J. and Williams, J. (1994). Living in the community: An examination of the philosophical and practical aspects. *Journal of Head Trauma Rehabilitation, 9*(2), 35-48.

Randolph, F., Laux, B., and Carling, P. (1987). *The search for housing: Creative approaches to financing integrated housing.* Burlington, VT: The Center for Community Change through Housing and Support, University of Vermont.

Rapp, C., Kisthardt, W., Gowdy, E., and Hanson, J. (1994). Amplifying the consumer voice: Qualitative methods, empowerment and mental health research. In E. Sherman and W. Reid (Eds.), *Qualitative research in social work* (pp. 381-395). New York: Columbia University Press.

Ratterman, D. (1987). *Reasonable efforts: A manual for judges.* Washington, DC: American Bar Association.

Reagles, K., Wright, G., and Thomas, K. (1972). Development of client satisfaction for clients receiving vocational rehabilitation counseling services. *Rehabilitation Research and Practice Review, 39*(2), 15-22.

Reason, P. (1994). Three approaches to participative inquiry. In N.K. Denzin and Y.S. Lincoln (Eds.), *Handbook of qualitative research* (pp. 324-339). Thousand Oaks, CA: Sage.

Redfield, R. (1953). Relations of anthropology to the social sciences and humanities. In A.L. Kroeber (Ed.), *Anthropology Today* (pp. 728-738). Chicago: University of Chicago Press.

Rehabilitation Research and Training Centers on Family and Community Living (1990). *Sharing the vision. . . . Meeting the challenge.* Washington, DC: Author.

Reiss, A.J. (1959). The sociological study of communities. *Rural Sociology, 24,* 118-130.

Research and Training Center (RTC) on Accessible Housing (1993). *A proposal for a national center on housing and support.* Raleigh, NC: North Carolina State University, Center on Accessible Housing.

Research and Training Center (RTC) on Community Integration (1990). *A proposal for a RTC on Community Integration.* Syracuse, NY: Syracuse University.

Reynolds, R., Dooley, J., and Parry, J. (1988, July/August) Court monitors and special masters in mental disability litigation: Variables affecting implementation of decrees. *MPDLR (Mental Disability Law Reporter), 12*(4), 322-332.

Reynolds, W. (1991). *Households and health services policy review: Policy for supportive services to families of traumatic brain injury patients.* Albany, NY: New York State Department of Health.

Reynolds, W. and Rosen, B. (1994). The impact of public policy on persons with traumatic brain injury and their families. *Journal of Head Trauma Rehabilitation, 9*(2), 1-11.

Rhoades, C. (1986). Self-advocacy. In J. Wortis (Ed.), *Mental Retardation and Developmental Disabilities* (Volume XIV) (pp. 69-90). New York: Elsevier.

Rhule, P. (1998). Dream home 2000: Houses that grow with you. *PARADE, USA Weekender*, April, 3-5, p. 8.

Richardson, A. and Higgins, R. (1990). *Case management in practice: Reflections on the Wakefield casemanagment project.* Leeds, UK: The Nuffield Institute for Health Services Studies, University of Leeds.

Ridgway, P. (1988). *The voice of consumers in mental health systems: A call for change: A literature review.* Burlington, VT: Center for Community Change through Housing and Support.

Riley, D. and Eckenrode, J. (1986). Social ties: Costs and benefits with differing groups. *Journal of Personality and Social Psychology*, 51(4), 770-778.

Rist, R. (1977). On the relationship among the educational paradigms. *Anthropology and Education*, 8(2), 42-50.

Rist, R. (1984). On the application of qualitative research to the policy process: An emergent linkage. In L. Barton and S. Walker (Eds.), *Social crisis and educational research* (pp. 153-170). London: Helen Croom.

Rist, R. (1994). Influencing the policy process with qualitative research. In N.K. Denzin and Y.S. Lincoln (Eds.), *Handbook of qualitative research* (pp. 545-557). Thousand Oaks, CA: Sage.

Rivara, J., Jaffe, K.M., Fay, G., Polissar, N., Martin, K.M., Shurtleff, H.A., and Liao, S. (1994). Family functioning and injury severity as predictors of child functioning one year following traumatic brain injury. *Archives of Physical Medicine, 74,* 1047-1055.

Robertson, R.M. (1988). Oneida educational planning: Assessing community needs today. In J. Campisis and L.M. Hauptman (Eds.), *The Oneida Indian experience: Two perspectives* (pp. 157-176). Syracuse, NY: Syracuse University Press.

Robinson, W.S. (1951). Logic structure of analytic induction. *American Sociological Review, 16,* 812-818.

Roecker, M.A. (1971). *Foster family homes for adults: Final report.* Olympia, WA: Washington Social and Health Services Department.

Roeher, G.A. (1975). Level 2 options. *Residential services: Community housing options for handicapped people* (pp. D2 to D6). Toronto: National Institute on Mental Retardation.

Rogan, P. (1992). *Employment for all.* Syracuse, NY: Syracuse University, Center on Human Policy, Research and Training Center on Community Integration.

Rogers, C. (1980). *A way of being.* Boston: Houghton Mifflin Company.

Rogers, P. and Hough, G. (1995). Improving the effectiveness of evaluations: Making the link to organizational theory. *Evaluation and program planning, 18*(4), 321-332.

Rose, M. (1995). *Possible lives: The promise of public education in America.* Boston: Houghton Mifflin Company.

Rose, S.M. and Black, B.L. (1985). *Advocacy and empowerment: Mental health care in the community.* Boston: Routledge and Kegan Paul.

Rosenbaum, E. (1996, November). Racial/ethnic differences in home ownership and housing quality, 1991. *Social Problems, 43*(4), 403-426.

Rosenberg, R. (1994). Capitol People First: Self advocacy and quality of life issues. In D. Goode (Ed.), *Quality of life for persons with disabilities: International perspectives and issues* (pp. 176-184). Cambridge, MA: Brookline Books.

Roseneau, N. and Provencal, G. (1981). Community placement and parental misgivings. *Canadian Journal of Mental Retardation, 31*(2), 3-11.

Rosenthal, C. (1986). The differentiation of multigenerational households. *Canadian Journal on Aging, 5*(1), 27-42.

Rosenthal, J., Motz, J., Edmonson, D., and Groze, V. (1991). A descriptive study of abuse and neglect in out-of-home placement. *Child Abuse and Neglect, 15,* 249-260.

Rosenthal, M. and Young, T. (1988). Effective family intervention after traumatic brain injury: Theory and practice. *Journal of Head Trauma Rehabilitation, 3*(4), 42-50.

Rossi, P.H. (1988). No good applied social research goes unpunished. *Special Feature: Society, 25*(1), 74-79.

Rossi, P.H. and Freeman, H. (1993). *Evaluation: A systematic approach.* Newbury Park, CA: Sage.

Rothman, D. and Rothman, S. (1984) *The Willowbrook wars.* New York: Harper & Row.

Ruckdeschel, R., Earnshaw, P., and Firrek, A. (1994). The qualitative case study and evaluation: Issues, methods and examples. In E. Sherman and W. Reid (Eds.), *Qualitative research in social work* (pp. 251-264). New York: Columbia University Press.

Rucker, L. (1986). *Life is just what you make it or a difference you can see: One example of services to persons with severe or profound mental retardation.* Lincoln, NE: Region V Mental Retardation.

Ryzin, G. (1996). The impact of resident management on residents' satisfaction with public housing: A process analysis of quasi-experimental data. *Evaluation Review, 20*(4), 485-506.

Sabatino, C.P., and Litvak, S. (1995). *Liability issues affecting consumer-directed personal assistance services, report and recommendations.* Oakland, CA: World Institute on Disability, Research and Training Center on Personal Assistance Services.

Sailor, W., Kleinhammer-Tramill, J., Skirtic, T., and Oas, B. (1996). Family participation in new community schools. In G. Singer, L. Powers, and A. Olson (Eds.), *Redefining family support: Innovations in public-private partnerships* (pp. 313-332). Baltimore, MD: Paul H. Brookes.

Salisbury, C. (1990). Characteristics of users and nonusers of respite care. *Mental Retardation, 28*(5), 291-297.

Salisbury, C.L., Palombaro, M., and Hollowood, T. (1993). On the nature and change of an inclusive elementary school. *Journal of the Association of Persons with Severe Handicaps, 18*(2), 75-84.

Salisbury, S., Dickey, J., and Crawford, C. (1987). *Individual empowerment and social services accountability.* Downsview, Ontario, Canada: The G. Allan Roehrer Institute.

Santiago, J.M. (1987). Reforming a system of care: The Arizona experiment. *Hospital and Community Psychiatry, 38*(3), 270-273.

Sapon-Shevin, M. (1996). Celebrating diversity, creating community: Curriculum that honors and builds on differences. In S. Stainback and W. Stainback (Eds.), *Inclusion: A guide to educators* (pp. 255-270). Baltimore, MD: Paul H. Brookes.

Sarason, S.B. and Doris, J. (1979). Old people, intermediate care facilities, and mentally retarded residents. In *Educational handicap, public policy and social history: A broadened perspective on mental retardation* (pp. 79-106). New York: The Free Press.

Schalock, R. (1995). *Outcome-based evaluation.* New York: Plenum Press.

Schalock, R.L. and Lilly, M.A. (1986). Placement from community-based mental retardation programs: How well do clients do after eight to ten years? *Journal of Mental Deficiency, 90*(6), 669-677.

Schein, E.H. (1969). *Process consultation: Its role in organizational development.* Reading, MA: Addison-Wesley Publishing Company.

Scheinost, T. (1988). Quotation cited in Smith, R. and Gettings, S. (1988). *An assessment of services to South Dakota's citizens with developmental disabilities.* Alexandria, VA: National Association of State Mental Retardation Program Directors.

Schleien, S., Meyer, L.H., Heyne, L.A., and Brandt, B.B. (1995). *Lifelong leisure skills and lifestyles for persons with developmental disabilities.* Baltimore, MD: Paul H. Brookes.

Schwartz, D.B. (1990). How regulatory control expands. In J. O'Brien, C. O'Brien, and D.B. Schwartz (Eds.), *What can we count on to make and keep people safe?* (pp. 18-23). Lithonia, GA: Responsive Systems Associates.

Schwartz, I. (1989). Hospitalization of adolescents for psychiatric and substance abuse treatment: Legal and ethical issues. *Journal of Adolescent Health, 10*, 473-478.

Schwartzman, H.B. (1993). *Ethnography in organizations (Qualitative research methods series 27).* Thousand Oaks, CA: Sage.

Schwier, K.M. (1990). *Speakeasy: People with mental handicaps talk about their lives in institutions and community.* Austin, TX: PRO-ED.

Scott, J.R., Ujcich, K., Nangle, D.W., Weigle, K., Ellis, J., Kirk, K., Vittimberga, G., Giacoletti, A., and Carr-Nangle, R. (1996). Evaluation of an HIV/AIDS education program for family-based foster care providers. *American Journal of Mental Retardation, 34*(2), 75-82.

Segal, R.M. (1970). Case studies of the establishment of three offices of mental retardation. In *Mental retardation and social action: A study of the Associations for Retarded Children as a force for social change* (pp. 108-151). Springfield, IL: Charles C Thomas Publishers.

Shank, H. and Turnbull, A. (1993). Cooperative family problem solving: An intervention for single parent families of children with disabilities. In G. Singer and L. Powers (Eds.), *Families, disability, and empowerment* (pp. 231-258). Baltimore, MD: Paul H. Brookes.

Shaw, B. (1994). *The ragged edge: The disability experience from the pages of the Disability Rag.* Louisville, KY: The Avocado Press.

Shaw, C.R. (1929). Case study method. *American Sociological Association, 21,* 149-157.

Sherman, E. (1994). Discourse analysis in the framework of the change process. In E. Sherman and W.J. Reid (Eds.), *Qualitative research in social work* (pp. 228-241). New York: Columbia University Press.

Sherman, P. and Porter, R. (1991, May). Mental health consumers as case management aides. *Hospital and Community Psychiatry, 42*(5), 494-498.

Shoultz, B. (nd). The self-advocacy movement. *Community integration report.* Arlington, TX: The ARC National Headquarters and the Center on Human Policy, Syracuse University.

Shoultz, B. (1992a). *Community integration report: A home of one's own.* Arlington, TX: The ARC of the United States.

Shoultz, B. (1992b). *Like an angel they came to help us: The origins and workings of New Hampshire's family support network.* Syracuse, NY: Syracuse University, Center on Human Policy, Research and Training Center on Community Integration.

Shoultz, B. (1995). My heart chose freedom: The story of Lucy Rider's second life. In S.J. Taylor, R. Bogdan, and Z.M. Lutfiyya (Eds.), *The variety of community experiences: Qualitative studies of family and community life* (pp. 155-174). Baltimore, MD: Paul H. Brookes.

Shoultz, B. and Racino, J. (1988). Supporting people with medical and physical needs in the community. In J. Racino (Ed.), *Resources in supporting people with extensive health care needs* (pp. 1-19). Syracuse, NY: Syracuse University, Center on Human Policy, Research and Training Center on Community Integration and the Community Integration Project.

Shoultz, B. and Ward, N. (1996). Self advocates becoming empowered: The birth of a national organization in the U.S. In G. Dybwad and H. Bersani (Eds.), *New voices: Self-advocacy by people with disabilities* (pp. 18-34). Cambridge, MA: Brookline Books.

Shreve, M. (1991). *Peer counseling in independent living centers: A study of service delivery variations.* Houston, TX: Research and Training Center on Independent Living.

Sieber, R.J. (1981). Many roles, many faces: Researching school-community relations in a heterogeneous community. In D. Messerschmidt (Ed.), *Anthropologists at home in North America* (pp. 202-220). London: Cambridge University Press.

Sigelman, C.K. and Parham, J.D. (1981). *Independent living and mentally retarded persons: The role of independent living programs.* Houston, TX: Independent Living Research Utilization.

Sigelman, C.K., Schoenrock, C., Winer, J., Sanhel, C., Hromas, S., Martin, P., Budd, E., and Bensberg, G. (1981). Issues in interviewing mentally retarded persons: An empirical study. In R. Bruininks, C.E. Meyers, B. Sigford, and K.C. Lakin (Eds.), *Deinstitutionalization and community adjustment of mentally retarded people* (pp. 114-129). Washington, DC: American Association on Mental Deficiency.

Silver, S.E., Duchnowski, A.J., Kutash, K., Bradenburg, M.A., and Greenbaum, P.E. (1992). A comparison of children with serious emotional disturbance served in residential and school settings. *Journal of Child and Family Studies, 1,* 43-59.

Simon-Rusinowitz, L. and Hofland, B. (1993). Adopting a disability approach to home care services for older adults. *The Gerontologist, 33*(2), 159-167.

Singer, G.H. (1987). Report on a working group on community-based housing options. In A.M. Covert and H.D.B. Fredericks (Eds.), *Transition for persons with deaf-blindness and other profound handicaps: State of the art* (pp. 51-54). Monmouth, OR: Teaching Research Publications.

Singer, G. and Nixon, C. (1990). *"You can't imagine unless you have been there yourself": A report on the concerns of parents of children with traumatic brain injury.* Eugene, OR: Oregon Research Institute.

Sinnema, G. (1988). The development of independence in adolescents with cystic fibrosis. *Journal of Adolescent Health,* 9, 61-66.

Skarnulis, E. and Lakin, C. (Eds.) (1990, Spring). Consumer controlled housing (Feature issue). *IMPACT* (University of Minnesota, Institute on Community Integration), *3*(1), 1-20.

Skodak-Crissy, M. and Rosen, M. (1985). *Institutions for the mentally retarded: A changing role in changing times.* Austin, TX: PRO-ED.

Skord, K. and Miranti, S. (1994). Towards a more integrated approach to job placement and retention for persons with traumatic brain injury and premorbid disadvantages. *Brain Injury, 8*(4), 383-392.

Smith, E. and Guthiel, R. (1988). Successful foster parent recruiting: A voluntary agency effort. *Child Welfare, LXVII* (2), 137-146.

Smith, G.W. (1990). Political activist as ethnographer. *Social Problems, 37*(4), 629-648.

Smith, G. (1990). *Supported living: New directions in services for people with developmental disabilities.* Alexandria, VA: National Association of State Mental Retardation Program Directors.

Smith, G. (1991, May 28). Supported employment expands in New Hampshire. *Bulletin No. 91-17.* Alexandria, VA: National Association of State Mental Retardation Program Directors.

Smith, G. (1994). *Medicaid PCA services in Massachusetts: Issues and options.* Alexandria, VA: National Association of State Directors of Developmental Disabilities Services.

Smith, G. (1995). *Supporting Connecticut citizens with disabilities to have a home of their own.* Littleton, CO: National Association of Directors of Developmental Disabilities Services.

Smith, G. and Alderman, S. (1987). *Paying for community services.* Alexandria, VA: National Association of State Mental Retardation Program Directors.

Smith, G. and Gettings, R. (1988). *An assessment of services to South Dakota's citizens with developmental disabilities.* Alexandria, VA: National Association of State Mental Retardation Program Directors.

Smith, G. and Gettings, R. (1991). *Supported employment and Medicaid financing.* Alexandria, VA: National Association of State Mental Retardation Program Directors.

Smith, G. and Gettings, R. (1994, October). *The HCB waiver and CSLA programs: An update on Medicaid's role in supporting people with developmental disabilities in the community.* Alexandria, VA: National Association of Directors of Developmental Disabilities Services, Inc.

Smith, G., Prouty, R., and Lakin, K.C. (1996, August). The HCB waiver program: The fading of Medicaid's "institutional bias." *Mental Retardation, 34*(4), 262-263.

Smith, J. and Polloway, E. (1993). Institutionalization, involuntary sterilization, and mental retardation: Profiles from the history of the practice. *Mental Retardation, 31*(4), 208-214.

Smith, P. (1994). All children belong. *Exceptional Parent, 24*(7), 36-38.

Smith, R. (1981). Implementing the results of evaluation studies. In S. Barrett, and C. Fudge (Eds.), *Policy and action: Essays on the implementation of public policy* (pp. 225-245). London: Methuen.

Smull, M. (1989). *Crisis in the community.* Alexandria, VA: National Association of State Mental Retardation Program Directors.

Smull, M.W. and Bellamy, G.W. (1991). Community services for adults with disabilities: Policy challenges in the new support paradigm. In L.H. Meyer, C.A. Peck, and L. Brown (Eds.), *Critical issues in the lives of people with severe disabilities* (pp. 527-536). Baltimore, MD: Paul H. Brookes.

Smull, M. and Harrison, S. (1992). *Essential lifestyle planning.* Alexandria, VA: National Association of State Mental Retardation Program Directors.

Snell, M. (1994). Replacing cascades with supported education. *The Journal of Special Education, 27*(4), 393-409.

Snow, J. and Racino, J. (1991). *Presentation on individualized financing of support and personal assistance services.* Oakland, CA: World Institute on Disability, World Rehabilitation Fund, and the Research and Training Center on Public Policy and Independent Living (International Personal Assistance Symposium).

Sobsey, D. (1994). *Violence and abuse in the lives of people with disabilities: The end of silent acceptance?* Baltimore, MD: Paul H. Brookes.

Stainback, S. and Stainback, W. (1990). Inclusive schooling. *Support networks for inclusive schooling: Interdependent integrated education* (pp. 3-23). Baltimore, MD: Paul H. Brookes.

Stainback, S. and Stainback, W. (1996). *Inclusion: A guide for educators.* Baltimore, MD: Paul H. Brookes.

Stainback, S., Stainback, W., and Ayres, B. (1996). Schools as inclusive communities. In W. Stainback and S. Stainback (Eds.), *Controversial issues confronting special education* (pp. 31-43). Boston: Allyn and Bacon.

Stainback, S., Stainback, W., and Jackson, H.J. (1992). Toward inclusive classrooms. In S. Stainback W. Stainback (Eds.), *Curriculum considerations in inclusive classrooms* (pp. 3-17). Baltimore, MD: Paul H. Brookes.

Stainback, W. and Stainback, S. (1989). Using qualitative data collection procedures to investigate supported education issues. *Journal of the Association for Persons with Severe Handicaps, 14*(4), 271-277.

Stake, R.E. (1988). Case study methods in educational research: Seeking sweet water. In R.M. Jaeger (Ed.), *Complementary methods of research in education* (pp. 253-270). Washington, DC: American Educational Research Association.

Stake, R.E. (1994). Case studies. In N.K. Denzin and Y.S. Lincoln (Eds.), *Handbook of qualitative research* (pp. 236-247). Thousand Oaks, CA: Sage.

State of New Hampshire (1989). *Family support legislation—1989 Laws of New Hampshire*, Chapter 255.

Stephens, S.A., Lakin, K.C., Brauen, M., and O'Reilly, F. (1990). *The study of programs of instruction for handicapped children and youth in day and residential facilities.* Washington, DC: U.S. Department of Education, and Mathematical Policy Research. Cited in Hallenbeck, B., Kauffman, J.M., and Lloyd, J.W. (1993). When, how and why educational placement decisions are made: Two case studies. *Journal of Emotional and Behavioral Disorders, 1*(2), 109-117.

Stewart, L. (1991). Personal assistance services for people with psychiatric disabilities. In J. Weissman, J. Kennedy, and S. Litvak (Eds.), *Personal and political perspectives on personal assistance services* (pp. 67-71). Oakland, CA: World Institute on Disability.

Stone, H.D. (1969). *Reflections on foster care: A report of a national survey of attitudes and practices.* New York: Child Welfare League of America.

Stone, H.D. (1989). *Ready, set, go: An agency guide to independent living.* Washington, DC: Child Welfare League of America.

Stoneman, Z. and Crapps, J. (1990). Mentally retarded individuals in family care homes: Relationships with families of origin. *American Journal on Mental Retardation*, 94(4), 420-430.

Strauss, A. and Corbin, J. (1994). Grounded theory methodology: A review. In N.K. Denzin and Y.S. Lincoln (Eds.), *Handbook of qualitative research* (pp. 273-285). Thousand Oaks, CA: Sage.

Strossberg, M.A. and Wholey, J.S. (1983). Evaluability assessment: From theory to practice in the Department of Health and Human Services. *Public Management Forum, 43,* 66-71.

Stroul, B. and Friedman, R. (1986). *A system of care for severely emotionally disturbed children and youth.* Washington, DC: Georgetown University Child and Development Center.

Stroul, B. and Goldman, S.R. (1996). Community-based service approaches: Home-based services and therapeutic foster care. In B. Stroul (Ed.), *Children's mental health: Creating systems of care in a changing society* (pp. 453-473). Baltimore, MD: Paul H. Brookes.

Strully, J. and Strully, C. (1991). Thinking differently about developing personal assistance support. In J. Weissmann, J. Kennedy, and S. Litvak (Eds.), *Personal perspectives on personal assistance services* (pp. 26-30). Oakland, CA: Research and Training Center on Public Policy in Independent Living, World Institute on Disability, Info Use, and the Western Health Consortium.

Struyk, R., Tuccillo, J., and Zais, J. (1982). Housing and community development. In J. Palmer, and I. Sawhill (Eds.), *The Reagan experiment* (pp. 393-417). Washington, DC: The Urban Institute.

Summers, J., Dell'Oliver, C., Turnbull, A., Benson, H., Santelli, E., Campbell, M., and Siegel-Causey, E. (1990). Examining the individualized family service plan process: What are family and practitioner preferences? *Topics in Early Childhood, 10*(1), 79-99.

Sunshine, J., Sunshine and Associates, Witkin, M., Atay, J., and Manderscheid, R. (1991, July). *Residential treatment centers and other organized mental health care for children and youth: United States, 1988. Mental health statistical note 1988.* Washington, DC: U.S. Department of Health and Human Services, National Institute of Mental Health.

Surles, R., Blanch, A., Shern, D., and Donahue, S. (1992). Case management as a systems strategy. *Health Affairs, 11,* 151-163.

Takanish, R. (Ed.) (1990). *Adolescence in the 1990s: Risk and opportunity.* New York: Teachers College Press, Columbia University.

Tanner, R. (Trans.) (nd). *The intellectually handicapped in Sweden—New legislation in a bid for normalisation.* Unpublished paper, pp. 2-10.

Tanzman, B. (1993). An overview of surveys of mental health consumers' preferences in housing and support. *Hospital and Community Psychiatry, 44*(5), 450-455.

Tate, D.G. and Chadderdon, L.M. (1982). *Independent living: An overview of efforts in five countires: Denmark, Federal Republic of Germany, Yugoslavia,*

Costa Rica and Japan. East Lansing, MI: Michigan State University, University Center for International Rehabilitation.

Taylor, S.J. (1982). From segregation to integration: Strategies for integrating severely handicapped students in normal school and community settings. *TASH Journal, 8,* 42-49.

Taylor, S.J. (1984, August). A man named August. *Institutions, Etc.* Syracuse, NY: Syracuse University, Center on Human Policy.

Taylor, S.J. (1985). *A site visit record on MacComb-Oakland Regional Center, Michigan (June 25-26, 1985).* Syracuse, NY: Syracuse University, Center on Human Policy, Community Integration Project.

Taylor, S.J. (1986a). *Memorandum to Linda Goodman and Charlie Galloway, State of Connecticut.* Syracuse, NY: Syracuse University, Center on Human Policy.

Taylor, S.J. (1986b). *On the issue of "small residential units" on the grounds of New York State institutions.* Syracuse, NY: Syracuse University, Center on Human Policy.

Taylor, S.J. (1987a, July). *A policy analysis of the supported housing demonstration project: Pittsburgh, PA.* Syracuse, NY: Syracuse University, Center on Human Policy, Research and Training Center on Community Integration.

Taylor, S.J. (1987b). Observing abuse: Professional ethics and personal morality in the field of research. *Qualitative Sociology, 10,* 288-302.

Taylor, S.J. (1987c). Review of institutions for mentally retarded: A changing role in changing times. *Journal of the Association of Persons with Severe Handicaps, 12*(1), 80-83.

Taylor, S.J. (1987d). "They're not like you and me": Institutional attendants' perspectives on residents. *Child and Youth Services: Qualitative Research and Evaluation in Group Care, 8*(3/4), 109-125.

Taylor, S. (1988). Caught in the continuum: A critical analysis of the principle of the least restrictive environment. *Journal of the Association of Persons with Severe Handicaps, 13*(1), 41-53.

Taylor, S.J. (1990). *A proposal for a Research and Training Center on Community Integration.* Syracuse, NY: Syracuse University, Center on Human Policy.

Taylor, S.J. (1991a). *"Children's division": The experiences of a family with disabilities with child protective agencies.* Syracuse, NY: Syracuse University, Center on Human Policy, Research and Training Center on Community Integration.

Taylor, S.J. (1991b). Community living in three Wisconsin counties. In S. Taylor, R. Bogdan, and J. Racino (Eds.), *Life in the community: Case studies of organizations supporting people with disabilities* (pp. 105-112). Baltimore, MD: Paul H. Brookes.

Taylor, S.J. (1991c). *Leisure and entertainment as participation in social worlds.* Syracuse, NY: Syracuse University, Center on Human Policy, Research and Training Center on Community Integration.

Taylor, S.J. (1991d). *"You're not a retard, you're just wise": The social meaning of disability.* Syracuse, NY: Syracuse University, Center on Human Policy, Research and Training Center on Community Integration.

Taylor, S.J. (1992). The paradox of regulations: A commentary. *Mental Retardation, 30*(3), 185-190.

Taylor, S.J. (1995). Deinstitutionalization. In A.E. Dell Orto and R.P. Marinelli (Eds.), *Encyclopedia of disability and rehabilitation* (pp. 247-249). New York: Macmillan Library, USA.

Taylor, S. and Biklen, D. (1980). *Understanding the law: An advocate's guide to the law and developmental disabilities.* Syracuse, NY: Human Policy Press.

Taylor, S.J., Biklen, D., and Knoll, J. (1987). *Community integration for persons with severe disabilities.* New York: Teachers College Press.

Taylor, S. and Bogdan, R. (1980). Defending illusions: The institution's struggle for survival. *Human Organizations, 39,* 209-218.

Taylor, S. and Bogdan, R. (1981). A qualitative approach to the study of community adjustment. In R.H. Bruininks, C.E. Meyers, B. Sigford, and K.C. Lakin (Eds.), *Deinstitutionalization and community adjustment of mentally retarded people* (pp. 71-81). Washington, DC: American Association on Mental Deficiency.

Taylor, S.J. and Bogdan, R. (1984). *An introduction to qualitative research methods* (Second Edition). New York: John Wiley.

Taylor, S. and Bogdan, R. (1989). On accepting relationships between people with mental retardation and non-disabled people: Towards an understanding of acceptance. *Disability, Handicap and Society, 4,* 21, 36.

Taylor, S.J. and Bogdan, R. (1990). Quality of life and individual's perspective. In R. Schalock (Ed.), *Quality of life: Perspectives and issues* (pp. 27-40). Washington, DC: American Association on Mental Retardation.

Taylor, S. and Bogdan, R. (1994). Qualitative research in community living. In M. Hayden and B. Abery (Eds.), *Challenges for a service system in transition* (pp. 43-63). Baltimore, MD: Paul H. Brookes.

Taylor, S.J. and Bogdan, R. (1998). *An introduction to qualitative research methods.* (Third Edition). New York: John Wiley.

Taylor, S., Bogdan, R., and Racino, J. (1991). *Life in the community: Case studies of organizations supporting people with disabilities in the community.* Baltimore, MD: Paul H. Brookes.

Taylor, S., Brown, K., McCord, W., Giambetti, A., Searl, S., Mlinarcik, S., Atkinson, T., and Lichter, S. (1981). *Title XIX and deinstitutionalization: The issue for the 80s.* Syracuse, NY: Syracuse University.

Taylor, S., Knoll, J., Lehr, S., and Walker, P. (1989). Families for all children: Value-based services for children with disabilities and their families. In L. Irvin and G. Singer (Eds.), *Support for caregiving families: Enabling positive adaptations* (pp. 41-53). Baltimore, MD: Paul H. Brookes.

Taylor, S., Lakin, K.C., and Hill, B. (1989). Permanency planning for children and youth: Out-of-home placement decisions. *Exceptional Children, 55*(6), 541-549.

Taylor, S., Lutfiyya, Z.M., Racino, J., Walker, P., and Knoll, J. (1986). *An evaluation of Connecticut's Community Training Home Program*. Syracuse, NY: Syracuse University, Center on Human Policy,Community Integration Project.

Taylor, S.J., McCord, W., and Searl, S.J. (1981). Medicaid dollars and community homes: The community ICF-MR controversy. *The Journal of the Association for the Severely Handicapped, 6*(1), 59-64.

Taylor, S. and Racino, J. (1987a). Common issues in foster care. *TASH Newsletter, 13*(2), 1-4.

Taylor, S. and Racino, J. (1987b, November). The clustered apartment model of services. *TASH Newsletter, 13*(11), 8-9.

Taylor, S.J. and Racino, J. (1989, January). "Supervision" in community living arrangements. *TASH Newsletter, 15*(1), 5-8.

Taylor, S.J., Racino, J., and Knoll, J. (1985). *Report to NIDRR on a literature review on community integration of people with the most severe disabilities*. Syracuse, NY: Syracuse University, Center on Human Policy, Community Integration Project.

Taylor, S., Racino, J., Knoll, J., and Lutfiyya, Z.M. (1986). *The non-restrictive environment: On community integration for people with the most severe disabilities*. Syracuse, NY: Syracuse University, Community Integration Project, field test version.

Taylor, S.J., Racino, J., Knoll, J., and Lutfiyya, Z.M. (1987a). Down home: Community integration for people with the most severe disabilities. In S. Taylor, D. Biklen, and J. Knoll (Eds.), *Community integration for persons with severe disabilities*. New York: Teachers College Press.

Taylor, S., Racino, J., Knoll, J., and Lutfiyya, Z.M. (1987b). *The nonrestrictive environment: On community integration for people with the most severe disabilities*. Syracuse, NY: Human Policy Press.

Taylor, S., Racino, J., and Rothenberg, K. (1988). *A policy analysis of private community living arrangements in Connecticut*. Syracuse, NY: Syracuse University, Center on Human Policy, Research and Training Center on Community Integration.

Taylor, S., Racino, J., and Shoultz, B. (1988). *From being in the community to being part of the community: The proceedings of a leadership institute on community integration for people with developmental disabilities*. Washington, DC: Syracuse University, Center on Human Policy, Research and Training Center on Community Integration.

Taylor, S., Racino, J., and Walker, P. (1992). Inclusive community living. In W. Stainback and S. Stainback (Eds.), *Controversial issues confronting special education* (pp. 279-290). Boston: Allyn and Bacon.

Taylor, S.J., Racino, J.A., Walker, P., Lutfiyya, Z.M., and Shoultz, B. (1992). *Permanency planning for children with developmental disabilities in Pennsylvania: The lessons of Project STAR*. Syracuse, NY: Syracuse University, Center on Human Policy, Research and Training Center on Community Integration.

Taylor, S. and Searl, S. (1987). The disabled in America: History, policy and trends. In P. Knoblock (Ed.), *Understanding exceptional children and youth* (pp. 5-64). Boston: Little Brown.

Thom, J.A. (1976, March). Indiana's self-reliant Uplanders. *National Geographic*, 149(3), 341-363.

Thomas, D. (1991a). *Making change effective: Report of a visit to Southport and Formby.* London: National Development Team.

Thomas, D. (1991b, July). Managing retraction and closure. In D. Thomas, *Making change effective: A report of a visit to Southport and Formby.* London: National Development Team.

Thomas, D. and Menz, F. (1990, Summer). Conclusions of a national think tank on issues relevant to community-based employment for survivors of traumatic brain injury. *American Rehabilitation*, 16(2), 20-33.

Thomas, K.R. (1993). Commentary: Some observations on the use of the word "consumer." *Journal of Rehabilitation, 59*(2), 6-12.

Thompson-Hoffman, S. and Storck, I.F. (1991). *Disability in the United States: A portrait from national data.* New York: Springer Publishing.

Tines, J., Rusch, F., McCaughrin, W., and Conley, R. (1990). Benefit cost analysis of supported employment in Illinois: A statewide evaluation. *American Journal on Mental Retardation, 95*(1), 44-54.

Tjosvold, D. (1989). Interdependence and the power between managers and employees: A study of the leader relationship. *Journal of Management, 18*(1), 49-62.

Towell, D. (1980, March). Large institutions reconsidered: An approach to the management of transition. *Hospital and Health Services Review, 76*(3), 87-90.

Towell, D. (1981). Developing better services for the mentally ill: An exploration of learning and change in complex agency networks. In S. Barrett and C. Fudge (Eds.), *Policy and action: Essays on the implementation of public policy* (pp. 183-205). London: Metheun.

Towell, D. (1988). *Enabling community integration: The role of public authorities in promoting an ordinary life for people with learning difficulties in the 1990s.* London: King Edward's Hospital Fund.

Towell, D. (1989a). *Managing psychiatric services in transition working papers.* London: King's Fund College.

Towell, D. (1989b). *Towards a new deal for people with learning difficulties and their families in Tower Hamlets.* London: National Development Team.

Towell, D. (1997). Promoting a better life for people with learning disabilities and their families: Disabilities and their families: A practice agenda for the new government. *British Journal of Learning Disabilities, 25*, 90-94.

Towell, D. and Beardshaw, V. (1991). *Enabling community integration: The role of public authorities in promoting an ordinary life for people with learning difficulties in the 1990s.* London: King's Fund College.

Towell, D., Racino, J., and Rucker, L. (1990). *Strategic planning for people with learning difficulties.* London: King's Fund College.

Transitional Living Services of Onondaga County (1979). *Oral history: Neighborhood and apartment complexes for people with psychiatric and developmental disabilities.* Syracuse, NY: Author.

Traustadottir, R. (1987). *"The answer to my prayers": A case study of the CITE Family Support Program, Cincinnati, Ohio.* Syracuse, NY: Syracuse University, Center on Human Policy, Research and Training Center on Community Integration.

Traustadottir, R. (1988, August). *Women and family care: On the gendered nature of caring.* Paper presented at the First International Conference on Family Support Related to Disability, Stockholm, Sweden. Syracuse, NY: Center on Human Policy, Research and Training Center on Community Integration, and the Community Integration Project.

Traustadottir, R. (1991). Mothers who care: Gender, disability and family life. *Journal of Family Issues, 12*(2), 211-228.

Traustadottir, R., Lutfiyya, Z.M., and Shoultz, B. (1994). Community living: A multicultural perspective. In M. Hayden and B. Abery (Eds.), *Challenges for a service system in transition* (pp. 405-426). Baltimore, MD: Paul H. Brookes.

Turnbull, A., Brotherson, M.J., and Summers, J.A. (1985). The impact of deinstitutionalization on families. In K.C. Lakin and R.H. Bruininks (Eds.), *Living and learning in the least restrictive environment* (pp. 115-140). Baltimore, MD: Paul H. Brookes.

Turnbull, A. and Rutherford, R. (1985). Developing independence. *Journal of Adolescent Health Care, 6,* 108-119.

Turnbull, H.R., Bateman, D., and Turnbull, A. (1991). *ADA, IDEA and families.* Lawrence, KS: The University of Kansas, Beach Center on Families and Disability.

Turnbull, H.R., Garlow, J., and Barber, P. (1991). A policy analysis of family support for families with members with disabilities. *The University of Kansas Law Review, 39*(3), 739-782.

Turnbull, H.R. and Turnbull, A. (1987). *The Latin American family and public policy in the United States: Informal support and transition into adulthood.* Lawrence, KS: University of Kansas, Beach Center on Families and Disability.

Turnbull, H., Turnbull, A., and Senior Staff (1989). *Report of a consensus conference on principles of family research.* Lawrence, KS: University of Kansas, Bureau of Child Research, Beach Center on Families and Disability.

Turner, E. (1995). Self-advocacy: A key to self-determination. *Journal of Vocational Rehabilitation, 5*(4), 329-336.

Tymchuk, A. (1992). Do mothers with or without mental retardation know what to report when they think their child is ill? *Children's Health Care, 21*(1), 53-57.

Tymchuck, A. and Andron, L. (1990). Mothers who do or do not abuse their children. *Child Abuse and Neglect, 14,* 313-323.

Ulciny, G. and Jones, M. (1988). Consumer management of attendant services: Benefits and obstacles. *NARIC Quarterly, 1*(2), Summer 1988.

Ulciny, G., White, G., Bradford, B., and Mathews, R.M. (1990, March). Consumer exploitation by attendants: How often does it happen and can anything be done about it? *Rehabilitation Counseling Bulletin, 33*(3), 240-246.

United Nations. (1993a). *Human Rights and Disabled Persons.* NY: Author.

United Nations. (1993b). UN standard rules on the equalization of opportunities for persons with disabilities. *Yearbook of the UN, 47,* 978-988.

U.S. Catholic Conference (1981). The right to a decent home: A pastoral response to the crisis in housing. In J.B. Benestad and F.J. Butler (Eds.), *Quest for justice* (pp. 298-318). Washington, DC: Author.

U.S. Congressional Committee on Government Operations. (1988). *From backwards to back streets: The failure of the federal government in providing services for the mentally ill.* Washington, DC: U.S. Government Printing Office.

U.S. Department of Health and Human Services (1991). *Services integration: A twenty year retrospective.* Washington, DC: Author, Office of the Inspector General.

U.S. Department of Housing and Urban Development (1991, December). *Affordable housing: A bibliography of selected periodical articles—1981-1991.* Washington, DC: HUD Law Library.

U.S. Department of Justice, Civil Rights Division and Equal Employment Opportunity Commission [USDOJ, CRD and EEOC] (1997, May). *The Americans with Disabilities Act: Questions and answers.* Washington, DC: Authors.

University of Illinois, Chicago (1991). *Overview of New Hampshire.* Chicago: University of Illinois, Chicago, Institute on Developmental Disabilities, draft.

University of Minnesota (1990). *Effective self advocacy: Empowering people with disabilities to speak for themselves.* Minneapolis, MN: University of Minnesota, Research and Training Center on Community Living, Institute on Community Integration.

The Urban Institute (1975). Architectural barriers. *Report of the comprehensive needs study* (pp. 242-266). Washington, DC: Department of Health, Education and Welfare.

Vail, D.J. and Miller, L. (1966). *Dehumanization and the institutional career.* Springfield, IL: Charles C Thomas.

Values in Action (1990, July). *Community integration and advocacy.* London: VIA, United Kingdom.

Van Willigen, J. (1986). Community development. Evaluation. *Applied Anthropology* (pp. 93-109, 173-189). New York: Bergin and Garvey.

Vanier, J. (1982). *The challenge of L'Arche.* London: Darton, Longman and Todd.

Varela, R.A. (1983). Changing social attitudes and legislation regarding disability. In N.M. Crewe and I.K. Zola (Eds.), *Independent living for physically disabled people* (pp. 28-48). London: Jossey-Bass Publishers.

Vaux, A. (1988). Limitations of family support programs to date. *Social support: Theory, research and intervention* (pp. 292-293). New York: Praeger.

Veldheer, L.C. (1990). Public policy issues related to head injury. In J. Kreutzer and P. Wehman (Eds.), *Community integration following traumatic brain injury* (pp. 313-325). Baltimore, MD: Paul H. Brookes.

Vidal, A.C. (1992). *Rebuilding communities: A national study of urban development corporations.* New York: New School of Social Research, Graduate School of Management and Urban Policy.

Vidich, A.J. (1955). Participant observation and the collection and interpretation of data. *The American Journal of Sociology, 60,* 59-61.

Vilhjalmsson, R. (1994, August). Effects of social support on self-assessed health in adolescence. *Journal of Youth and Adolescence, 23*(4), 437-453.

Virginia Department of Education (1992). *Guidelines for educational services for students with traumatic brain injury.* Richmond, VA: Rehabilitation Research and Training Center on Severe Traumatic Brain Injury with Virginia Department of Education.

Vivona, V. and Kaplan, D. (1990). *People with developmental disabilities speak out on quality of life: A statewide agenda for enhancing the quality life of people with disabilities.* Oakland, CA: World Institute on Disability.

Vocational Consulting Services (1994). *Facts on disabilities.* Madison, WI: Author.

Voeltz, L.M. and Evans, I.M. (1983). Educational validity: Procedures to evaluate outcomes in programs for severely handicapped learners. *Journal of the Association of Persons with Severe Handicaps, 8,* 3-15.

Wagner, B.R., Long, D.F., Reynolds, M.L., and Taylor, J. (1995, October). Voluntary transformation from an institutionally-based to a community-based service system. *Mental Retardation, 33*(5), 317-321.

Walker, P. (1989). *Family supports in Montana: Region III: Special training program for exceptional people (STEP).* Syracuse, NY: Syracuse, University, Center on Human Policy, Research and Training Center on Community Integration.

Walker, P. (1991). Anything's possible: Project Rescue, Georgia. In S. Taylor, R. Bogdan, and J. Racino (Eds.), *Life in the community: Case studies of organizations supporting people with disabilities* (pp. 171-183). Baltimore, MD: Paul H. Brookes.

Walker, P. (1992). *From deinstitutionalization to supporting people in their own homes in Region VI, New Hampshire.* Syracuse, NY: Syracuse University, Center on Human Policy, Research and Training Center on Community Integration.

Walker, P. (1993). "We don't put up the roadblocks we used to": Agency change through the citizenship project. In J. Racino, P. Walker, S. O'Connor, and S. Taylor (eds.), *Housing, support and community: Choices and strategies for adults with disabilities* (pp. 299-312). Baltimore, MD: Paul H. Brookes.

Walker, P. (1995). Community based is not community: The social geography of disability. In S. Taylor, R. Bogdan, and Z.M. Lutfiyya (Eds.), *The variety of community experiences* (pp. 175-192). Baltimore, MD: Paul H. Brookes.

Walker, P. and O'Connor, S. (1997). *Not just a place to live: Building community in Toronto.* Syracuse, NY: Syracuse University, Center on Human Policy.

Walker, P., Salon, R., and Shoultz, B. (1987). *Evaluation of the host home program—Colorado.* Syracuse, NY: Syracuse University, Center on Human Policy, Research and Training Center on Community Integration.

Walker, P., Taylor, S., Searl, J., Shoultz, B., Hulgin, K., Harris, P., and Handley, M. (1996). *Evaluation of the self-directed personal services program operated through ENABLE.* Syracuse, NY: Syracuse University, Center on Human Policy, Research and Training Center on Community Integration.

Wandersman, A., Valois, R., Ochs, L., Dela Cruz, O., Adkins, E., and Goodman, R. (1996). Toward a social ecology of community coalitions. *American Journal of Health Promotion, 10*(4), 299-307.

Warren, C. (1981). New forms of social control: The myth of deinstitutionalization. *American Behavioral Scientist, 24*(6), 724-740.

Warren, D. (1980). Support systems in different types of neighborhoods. In J. Garbarino and S. Stocking (Eds.) *Protecting children from abuse and neglect* (pp. 61-93). San Francisco, CA: Jossey-Bass.

Warren, J.L. (1990). *School age parents: The challenge of three generational living.* Buena Park, CA: Morning Glory Press.

Warren, R.L. (1977). *Social change and human purpose: Toward understanding social action.* Chicago: Rand McNally College Publishing Company.

Warren, R. and Cohen, S. (1985). *Respite care: Principles, programs and policies.* Austin, TX: PRO-ED.

Warren, R. and Dickman, I.R. (1981). *For this relief, much thanks.* New York: UCPA, Inc.

Wasik, B.H. and Roberts, R. (1994). Survey of home visiting programs for abused and neglected children and their families. *Child Abuse and Neglect, 18*(3), 271-283.

Watson, S. (1991). PAS and head injury. In J. Weissman, J. Kennedy, and S. Litvak (Eds.), *Personal perspectives on personal assistance services* (pp. 72-75). Oakland, CA: Research and Training Center on Public Policy and Independent Living, World Institute on Disability.

Watson, S. (1993). *Public responsibility, personal choice: Providing personal assistance services in Montana.* Cambridge, MA: Case Program, John F. Kennedy School of Government.

Wayne Community Living Services (1987). *Self advocates: "Give us a chance to try."* Northville, MI: Wayne Community Living Services.

Webb, A. (1988). *Closing institutions: One state's experience.* Albany, NY: New York State Office of Mental Retardation and Developmental Disabilities.

Wehman, P. (1993). *The ADA: Mandate for social change.* Baltimore, MD: Paul H. Brookes.

Wehman, P. (1996). *Life beyond the classroom: Transition strategies for young people with disabilities.* Baltimore, MD: Paul H. Brookes.

Wehman, P., Booth, M., Stallard, D., Mundy, A., Sherron, P., West, M., and Cifu, D. (1994). Return to work for persons with traumatic brain injury and spinal cord injury: Three case studies. *International Journal of Rehabilitation Research, 17,* 268-277.

Wehman, P. and Kregel, J. (1990). Supported employment for persons with severe and profound mental retardation: A critical analysis. *International Journal of Rehabilitation Research, 13,* 93-107.

Wehman, P. and Kregel, J. (1998). *More than a job: Securing satisfying careers for people with disabilities.* Baltimore, MD: Paul H. Brookes.

Wehman, P., Revell, G., Kregel, J., Kreutzer, J., Callahan, M., and Banks, D. (1991). Supported employment: An alternative model for vocational rehabilitation of persons with neurologic, psychiatric, or physical disability. *Archives of Physical Medicine and Rehabilitation, 72,* 101-105.

Wehman, P., Sale, P., and Parent, W. (1992). Program evaluation: Toward quality assurance. *Supported employment: Strategies for integration of workers with disabilities* (pp. 215-240). Boston: Andover Medical Publishers.

Wehman, P., West, M., Sherron, P., Groah, C., and Kreutzer, J. (1993). Return to work: Supported employment strategies, costs and outcome data. In D.F. Thomas, F. E. Menz, and D.C. McAlees (Eds.), *Community-based employment following traumatic brain injury* (pp. 227-250). Menomie, WI: University of Wisconsin, Stout.

Wehmeyer, M., Kelchner, K., and Richards, S. (1995). Individual and environmental factors related to self-determination of adults with mental retardation. *Journal of Vocational Rehabilitation, 5,* 291-305.

Wehmeyer, M. and Metzler, C. (1995). How self-determined are people with mental retardation? The national consumer survey. *Mental Retardation, 33*(2), 111-119.

Weil, M.O. (1996). Community building: Building community practice. *Social Work, 41*(5), 433-576.

Weintraub, F. and Abeson, A. (1976). New education policies for the handicapped: The quiet revolution. In F.J. Weintraub, A. Abeson, J. Ballard, and M. LaVor (Eds.), *Public policy and the education of exceptional children* (pp. 7-13). Reston, VA: Council on Exceptional Children.

Weiss, C. (1970). "The politicalization of evaluation research." *Journal of Social Issues, XXVI,* 57-68.

Weiss, C.H. (1972). *Evaluation research: Methods for assessing program effectiveness.* Englewood Cliffs, NJ: Prentice-Hall.

Weiss, C.H. (1978). Improving the linkage betwen social research and public policy. In L. Lynn (Ed.), *Knowledge and policy: The uncertain condition* (pp. 23-81). Washington, DC: National Academy of Sciences.

Weiss, C.H. (1995). There's nothing as practical as good theory: Exploring theory-based evaluation for comprehensive community initiatives for children and families. In J. Connell, A. Kubish, L. Schorr, and C.H. Weiss (Eds.), *New approaches to evaluating community initiatives: Concepts, methods and contexts* (pp. 65-92). Washington, DC: Aspen.

Weiss, H.B. (1989). State family support and education programs: Lessons from the Pioneers. *Journal of Orthopsychiatry, 59*(1), 32-48.

Weissman, J., Kennedy, J., and Litvak, S. (1991). *Personal perspectives on personal assistance services.* Oakland, CA: Research and Training Center on

Public Policy and Independent Living, World Institute on Disability, InfoUse, and Western Public Health Consortium.

Wells, K. and Biegel, D. (1991). *Family preservation services.* Newbury Park, CA: Sage.

West Virginia Medley Project (1988). *The Medley project status report as of June 1988.* Charleston, WV: U.S. Department of Health, Human Services and Education.

Westat (1988). *A national evaluation of the Title IV-E foster care/independent living programs for youth.* Phase I: Final report. Rockville, MD: Westat, Inc.

Western Regional Resource Center, University of Oregon (1993, May). *Traumatic brain injury: The role of schools in assessment.* Eugene, OR: University-Affiliated Program, University of Oregon.

Wetzel, M., McNabe, C., and McNaboe, K. (1995). A mission based ecological evaluation of summer camp for youth with disabilities. *Evaluation and program planning, 18*(1), 37-46.

White, C., Lakin, K.C. and Bruininks, R.H. (1989). *Persons with mental retardation and related conditions in state-operated residential facilities: Year ending June 30, 1988 with longitudinal trends from 1950 to 1988 (Report #30).* Minneapolis, MN: University of Minnesota, Research and Training Center on Residential Services and Community Living.

White, F., Gutierrez, R., and Seekins, T. (1996). Preventing and managing secondary conditions: A proposed role for independent living centers. *Journal of Rehabilitation, 62*(3), 14-21.

White House Domestic Policy Council (1993). *The President's health security plan: The Clinton blueprint.* New York: Times Books, Random House.

Whitehead, S. (1990, January). *Moving home: Making changes work particularly for people who are moving from hospitals.* London: National Development Team, Great Britain.

Whittico, P. with Racino, J. (1994, May). *Advocacy and personal assistance services.* Presentation at the Ohio Statewide Community Living Conference on Personal Assistance Services and Advocacy. Columbus, Ohio.

Wholey, J. (1983). *Evaluation and effective public management.* Boston: Little, Brown and Company.

Whyte, J. and Rosenthal, M. (1993). Rehabilitation of the patient with traumatic brain injury. In J. DeLisa and B. Gans (Eds.), *Rehabilitation medicine: Principles and practice* (pp. 825-860). Philadelphia, PA: Lippincott Company.

Whyte, W.F. (1991). *Social theory for action: How individuals and organizations learn to change.* Newbury Park, CA: Sage.

Wickham-Searl, P. (1992). Mothers with a mission. In D. Ferguson, P. Ferguson, and S. Taylor (Eds.), *Interpreting disability* (pp. 251-274). New York: Teachers College Press.

Widrick, G., Hasazi, J., and Hasazi, S. (1990). Citizen advocacy relationships: Advocates, proteges and relationship characteristics and satisfaction ratings. *Journal of the Association of Persons with Severe Handicaps, 15*(3), 170-176.

Wilcox, D. (1991, March). Heather's story: The long road for a family in search of a diagnosis. *Exceptional Parent, 21*(2), 92-94.

Willer, B. and Intagliata, J. (1982). Comparison of family-care and group homes as alternatives to institutions. *American Journal of Mental Deficiency, 80*(6), 588-595.

Willer, B. and Intagliata, J. (1984). *Promises and realities of mentally retarded citizens*. Baltimore, MD: University Park Press.

Willer, R., Linn, R., and Allen, F. (1994). Community integration and barriers to integration for individuals with brain injury. In M.A.J. Finlayson and S. Garner (Eds.), *Brain injury rehabilitation: Clinical considerations* (pp. 355-375). Baltimore, MD: Williams and Wilkins.

Williams, J. (1996). The relative nature of brain injury. In G.H. Singer, L. Powers, and A. Olson (Eds.), *Redefining family support: Innovations in public-private partnerships* (pp. 225-238). Baltimore, MD: Paul H. Brookes.

Williams, J. and Kay, T. (1991). *Head injury: A family matter*. Baltimore, MD: Paul H. Brookes.

Wilner, D.M., Walkley, R.P., Pinkerton, T.C., and Tayback, M. (1962). *The housing environment and family life: A longitudinal study of the effects of housing on morbidity and mental health*. Baltimore, MD: Johns Hopkins Press.

Wisconsin Department of Health and Social Services (1983). *Community integration program: Guidelines and procedures*. Madison, WI: Author.

Wisconsin Department of Health and Social Services (1985, November). *Family support protgam. Guidelines and procedures—Support to families who have a child with a severe disability*. Madison, WI: Author.

Wojdyla, P. (1990). *Parent involvment project: Final evaluation report*. Syracuse, NY: Parents' Information Group for Exceptional Children, Inc.

Wolcott, H. (1982). Differing styles of on-site research, or "If it isn't ethnography, what is it?" *Review Journal of Philosophy and Science, 1*(2), 154-169.

Wolf, J. (1990). A chronicle of change: A case study of the Connecticut mental health system. *Administration and Policy in Mental Health, 17*(3), 151-164.

Wolfensberger, W. (nd). How to exclude mentally retarded children from school. *Mental Retardation*, 30-31.

Wolfensberger, W. (1969). A new approach to decision making in human management services. In R.B. Kugel and W. Wolfensberger (Eds.), *Changing patterns in residential services for the mentally retarded* (pp. 367-381). Washington, DC: President's Committee on Mental Retardation.

Wolfensberger, W. (1972). *The principle of normalization in human services*. Toronto: National Institute on Mental Retardation.

Wolfensberger, W. (1975). *The origin and nature of our institutional models*. Syracuse, NY: Human Policy Press.

Wolfensberger, W. (1976). "Will there always be an institution? II. The impact of new service models." In M. Rosen, G. Clark, and M. Kivitz (Eds.), *History of mental retardation* (Volume 2) (pp. 415-432). Baltimore, MD: University Park Press.

Wolfensberger, W. (1977). *Course in residential services.* Syracuse, NY: Syracuse University, School of Education.

Wolfensberger, W. (1983). Social role valorization: A proposed new term for the principle of normalization. *Mental Retardation, 21*(6), 234-239.

Wolfensberger, W. (1985). Social role valorization: A new insight, and a new term for normalization. *Australian Association for the Mentally Retarded Journal, 9*(1), 4-11.

Wolfensberger, W. and Glenn, L. (1975). *PASS 3: A method for the quantitative evaluation of the human services field* (Third Edition). Toronto, Canada: National Institute on Mental Retardation.

Wolfensberger, W. and Thomas, S. (1983). *PASSING: Program Analysis of service systems implementation of normalization goals.* Canada: National Institute on Mental Retardation.

Wolfensberger, W. and Zuaha, H. (1973). *Citizen advocacy and protective services for the impaired and the handicapped.* Toronto: National Institute on Mental Retardation.

Wolins, M. (1963). *Selecting foster parents: The ideal and the reality.* New York: Columbia University Press.

Wong, H. and Millard, R. (1992). Ethical dilemmas encountered by il (independent living) service providers. *Journal of Rehabilitation, 58*(4), 10-15.

World Health Organization (1997). *ICIDH-2: International classification of impairments, activities, and participation. A manual of dimensions of disablement and health. Beta-1 draft for field test trials.* Geneva: World Health Organization.

World Institute on Disability (1991a). *Meeting on goals and objectives, and project status.* Oakland, CA: Research and Training Center on Public Policy and Independent Living, World Institute on Disability.

World Institute on Disability (1991b). *Personal assistance services: A guide to policy and action.* Oakland, CA: Research and Traing Center on Public Policy and Independent Living, World Institute on Disability, InfoUse, and the Western Public Health Consortium.

World Institute on Disability (1991c). *Resolution on personal assistance services.* Oakland, CA: Author.

World Institute on Disability (1993). *A proposal for a RTC on personal assistance services.* Oakland, CA: Author.

Worth, P. (1992, April). Guardianship. *Rights: People First of Canada National Organizer, 24,* 9.

Wright, B. (1993, February). *What legislators need to know about traumatic brain injury.* Denver, CO: National Conference of State Legislators.

Wright, B., King, M.P., and the National Conference on State Legislators (1991, February). *Americans with developmental disabilities: Policy directions for the states.* Washington, DC, and Denver, CO: National Conference on State Legislators.

Yang, H., Leung, P., Wang, J. and Shim, N. (1996). Asian Pacific Americans: The need for ethnicity-specific disability and rehabilitation data. *Journal of Disability Policy Studies, 7*(1), 33-54.

Yates, J. (1991, Spring). Deinstitutionalization and deception: The United States has the highest rate of imprisonment in the world. *Community,* 12-13.

Yin, R. (1989). *Case study research: Design and methods.* Newbury Park, CA: Sage Publications.

Yuan, S., Baker-McCue, T., and Witkin, K. (1996). Coalitions for family support and creation of two flexible funding programs. In G. Singers, L. Powers, and A. Olson (Eds.), (1996). *Redefining family support: Innovations in public-private partnerships* (pp. 357-388). Baltimore, MD: Paul H. Brookes.

Yucker, H.E. (1983). The lack of a stable order of preference for disabilities: A response to Richardson and Ronald. *Rehabilitation Psychology, 28*(2), 93-103.

Yukl, G. (1989). Managerial leadership: A review of the theory and research. *Journal of Management, 15*(2), 251-289.

Zald, M.N. (1965). Organizational control structures in five correctional institutions. In M.N. Zald (Ed.), *Social welfare institutions* (pp. 451-465). New York: John Wiley and Sons, Inc.

Zand, D. and Sorensen, R. (1975). Theory of change and effective use of management science. *Administrative Science Quarterly, 20,* 208-219.

Ziegler, M. (1988). Parent to parent support: A federal program. *Family Resource Coalition Report, 7*(2), 8.

Zigler, E. and Weiss, H. (1985). Family support systems: An ecological approach to child development. In R.N. Rapoport (Ed.), *Children, youth and families: The action research relationship* (pp. 166-205). Cambridge, MA: Cambridge University Press.

Zito, J. M. (1974). Anonymity and neighboring in urban, high rise complex. *Urban Life and Culture, 3*(3), 243-263.

Zola, I. (1987). The politicalization of the self help movement. *Social Policy, 18*(2), 32-33.

Zola, I.K. (1989). Toward the necessary universalizing of disability policy. *Milbank Quarterly, 67* (Suppl. 2, Part 2), 401-428.

Zola, I.K. (1992). *Working group on disability studies.* Washington, DC: National Council on Disability.

Zola, I. (1994). Toward inclusion: The role of people with disabilities in policy and research issues in the United States—A historical and political analysis. In M.H. Rioux and M. Bach (Eds.), *Disability is not measles: New research paradigms in disability* (pp. 49-66). North York, Ontario, Canada: Roeher Institute.

Organizations, Departments, and Associations Index

Page numbers followed by the letter "t" indicate tables.

Subject Index

Page numbers followed by the letter "t" indicate tables.

Access, 142t
  architectural, and housing,
    274-275
  community, 6, 175-176
  information, 174-175, 211-212
  systems barriers to, 210, 340
  universal, 14, 97, 169-170,
    173-174, 210, 275
Administration. *See also* Community
    integration; Medicaid
  community agency,
    administration, 255-261,
    289-290, 293-294, 327, 328,
    329
  and community services spending
    and family support initiatives,
      253-254, 256
    institutional spending, 26
    state, 33
  county administration, 256, 282,
    284, 289-290, 316
  shift to family support, 242
    and families as customers, 46
  state funding processes, 260,
    280t-281t, 284
  state offices, 42, 267-269,
    280t-281t, 315
  state operation of foster/personal
    care, specialized, and child
    welfare, 299-314
  state operation of public
    institutions, 26, 71-84, 268,
    289

Administration *(continued)*
  state-regional and county offices,
    289-290, 301t
Adolescents, 250t
  advocacy and safeguards, 167
  and brain injury research, 191, 202
  growth and development, 216-217
  transition to adulthood, 105t, 292
  youth and family support, 209t
  youth in out-of-home care, and
    independent living, 299, 304,
    308, 317-318
  youth with disabilities, and
    personal assistance services,
    207-224, 209t
Adults with disabilities, 85-90, 101,
    119-137, 144-149, 153-169,
    171-187, 189-205, 230-231,
    240-243, 263-287, 300-303,
    305-313, 317-319
Advocacy, and advocacy groups. *See
    also* Leadership;
    Self-advocacy
  citizen, 132, 186, 269
  legislative
    New Hampshire legislature, 44,
      46
    and self-advocacy, 87
    task force, and family support,
      NH, 44
  and media, 45, 63
  organizations, 42-43, 44-45

Businesses. *See also* Employment,
   and disability
   beauty parlors, stores, and local
      businesses, 122, 125
   disability as an industry, 4-5
   Dunkin' Donuts, 75
   as employment sites, 64, 114
   Mexican restaurant, NH, 122

Case management, 123t
   community and institution, 79-80
   family support and service
      coordination, 260, 345
   federal demonstration region, 38,
      106t
   flexible funds for case managers,
      345
   foster care, 294-295
   opposition to in mental health,
      144-145, 159-160
   as systems change, 344
Case studies. *See also* Evaluation
      research; Family research
   multi-case studies, 321, 324
   and comparative designs, 326
Cerebral palsy, 121
Change. *See also* Leadership;
      Systems change
   case studies and, 325-326
   and community integration, 8-9,
      25-30, 31-51, 37t, 53-70,
      71-84, 85-100, 101-117,
      119-137, 141-151, 227-233,
      235-261, 263-287, 289-314,
      315-334, 339-340
   concerns, 39t-40t
   practices, 38t
   and personal assistance services,
      141-151, 153-224
   perspectives on state change,
      46-49
      comparative roles in change
         process, 44-46
      key events timeline, 41t

Change *(continued)*
   state characteristics supporting
      change, 37t
   state leadership, 42-44, 65-67
   values-based training and
      leadership, 3-4, 7-9, 11, 12t,
      28-30, 31, 37, 43, 47-48,
      64-65, 72-74, 106t, 120,
      142t-144t, 146, 173, 184,
      190-191t, 210, 227-233, 267,
      279, 298-299, 314
Child care. *See also* Families
      and family support
   integrated day care, 269
   and rural unavailability, 260
Child welfare. *See also* Foster care
   abuse and neglect, 313
   Adoption Assistance and Child
      Welfare Act of 1980, 297-298
   coordination and comparison to
      specialized systems, 300, 302
   and room and board, 303
   and family preservation, and crisis
      intervention, 298-299, 310,
      314
      homebuilders, and children's
         mental health, 308
   Family Preservation and Support
      Services Act, 298
   and generic foster care, 299
   and independent living from
      out-of-home care, 299, 304
Children with medical and physical
      needs. *See* Assistive
      technology; Community
      support services
Children's mental health, 156-157,
      240-243, 297-299, 304,
      308-310, 313-314, 336-337
Choice, 121, 127-137, 230. *See also*
      Guardianship; Personal
      assistance services; Personal
      autonomy
   as central principle, 7, 10, 13,
      142t, 146t, 279t

Program evaluations *(continued)*
  formative and summative
    evaluations, 15, 255-261,
    263-270, 289-297, 315-319
  outcome and process evaluations,
    15-16
Psychiatric hospitals. *See also*
    Institutions
  costs of hospitalization, 155
  involuntary commitment, 164,
    167, 168
  and voluntary, 157
  loss of rights, 157
  prevention of admissions, PAS, 166
  treatment as punitive and arbitrary,
    157
  use of, in developmental disabilities
    services system, 122, 124
Psychiatric service systems, 144-146.
    See also Case management;
    Children's mental health;
    Psychiatric hospitals;
    Psychiatric survivors;
    Supported housing
  community approaches to PAS, 166
  consumer-controlled housing, 277
  and services, 170
  housing certificates, and chronic
    mental illness, 273
  institutional and medical bias, 141
  and psychiatric rehabilitation, 160
  recipient-run crisis teams, 163
  single-room occupancy,
    and boarding homes, 277
  treatment vs. PAS, 157, 163-164
Psychiatric survivors, 4, 5, 141,
    144-146. *See also* Personal
    assistance services
  abuse, trauma, and victimization,
    156-157
  advance directives, and self-help
    strategies, 164-165
  advocacy, peer support, and PAS,
    166
  commitment, and oppression, 164

Psychiatric survivors *(continued)*
  competency and decision making,
    167-168
  case management, concerns about,
    159-160
  consumer run drop-in centers, 160
  diagnoses, vs. individualization,
    15
  and independent living centers,
    158-159, 169
  PAS as a nonprofessional service,
    170
  peer counseling and benefits
    advocacy, 160
  self-help movement,
    and politicalization
    of language, 156
  psychological distress, and
    assistance, 161, 162t
  stigmatization, treatment, and
    hospitalization, 157
  supported housing, 160
  user-directed personal assistance,
    153-170
Public policy. *See also* Service
    systems
  community integration,
    and segregation, 6-7, 8-9, 10,
    25-30, 337-340
  deinstitutionalization, 9, 25-28,
    31-137
    toward support, 10-11, 12t,
    337-338
  and disability politics, 4-6
  diversity, and democracy, 9,
    335-336
  economic, 6
  education, 6, 335
  elders, 6
  employment, 335
    income support
    and employment
    disincentives, 6
  family, 240-241, 260-261
    and family support, 13

Qualitative research *(continued)*
  snowballing techniques,
      and purposeful sampling,
      256, 321, 351-352
  tape recordings and transcriptions,
      352, 361
  telephone interviews, 352
    and conversations, 236
  trustworthiness of observations,
      interpretations
      and generalizations, 323
  writing up findings
      and publishing, 353
Quality of life. *See also* Advocacy
      and Advocacy groups;
      Values-based principles
  and accreditation standards, 269
  and housing quality, 275
    and life outcomes, 15
  and relationship to services
      and values, 13
  research and, 9-11
  standards, 269
  systemic quality safeguards
    appeals procedures, 144t
    and independent evaluations,
      346
Quantitative research, 14-19. *See
      also* Evaluation research;
      Policy research; Qualitative
      research
  exploratory research and pilots, 16
  inductive and deductive reasoning,
      255
  qualitative analyses of quantitative
      designs, 17
  qualitative vs. quantitative, 255
  quantitative, longitudinal studies,
      compared to ethnographies, 18
  quasi-experimental
      and experimental, 17
  survey research, 18

Recreation
  activities, hobbies, and sports,
      124, 125
  of child as parental respite, 243
  family activities, and recreation,
      236, 250, 252, 302-303
  and friendships, 123t, 126
  holidays, birthdays, and parties,
      125, 126, 134
  integration and recreation, 338
  places, and restaurants, 123t, 125
  social activities, self-advocacy, 93
  teenage, 215-216
  therapy and, 250
  travel, 124
Regions. *See also* Area agencies, NH
  Nampa-Caldwell-Boise area,
      Idaho, 306
  regional agencies, Adjustment
      and Training Centers, South
      Dakota, 265-269
  regional offices of the state
      departments of health, social
      services, and vocational
      rehabilitation, South Dakota,
      268
  state-regional structures, 42,
      101-117, 136, 266
Regulations. *See also* Legislation
  and accreditation standards, 269
  approaches to regulations, 115-117
  certification and monitoring,
      295-296
  federal regulations, 115-117, 135
  and foster care, 296
    and personal care, 305-308
  housing quality, and community
      standards, 275
  and liability, 343
  life safety codes, state,
      and apartments, 134
  state priorities, 81
  state regulations, centralized
      control, 108, 281

Residential services *(continued)*
 neighborhoods, and neighbors,
  126, 134-135, 285, 271t
 normalization, and PAS training,
  120, 267
 personal choice, 130-132
 personal commitment, and
  celebrations, 134
 organizing for support
  financing, individualized
   services, 136-137, 271t
  paid roommates and neighbors,
   134
  and roommate options, 292
  staff, support, 132-134
 self-determination initiatives, New
  Hampshire, 179t
 supervised, independent,
  and monitored apartments,
  265
 supporting people, 128-129
  differing values, 130
  making mistakes, 129-130
 valued and paid work, 135-136
 waiting lists for residential
  services, 120, 268, 290, 342
Rett's Syndrome, 250t, 251t. *See
 also* Low incidence disorders
Rights. *See also* Advocacy;
  Americans with Disabilities
  Act; Citizenship; Institutional
  closure; Legislation
 constitutional rights, 230
 constitutional theory, Fourteenth
  Amendment, 61
 legal rights, adults, 6, 336-337
Rogers, Carl, 245, 267

Schools. *See also* Community
  integration; Education
 exclusion
  children with emotional
   and behavioral needs,
   exclusionary practices, 240

Schools, exclusion *(continued)*
 and family support, 235-243
 residential school placements,
  institutions, 235-240
 variance by state, and localities,
  240
 inclusion, 6-7, 9, 61, 191, 239-240,
  338
  definition of, and principles, 7,
   240
  practices and policies, 240
  segregation and inclusion
   in public policy, 6
 integration, 6-7, 240, 252t, 296
  children with brain injuries,
   return to schools, 197
  integrated placements, 240
   vs. segregation, 252t, 296
  placements in regular classes,
   240
 support services in,
  and extracurricular activities,
  213-214
Segregation. *See also* Community
  integration
 in day programs, school,
  residential facilities,
  and institutions, *xvii*
 exclusion of people with severe
  disabilities, 10
 as opposed to integration, 8
 and public policy, 6-7
Self-advocacy. *See also* Choice;
  Guardianship; Independent
  living
 and Congress, 87
 desired outcomes of self-advocacy,
  88-91
 development in New Hampshire,
  41t, 91-92, 130-132
  and South Dakota, 268, 270
 education, 88-89
 and family services, 96, 130-131
 future issues in self-advocacy,
  95-97, 131, 132